An Ethical Ri

A Formulation from a Buberian Diological Perspective

Manfred H. Vogel

Hamilton Books
an imprint of
University Press of America,® Inc.
Lanham · Boulder · New York · Toronto · Oxford

Hamilton Books
4501 Forbes Boulevard
Suite 200
Lanham, Maryland 20706
UPA Acquisitions Department (301) 459-3366

PO Box 317
Oxford
OX2 9RU, UK

Printed in the United States of America
British Library Cataloging in Publication Information Available

Library of Congress Control Number: 2004109679
ISBN 0-7618-3008-1 (paperback : alk. ppr.)

™ The paper used in this publication meets the minimum requirements of American National Standard for Information Sciences—Permanence of Paper for Printed Library Materials, ANSI Z39.48—1984

Dedicated to the memory of Edmund Perry,
a dear friend and a wonderful human being.

Contents

Introduction

Our objective in this work is to examine and analyze from the ethical perspective the issues of abortion, infanticide, euthanasia, suicide, assisted suicide, and capital punishment, and formulate an ethical position with respect to these issues that would be rationally persuasive. Clearly, if this objective is carried out successfully it would be of substantial significance. For there is no denying that these issues are presently tearing our society apart precipitating a profound divisiveness within it which manifests itself in the social, political and legal spheres. Still, in their essence these issues and the divisiveness that they precipitate are not primarily social, political or legal but ethical. This can be seen in the fact that for most people the issues will have to be decided, in the last analysis, not on the basis of considerations that are socially, politically or legally justifiable, but on the basis of considerations that are ethically justifiable. And clearly, the highly charged and profound emotional divisiveness that one encounters with respect to these issues is precipitated primarily by basic disagreements with respect to the ethical assessment of these issues. Thus, any advance towards formulating an ethical assessment of these issues that would be rationally persuasive is to be highly desired and valued as it would hopefully help us overcome this debilitating divisiveness by advancing us towards an ethical assessment that would command universal acceptance by all rational people. It is, indeed, in the hope of contributing to such an advance (and no matter how modest a contribution this may, in all probability, turn out to be) that the examination and the analysis of these specific issues is undertaken here.

Before proceeding, however, to deal with these specific issues, we must turn our attention to two additional issues that impinge most significantly and directly on all of the aforementioned specific issues. The first issue that we must address is the issue of how to define and delineate the parameters of the ethical enterprise. What is one to mean (or, more precisely, what do we mean) by the notion of ethics? It is important that we clarify what the ethical enterprise is to signify for us, seeing that we propose to assess the aforementioned specific issues from the ethical vantage point (inasmuch as we propose to examine whether their perpetration is ethically justifiable and, if yes, whether it is justifiable in all circumstances or only in some but not others and, if the latter, what these circumstances would be) and that there is by no means clarity, leave alone unanimity, as to what the notion of ethics is to signify.[1]

The other issue to which we must turn our attention is the issue of an ethical right to life. For, in the last analysis, this issue underlies our assessment of the aforementioned specific issues. Namely, our assessment of the issues of abortion, infanticide, euthanasia, suicide, assisted suicide, and capital punishment must per force reduce itself to this issue—in the last analysis its outcome revolves around the issue of whether or not the entity in question, i.e., the entity implicated in these specific issues (thus, for example, the entity to be aborted or put to death), can justifiably put forth a claim to possess an ethical right to its life. Indeed, in principle, our task of assessing the ethical justifiability of the aforementioned specific issues would essentially have been determined by the answer we can secure to the issue of the ethical right to life, namely, establishing an ethical right to life would in essence preempt the question of the ethical justifiability of the aforementioned specific issues. As such, addressing the issue of an ethical right to life is to be pivotal to our whole enterprise.[2] By this, however, we do not

---

1. Clearly, different people use the notion to signify different things, not to mention the fact that for a good number of people the notion remains fuzzy and imprecise and that, in the last analysis, they do not really know what they mean to say when using the notion of the ethical (except that it is something which ought to be viewed as commendable).

2. But, of course, it is all-important for us to note that the context in which the issue of a right to life arises for us here determines, in a number of significant ways, the more specific signification by which the issue is to be taken here. Thus, first, "life" as it appears in this issue is but the specification that would be applicable here of the more fundamental and general notion of existence. The issue in its most fundamental and general signification is that of a right to exist (although evidently, with respect to an entity that is living, its existence would be commensurate with life). Secondly, seeing that we are concerned with the assessment of this issue from an ethical vantage point rather than from some other vantage point (as for example, from the legal or political vantage point), the claim to a right to life, i.e., to existence, is a claim that implicates here a right that is an ethical right rather than a legal or a political right. Thirdly, and lastly, to spell out more precisely the signification of the ethical right to life (i.e., to exist) with which we are concerned here, it is specifically and exclusively the ethical right of an entity not to have its life, its existence, terminated; it is not a signification which articulates an ethical right to be brought into life (i.e., into existence) or to be sustained in life (i.e., in existence). Indeed, it is precisely because of this specification (i.e., taking the right here to signify exclusively the right not to have one's life terminated

mean to suggest that a settling of the issue of an ethical right to life would comprehensively settle the aforementioned specific issues in their totality thus precluding the possibility of any further discussion with regard to them. Far from it. For clearly, there are any number of possible additional considerations that can impinge on these issues and modify our final assessment of them (as, for example, the consideration of human life *in potentia* in connection with the issue of abortion or the consideration of the quality of life in connection with the issue of euthanasia). Indeed, in coming to deal with the aforementioned specific issues we want to pay attention to these possible additional considerations and try to determine the modifications which they would introduce into our original assessments of these issues.

Thus, in view of the foregoing considerations, the format by which we propose to proceed is as follows: we start, first, by trying to delineate, as briefly and schematically as we can, what, according to our understanding, the enterprise of ethics is all about, thus attempting to clarify what the appellation of the term "ethical" signifies for us. Here, while not denying the feasibility and, indeed, the validity of the relativistic approach that perceives the ethical enterprise as grounding itself in the ethos or mores of the society to which the individual belongs (these, indeed, being the original significations from which the terms "ethics" and "morality" are respectively derived), our formulation pursues the alternative approach that would claim that in addition to, though not necessarily in place of, the approach that takes all ethical evaluations as being relative to the societies in which they are formulated, there can be ethical evaluations that are absolute in the sense of being universal as to space and time. Such moral evaluations ground themselves not in the mores of certain societies or in the arbitrary likes and dislikes of the individual but in some aspect of the ontological constitution of the human entity as, for example, its rational capacity, its desire for happiness or for pleasure, seeing that the ontological constitution of the human entity transcends the relativism of space and time (true, an alternative grounding that can also claim to transcend the relativism of space and time is the grounding of ethical evaluation in a divine revelation, but such grounding, aside from the

---

rather than the right to be brought into life or to be sustained in life) that we are not dealing in this work with such issues as birth control or transplantation of organs, even though these issues may give rise to as much contention in our society as the issues with which we propose to deal here.

fact that it leads us away from the domain of philosophy to that of religion, precipitates, as we shall see below, some difficult problems).

Still, stopping at this point as regards the placement of our formulation relative to the placement of other formulations would not be satisfactory, and this because of two further considerations. First, grounding the ethical evaluations in any of these particular aspects of the ontological constitution of the human entity does not delve deep enough to come in contact with the fundamental "stuff" in terms of which the ontological constitution of the human entity constitutes itself—it merely stops at some of its expressions or manifestations. Second, in grounding the ethical evaluation in a single aspect of the ontological constitution of the human entity, it devoids it from proceeding beyond the evaluation of the act as such to the evaluation of its agent inasmuch as it does not provide for the agent the possibility of choosing and thus of bearing responsibility. Indeed, the ethical evaluation of the act itself becomes a forgone conclusion and thus fully predictable (an in this sense "empty"), seeing that no alternative way of acting is available to its agent inasmuch as the agent can only act in conformity with its ontological constitution, and in this case the ontological constitution precludes any other option of activity. To overcome this difficulty, the ontological constitution of the agent must be such as to allow it alternative modes of acting. It is precisely here, we would submit, that our formulation gains its advantage in that it manages to provide us with the possibility of an alternative way of acting. It does this by resorting to the Buberian It-Thou bifurcation, the bifurcation between acting in terms of utilization and acting in terms of affirmation and, indeed, by ultimately grounding this bifurcation in the fundamental ontological bifurcation between power, the "stuff" in terms of which the It-dimension constitutes itself, and consciousness, the "stuff" in terms of which the Thou-dimension constitutes itself, and by pointing out further that such a bifurcation is available not only in theory but in actuality, to wit, in the ontological constitution of the human entity. Namely, it claims to show that in contra-distinction to the entities of nature that are ontologically constituted exclusively in terms of the It-dimension and the biblical divine entity that ideally would, in the last analysis, ontologically constitute itself as a pure Thou entity, the human entity is ontologically constituted as an It/Thou entity, an entity that is ontologically constituted both in terms of power and in terms of consciousness.

Second, we move to analyze the notion of an ethical right to life, trying in the process to identify the attribute that can endow an entity with such an ethical right. After examining any number of alternative possibilities that have been put forth in the literature (trying to assess their respective strengths and weaknesses so as to incorporate the former and, hopefully, avoid the latter in our formulation), we put forth the claim that a persuasive rationale and thus justification for arrogating to an entity an ethical right not to have its existence terminated can be provided only on behalf of an entity that possesses self-consciousness—only the attribute of self-consciousness can endow an entity with such an ethical right (the possession of sensation, reason, or even consciousness as such fails to provide us with a satisfactory rationale).

Third, we conclude by turning our attention to examining the various specific issues that implicate the termination of life. Although as pointed out above, our fundamental position with respect to these issues has been, in principle, already determined by the conclusion at which we have arrived in the previous section, to wit, that an entity that possesses self-consciousness has by virtue of this an ethical right to claim that its existence be not terminated, these issues call nonetheless for further examination in view of, again as already pointed out, the extenuating factors that enter the picture in relation to them. Now, in pursuing this examination we try to address the many positions that have already been put forth with respect to these issues and in the process formulate our position with respect to any modifications, if any, that may be called for in response to these extenuating factors.

A final observation may perhaps be in order. Although the work here undertakes to examine and assess at some length various formulations that have been put forth, it is not to be taken as being principally a descriptive or a critical work a propos these alternative formulations. Rather, the principal thrust of the work here lies in its being "constructive," it attempts to advance innovative considerations and arguments regarding the difficult issues that arise within the various facets of the topic that is before us here.

I
The Nature and Parameters of the Ethical Enterprise

1) According to our understanding, the ethical enterprise, unlike the scientific enterprise, is to be delineated as an enterprise whose task is not one of the discovery or of description, but rather one of evaluation. The enterprise of ethics is engaged and concerned with the evaluation of things, not with their discovery or description. As such, indeed, it is much more similar to such an enterprise as that of esthetics (indeed, the two belong to the same class of enterprises, namely, the class that belongs to the axiological domain) than to such enterprises as those of chemistry, biology or sociology (enterprises that belong to the epistemological domain). Of course, for the ethical enterprise to be able to carry out its task of evaluation its object, i.e., that which is to be evaluated, must be present. It is not, however, the concern or the task of the ethical enterprise to bring about its presence or to establish its validation. Rather, the ethical enterprise takes the presence of its object as a given and proceeds from there its task of evaluating it.[1]

2) Evaluation, however, clearly implicates, of necessity, judgment. The act of evaluation is at one and the same time an act of judgment—to evaluate something is to judge that something. Thus, an evaluation that is positive necessarily implicates a judgment of approval and conversely an evaluation that is negative necessarily implicates a judgment of disapproval. Evaluation and judgment hang together—they are inseparable siamese twins. So, in claiming that the undertaking of the ethical enterprise is to evaluate, we inescapably and of necessity must also claim that it is to judge—the undertaking of the ethical enterprise is to evaluate/judge.

But the act of evaluation/judgment necessarily implicates, in turn, yet one more act, to wit, the act of prescription. For clearly, if something is evaluated positively and thus judged approvingly, this something would per force lend itself to being affirmatively prescribed, i.e., to being an act that ought to be done; and if it is evaluated negatively and thus judged disapprovingly, it would per force lend itself to being negatively prescribed, i.e., to being an act that ought not to be done. True, the implication here between evaluation/judgment and prescription is not semantic as is the case regarding the implication between evaluation and judgment. Namely, unlike the latter implication where the very meaning of the notion of the evaluation implicates the notion of judgment, here the meaning of the notion of evaluation or of the notion of judgment does not implicate the notion of prescription. Rather, the implication here is merely logical. Namely, logic dictates that a positive evaluation or a judgment of approval would entail an affirmative prescription while a negative evaluation or a judgment of disapproval would entail a negative prescription. Still, given our concerns here, the implicating force of the logical implication is, for all intents and purposes, equivalent to the implicatory force of the semantic implication. It would certainly strike us as highly inconsistent if one were to evaluate/judge that an act is right/good (i.e., evaluate/judge the act approvingly) and at the same time maintain that it ought not to be done or, conversely, evaluate/judge that an act is wrong/bad (i.e., evaluate/judge the act disapprovingly) and at the same time maintain that it ought to be done.

Thus, the ethical enterprise, by its very essence, implicates not only the act of evaluating/judging but also the act of prescribing; these three acts (or, more precisely, these two acts, seeing that the act of evaluating and the act of judging coincide semantically) constitute the essence of the enterprise. Indeed, we can now broaden our previous claim and say that, unlike the enterprise of science, the enterprise of ethics is not in the business of discovering and describing but in the business of evaluating/judging and prescribing; and commensurate with this, we can further say that, again, unlike the enterprise of science, it articulates itself not in propositional statements but in commands. And as such, it would follow, of course, that while indeed in the context of the scientific enterprise the issue of truth cannot not arise, in the context of the ethical enterprise it cannot, in principle, ever arise.[2] The enterprise of ethics has nothing to do with truth—it does not establish nor does it discover it.

3) But now what is this thing, this something, whose evaluation/judgment and prescription constitute the very task and raison d'être of the ethical enterprise? We would submit that primarily and essentially it is the acts perpetrated (and thus the conduct, the

behavior, manifested) by one entity towards another entity. Entities act on each other and it is precisely the evaluation/judgment and indeed prescription (either positive or negative) of these acts that constitutes the primary and essential task of the ethical enterprise. Thus, at this point we would have to say that, in its broadest and most basic sense, the task of the ethical enterprise is to evaluate/judge and prescribe any and every act that may be perpetrated by any and every entity.[3]

4) An act, however, necessarily implicates on a subject and an object, i.e., an entity perpetrating the act and an entity on the receiving end of the act. For in its most fundamental sense an act is but a movement from an active entity (i.e., the subject) to a passive entity (i.e., the object). But this, in turn, means that an act necessarily implicates a relation—a relation between the subject and the object of the act (the subject and the object being linked to each other by virtue of the set). And this being the case, it would follow that the ethical enterprise impinges not only on the acts perpetrated by one entity on another but also on the relations that obtain between them. The ethical enterprise in encompassing the evaluation/judgment and the prescription of the acts form subject to an object also per force encompasses the evaluation/judgment and prescription of the relations that should subsist between them. Thus, our delineation of the ethical enterprise must be stretched somewhat to encompass the evaluation/judgment and prescription not only of acts but, at one and the same time, also of relations.[4] Is there, then, a way by which the notion of the act can implicate a notion of the relation that would include also the relation of mutuality? Theoretically, the answer would seem to be "no," for as we have seen the notion of the act implicates exclusively a one-way relation and not a relation of mutuality. Still, practically speaking (and it is after all the practical rather than the theoretical aspect that is the determining consideration for encompassing the relation of mutuality within the ethical domain), a way of moving from a notion of the act to that of a relation that would include also the relation of mutuality may be feasible. This is so inasmuch as in the context of concrete experience the relation of mutuality almost inevitably reduces itself to being viewed from the vantage point of one of its poles rather than from its primary authentic vantage point, which is the vantage point of the in-between and as such it too, for all practical intents and purposes, presents itself as a relation constituted by the imposition of two opposite one-way relations, i.e., relations that move from the one pole to the other. But if this be the case, the act can (albeit in a practical

though not in a theoretical sense) implicate after all also a relation of mutuality.

5) This "stretching" of the evaluation/judgment of the act to encompass the relation can also be further "stretched," so to speak, in the opposite direction to encompass the agent that perpetrates the act or the subject that establishes the relation. Namely, in evaluating/judging a relation/act as good/right (and thus prescribing that it should be done), we inevitably and per force evaluate/judge its agent/subject as being good (and thus prescribe to it that it ought to perform/establish the act/relation. This is basically what can be meant when one evaluates/judges an agent/subject as being good—what is meant is that it is the agent/subject of an act/relation that is right/good. Thus, in our approach the evaluation/judgment of the agent/subject is derived from and is directly dependent on the evaluation/judgment of the act/relation of which it is the agent/subject.[5]

True, we often judge/evaluate an agent/subject not in relation to any of its specific acts/relations but in what may appear to be its own terms. Namely, we may appear to want to say that the agent/subject is ethically good in its own terms, i.e., by virtue of what it is, which is to say, by virtue of its possessing certain qualities, certain characteristics, that in themselves we can somehow evaluate/judge as ethically good or, as we might say, by virtue of its possessing certain virtues. But this is not what really takes place and any such claims to this effect would not be quite valid. For, we would submit that we really cannot evaluate/judge any qualities or characteristics of any entity as being themselves, in their own terms, ethically good. When we do evaluate/judge the agent/subject in itself as being ethically good we are engaged in a generalization and what we are really saying is that the agent/subject is an agent/subject that on the whole and as a rule perpetrates/establishes acts/relations that are ethically right/good. By saying that the entity is ethically good we are saying that as a rule and on the whole it would be an agent/subject of acts/relations that are ethically good; and by saying that is possesses virtues we mean to say that it possesses predilections, inclinations, to perpetrate/establish acts/relations that are ethically right/good, that it has qualities and characteristics that would incline it and lend it to perpetrate/establish to perpetrate/establish acts/relations that are ethically right/good.

6) It should be noted, however, that while the evaluation/judgment of an act/relation (and thus also of its prescription) with respect to its agent/subject, the same cannot be said with respect to its object. Indeed,

such an implication is not possible, seeing that the object is a passive recipient of the act/relation and, therefore, unlike the agent/subject of the act/relation, it does not play any role in constituting the act/relation, which, in turn, leads to the fact that, again, unlike the situation regarding the agent/subject, but in the situation regarding the object no implicatory relation from the act/relation to the object is feasible. This being the case, the evaluation/judgment of the act/relation cannot be extended and made to impinge also upon the object as is the case with the agent/subject.

7) Still, although the evaluation/judgment of the act/relation has no bearing whatsoever on the evaluation/judgment of its object, this is not to say that the object is not implicated in the process of evaluation judgment. Indeed, the object is very much implicated in the process of evaluation/judgment, except that it is implicated not as a recipient of the evaluation/judgment accorded to the act/relation in question but, just the opposite, as a determining factor in the constituting of the evaluation/judgment of the act/relation in question. For the kind of entity the object is will play an important role in determining what kind of act/relation is right/good with respect to it.

The relation here between an act/relation and its object is analogous to the relation that obtains between a key and its lock. Thus, in the same way that the evaluation/judgment of whether or not a key is the right key (i.e., the key that fits) depends on what kind of lock it is supposed to unlock (it being the contours of the lock that determine whether or not the key would fit as such whether or not it is the right key), so the evaluation/judgment of whether or not an act/relation is ethically right/good would depend on the kind of object to which it is directed. And by the same token that a key is not right (i.e., fitting) regarding one kind of lock may well be right (i.e., fitting) regarding another kind of lock, so an act/relation that is evaluated/judged ethically wrong with respect to one kind of object may well be evaluated/judged ethically right with respect to another kind of object. And clearly, as such, the kind of lock or object that is implicated will determine the evaluation/judgment of the rightness of the key or of the act/relation respectively that are involved here.

8) But, to turn back to the agent/subject of the act/relation, we should note that the commensurateness established above between the ethical evaluation/judgment of the act/relation and the ethical evaluation/judgment of its agent/subject (to wit, the extension of the

ethical evaluation/judgment from its act/relation that is evaluated/judged as ethically good is commensurately evaluated/judged as ethically good and, conversely, the agent/subject of the act/relation that is evaluated/judged as ethically bad is commensurately evaluated/judged as ethically bad) implicates an evaluation/judgment of the agent/subject that is not in terms of the agent/subject itself but merely in terms of the acts/relations that it has perpetrated/established. The evaluation of the agent/subject here is thus but a reflection of the evaluation of its acts/relations—it is but the mirror image of the evaluation/judgment of the acts/relations involved. As such, while the procedure by which the evaluation/judgment of the agent/subject is established is certainly valid and indeed the evaluation/judgment can be delineated as an ethical evaluation/judgment (namely, it is valid to deduce from the evaluation/judgment of an act/relation that is ethically good, that is, that its agent/subject is to be evaluated/judged as being, commensurately, also ethically good), such an evaluation/judgment is, in the last analysis, rather "thin" inasmuch as it is an automatic, foregone conclusion that inevitably ensues from the ethical evaluation/judgment of an act/relation and that as such does not ethically evaluates/judges the agent/subject in any sense that goes beyond the ethical evaluation/judgment of the act/relation in question itself.

But to evaluate/judge in an ethical sense the agent/subject in its own terms, thus giving us with respect to such an agent/subject an ethical evaluation that signifies something more than the mere fact that it is the agent/subject that is perpetrated/established (and to that extend appropriating the ethical evaluation accorded to the latter), it must be possible to hold the agent/subject accountable, i.e., responsible, for the acts/relations that it has perpetrated/established and that have been ethically evaluated/judged. For clearly, if the agent/subject cannot be held accountable, responsible, for the acts/relations that it has perpetrated/established, it cannot be, in a full sense and in its own terms, ethically evaluated/judged with respect to these acts/relations—it cannot really be evaluated/judged as ethically bad if they are evaluated/judged as ethically bad, nor can it be evaluated/judged as ethically good if they are evaluated/judged as ethically good (though, as we have tried to argue above, in a minimal and derived sense, merely by virtue of being their agent/subject, it can be ethically so evaluated/judged and this irrespective of whether or not it can be held accountable, responsible, for them).

But for it to be possible to hold the agent/subject accountable, responsible, for the acts/relations that it has perpetrated/established, the agent/subject must meet three conditions. First, the agent/subject must be an entity that is endowed with rationality. For clearly, it is only by virtue of possessing rationality that an entity can become aware of and discern between the ethically good and the ethically bad. But without the ability to become aware of and to discern between the ethically good and the ethically bad, an entity cannot be held accountable, responsible, for perpetrating/establishing one kind of act/relation rather than another. Clearly, the possession of rationality is a necessary condition for holding the agent accountable, responsible, for perpetrating/establishing its acts/relations. But just as clearly, this in itself is not yet a sufficient condition. The satisfying of a second condition must be added. Namely, the agent/subject must be an entity endowed with the capacity to choose its acts/relations freely, which is to say, that its choice of acts/relations is determined exclusively by itself and not by any factor outside itself. For clearly, it is not possible to hold an agent/subject accountable, responsible, for the acts/relations that it has perpetrated/established if the perpetration/establishment of the acts/relations is determined by any factor outside the agent/subject itself and this is the case irrespective of the fact that the agent/subject may be endowed with rationality. The satisfying of this second condition is clearly also a necessary condition for holding the agent/subject accountable, responsible, for perpetrating/establishing its acts/relations and thus for holding it to ethical evaluation/judgment in its own terms and in the full sense. But even so, it still fails to provide us with a sufficient condition for holding the act/subject accountable, responsible, for all its acts/relations. It merely adds another necessary condition but not a sufficient condition. We are still dealing with two conditions that are necessary but that either by themselves or together fall short of constituting a sufficient condition. To attain the state of affairs that would provide us not only with the necessary conditions but with an array of conditions that can constitute the sufficient condition, a third condition must be satisfied, namely, the condition that stipulates that the agent/subject must have the option of alternative acts/relations available to it. For only by having the stipulation of this third condition satisfied can there be the stipulation of the second condition, to wit, the stipulation whereby the agent/subject is to be endowed with the capacity to choose freely, be carried out and realized. Without having the option of alternative acts/relations available to itself, the agent/subject clearly cannot express and thus realize its capacity for choosing freely (or, for that matter, its possession of rationality);[6] for all intents and purposes, its act/relation is pre-determined for it outside its capacity to choose freely and its possession of rationality—the only act/relation that it can perpetuate/establish is the one available to it.[7] Thus, for an entity to be ethically evaluated/judged (in its own terms and in the fullest sense), all three foregoing conditions must be satisfied, each in itself constituting a necessary condition but only all three taken together constituting the sufficient condition.[8]

9) Now, this brings us to what is most likely the most fundamental issue in our whole undertaking here, which is to say, in the whole undertaking of trying to delineate and clarify the nature of the ethical enterprise and the way it comes to constitute itself, namely, it brings us to the issue of the criterion by virtue of which an ethical evaluation/judgment of an act/relation can be made.[9] For, if the ethical enterprise is to be delineated (as indeed, it is proposed here) as that enterprise that, by its very essence, undertakes to evaluate/judge acts/relations, then clearly the issue of what kind of criterion is to be involved must be introduced. For it is self-evident that an evaluation/judgment must per force implicate a criterion, seeing that it is only with reference to a criterion that an evaluation/judgment can formulate itself—if there is no criterion, evaluation/judgment is not feasible (no ticket, no laundry). So, the question that must arise for us is: what kind of criterion must be implicated in order for the evaluation/judgment that formulates itself in terms to be characterized as ethical rather than as something else, e.g. as esthetic or as technological? We would submit that what would constitute the criterion that would characterize an evaluation/judgment that is carried out in its terms as an ethical evaluation/judgment is the ontological structure of the agent/subject of the act/relation that is evaluated/judged. Thus, we would submit that an act/relation would be evaluated/judged as being ethically good/right in as much as it expresses, realizes, the ontological structure of its agent/subject.

10) But clearly, alternative delineations of the criterion that is to characterize the evaluations/judgments that are carried out in its light as being ethical have been put forth and this being the case we are clearly obliged to provide a rationale, a justification, why the delineation proposed by us, i.e., the delineation of the criterion in terms of the ontological structure of the agent/subject is to be preferred over the alternative delineations. Of course, in order to be able to provide such a rationale, a justification, an agreement must be available as to which aspects are taken as being essential to ethical evaluation/judgment, namely, as to which aspects must be satisfied as the condition *sine qua*

non for an evaluation/judgment to be characterized as ethical rather than as something else. For only as such can one have a benchmark by which to make the case in favor of a certain delineation over the various other alternative delineations that have been put forth that can provide us the criterion by which evaluations/judgments made in its light can be validly characterized as ethical. So, what are the aspects over which there may be agreement that they are essential (i.e. that they are a condition sine qua non), which is to say, that they must be satisfied if an evaluation/judgment is to be validly characterized as ethical? We would submit that there are, in principle, three such aspects. First, the evaluation/judgment must be universally applicable in the sense that it might apply indiscriminately to every individual member of the collectivity whose acts/relations are to be subjected to ethical evaluation/judgment, which is to say that if it applies to Tom then per force and inescapably it must also apply to Dick and Harry and every other individual member in the collectivity. Secondly, it must be absolute in its formulation in the sense that the validity of the evaluation is in no way contingent on time and space, which is to say that if an act/relation is evaluated/judged to-day in place A as ethically right/good, then (assuming, of course, that the act/relation and the circumstances in which it takes place remain the same) this evaluation must per force remain valid at all other imaginable points of time in the past and in the future and all places within this universe.[10] And thirdly, its justification ultimately must be grounded in processes of reflection (argumentation) that abide by the canons of rationality, which is to say that the justification for an evaluation/judgment that claims to be a *moral* evaluation/judgment must be in terms of reason, namely, it must resort to rational considerations in order to make a case for itself.[11]

But if this be the case, then the third stipulation that we have put down does also bear a significance. Indeed, the significance it bears is even more fundamental than that borne by the preceding two stipulations; for while the preceding two stipulations safeguard for us the ethical status of the evaluations/judgments in question, this third stipulation safeguards for us the very viability of the ethical enterprise itself. This is so in as much as a good case can be made that the ethical enterprise would not really be feasible if its evaluations/judgments were appropriated by only a segment, a fraction, of the members of the class of moral entities and not by the totality of the members. The ethical enterprise cannot be functional with respect to only one part of the moral community and still be viable; to be viable, the ethical enterprise must be capable of encompassing the totality of the moral community.

And it is precisely this capacity that the third stipulation delivers and safeguards, seeing that reason is a common denominator that underlies the totality of the moral community (indeed, it and free will are the only characterizations that can lend themselves here as common denominators; free will, however, has not been implicated here because, in contrast to reason, it does not apply to the issue of justification). Thus, all three stipulations presented above bear significantly on the viability of the ethical enterprise and, indeed, must be satisfied if that viability is to be safeguarded.

And now, having these three stipulations to serve as a standard, as a bench-mark, by which to determine the viability of any formulation that is being put forth (there being various formulations by virtue of the fact that there are any number of factors or considerations that may suggest themselves as the criterion in the light of which an ethical evaluation/judgment can be carried out), we can proceed to show how formulations that have been put forth thus far all fail, in the last analysis, to satisfy one or another of these three stipulations and consequently cannot really be viable and that, in contrast, the formulation that we propose to put forth will succeed in fully satisfying all three stipulations and will therefore be a viable formulation.

Thus, it should be clear that all subjectivist formulations, namely, all formulations that place the criterion for moral evaluation/judgment in one or another particular aspect or property possessed exclusively by an individual moral entity/agent,[12] cannot be viable. For such formulations cannot possibly satisfy the first two stipulations established above, i.e., the stipulations whereby moral evaluations/judgments must be universal in their applicability and absolute in their constitution, seeing that moral evaluations/judgments whose criterion is placed in some particular aspect or property possessed exclusively by an individual moral entity/agent can be applicable only to that single individual moral entity/agent but not necessarily to other prospective moral entities/agents (thus it is not universalizable) and that in as much as it is linked to a single individual moral entity/agent that by its very constitution is per force finite in the duration of its existence,[13] its viability cannot be established in an absolute sense, i.e., it cannot be established that it was applicable from time immemorial or that it would be applicable to the end of days. Thus, such formulations as, for example, the emotivist or the existentialist formulation cannot, in the light of the foregoing considerations, be taken as formulations that validly capture and represent the ethical enterprise. For clearly in both formulations the criterion, in the light of which the ethical evaluation/judgment is to be made, is placed in some subjective aspect of the prospective individual moral entity/agent—in the emotivist formulation it is placed in the emotion/attitude that the entity/agent happens to possess at the moment, while in the existentialist formulation it is placed in the absolute freedom (i.e., in the total lack of determination either by factors outside or by factors inside the entity/agent) by which the entity/agent makes its choices and acts. Thus, in both formulations here the ethical evaluation/judgment is to be carried out in terms of a criterion that is totally subjective, seeing that the criterion is located either in the feelings of the moment of the prospective moral entity/agent (in the emotivist formulation) or in its totally free and, as such, arbitrary choices (in the existentialist formulation).[14] And, of course, as such, these formulations could not possibly satisfy either the stipulation of universality or that of absoluteness and consequently cannot provide us with an evaluation/judgment that would be ethically valid.

To secure a formulation that would be ethically viable, i.e., that would be capable of satisfying the stipulations submitted above, we must forsake the formulations that are subjectivist and turn to formulations that are objectivist, i.e., to formulations that place the criterion whereby an ethical evaluation/judgment is to be made in some entity or factor outside the prospective individual moral entity/agent, this being the only alternative kind of formulation available to us. For only in escaping the subjectivist kind of formulation does the possibility of satisfying the stipulations of universality and absoluteness avail itself and, seeing that there is no other alternative kind of formulation available except the objectivist kind, this means, in turn, that the possibility of satisfying the stipulations of universality and absoluteness will avail itself only in the context of an objectivist formulation. And, of course, as such, the requirement that a formulation be objectivist constitutes itself as a necessary condition for an evaluation/judgment to be an *ethical* evaluation/judgment—an ethical evaluation/judgment can avail itself only with respect to objectivist formulations. But, at the same time, this is not to say that the requirement for an objectivist formulation is also a sufficient condition. Indeed, it is not, seeing that we can have objectivist formulations that nonetheless may fail to satisfy one or another of the three stipulations put forth above and that therefore could not qualify as being a moral formulation rather than, for instance, a legal formulation or a custom.

Thus, for example, two of the more substantial and prominent objectivist formulations may well fall into this category. We have in mind what may be referred to as the communal/social or nation/state formulation (e.g., Hegel's ethics) and the religious formulation (e.g., Judaism's or Christianity's ethics). These two formulations are clearly objectivist, seeing that in both the criterion in terms of which the moral evaluation/judgment is made is placed outside the prospective individual moral entity/agent—in the former it being placed in the interests and/or values of the community to which the prospective individual moral entity/agent belongs[15] (thus an act is to be evaluated/judged positively when it conforms to these interests and/or values and negatively when it diverges from them) while in the latter it being placed in the dictates emanating from a divine being as communicated through an act of revelation (thus an act is to be evaluated/judged positively when it conforms to these dictates and negatively when it diverges from them). Still, these two formulations, we would submit, fail to provide us with evaluations/judgments that are morally viable. This is so with respect to the communal/social formulation, seeing that the formulation here fails to satisfy the stipulations of universality and absoluteness. It fails to satisfy the stipulation of universality in as much as it places the criterion for the evaluations/judgments in the interests and/or values of one community/society to the exclusion of all others and consequently its evaluations/judgments can be ethically viable only in the context of this one community/society but not necessarily in the context of other communities/societies (an act that is evaluated/judged as morally right in the context of one community/society may not, and in all likelihood will not, be so evaluated/judged when the evaluation/judgment is carried out in the context of another community/society). And it fails to satisfy the stipulation of absoluteness in as much as no community/society is likely to exist forever;[16] and, indeed, even during the duration of its existence a community/society may well over time change its values and/or interests. Thus, clearly, if the evaluation/judgment of an act as morally right is to be determined by its conformity to the interests and/or values of the community/society to which its subject belongs, then the moral rightness so evaluated/judged here is neither universal nor absolute and as such the rightness here cannot be a moral rightness, and the evaluation/judgment cannot be ethically viable.[17] But this failure to satisfy the stipulation of universality and/or of absoluteness clearly cannot be raised with respect to the religious formulation (this is so particularly with respect to a religious formulation that formulates itself in monotheistic terms, a formulation that is most likely to be the case here, seeing that it is particularly in the context of a monotheistic formulation that the religious dimension is most likely to impinge upon the ethical). For in placing the criterion in the will of a monotheistic divine being the formulation here can satisfy the stipulations of absoluteness and of universality and, indeed, it can satisfy these stipulations in the maximal and the most uncompromising manner, more than any other conceivable formulation bar none (for what other entity or factor can possibly compete with the monotheistic divine being regarding absoluteness of being and universality of application?). Indeed, if ethical viability required the satisfaction of only the stipulations of universality and absoluteness, the religious formulation would have clearly proven itself to be ethically viable. But as we have seen, ethical viability requires also satisfying the stipulation of rationality (which here, as we have also seen, implicates the empirical dimension, i.e., the assertion that the claims made by the formulation will be ultimately accessible to our sense experience) and here, alas, the religious formulation runs into difficulties. For clearly the existence of a monotheistic divine being or the occurrence of revelation is not accessible to ordinary sense experience that as such would have, indeed, made it available to all the members of the class of prospective moral entities/agents. The existence of a monotheistic divine being or the occurrence of revelation is accessible only to faith, i.e., to an act of trust, and consequently can be available only to members of the subclass of the faithful but not to other members of the class of prospective moral entities/agents who do not share in this faith. But this means that there is no prospect of attaining a consensus within the class of prospective moral entities/agents with regard to what would constitute a viable moral evaluation/judgment (seeing that there is no way of persuading members of the class of prospective moral entities/agents, who, however, do not also belong to the sub-class of the faithful, of the validity of the criterion that is to underlie here the moral evaluation/judgment, i.e., the criterion of the divine command—there is no common ground on which the faithful and unfaithful can hope to attain a meeting of the minds). And this, in turn, means that the ethical enterprise cannot be viable in such a context.

To secure a formulation that would satisfy all three stipulations (and thus safeguard the viability of the ethical enterprise) the criterion in terms of which the ethical evaluation/judgment is to be made, would have to be placed, in our judgment, in the very ontological constitution that characterizes the perspective moral entity/agent.[18] Only as such, can the three stipulations be satisfied. Thus, placing the criterion in the ontological constitution should satisfy the universalist stipulation, seeing that the criterion here would apply to *all* members of the class of moral entities/agents—they all would have the same ontological constitution; it would not be possible to have here a prospective moral entity/agent that would not be characterized by this ontological constitution. Likewise, it should satisfy the stipulation of absoluteness, seeing that the factor of ontological constitution is per force present with respect to any conceivable entity/agent (there cannot be any entity/agent that would not be characterized by an ontological constitution) and as such its presence is permanent, unchanging, which is tantamount to saying that it is absolute (the factor of ontological constitution would always be available to provide the criterion for an ethical evaluation/judgment). Finally, it should satisfy the stipulation of empirical/rational validation, seeing that the ontological constitution of all conceivable entities/agents would have to be within the grasp of our natural sense-perception experience or (as in the case of a singular exception, i.e., the case of a divine entity) available to being rationally projected/inferred from such experience. But this is not to say that any formulation that places its criterion for evaluation/judgment in the ontological constitution of the entity/agent would *ipso facto* succeed in satisfying all three stipulations and as such be a valid and acceptable formulation. Whether or not a formulation succeeds in satisfying all three stipulations and as such qualifies itself as valid would clearly have to depend on the further determination of whether or not the ontological constitution that is implicated, i.e., that is put forth and utilized, by the formulation is acceptable, which, in turn, would depend on a) whether or not the ontological constitution conforms to our empirical/rational experience, and b) whether or not it, i.e., the ontological constitution, establishes itself in terms of the most fundamental and primary, i.e., ultimate, ontological elements available.[19] A formulation that implicates an ontological constitution that fails to meet these two specifications would fail to satisfy all three stipulations put forth above and would therefore, not withstanding the fact that it places its criterion for evaluation/judgment in the ontological constitution of the entity/agent, be unacceptable. Placing the criterion in the ontological constitution is indeed a necessary precondition but in itself it is not yet a sufficient pre-condition. To be also sufficient, the implicated ontological constitution must correspond to our empirical/rational experience (i.e., it must be available to empirical/rational validation) and it must constitute itself in terms of the ultimate ontological elements available and not in terms of some secondary, derivative, ontological elements, i.e., elements that are but the expression, manifestation, of some more fundamental, primary, ontological elements.

Indeed, one can encounter a number of formulations that, although placing the criterion for evaluation/judgment in the ontological constitution of the subject/agent of the act, fail to satisfy one or the other of the two preconditions and consequently must fail to satisfy one or another of the three stipulations put forth above making them, in our judgment, invalid as formulations that can provide us with a viable ethical evaluation/judgment. Thus, for example, G. E. Moore's formulation can exemplify for us the case of a formulation that while satisfying the second pre-condition fails to satisfy the first pre-condition set forth above. For as will be recalled the formulation posits a *sui generis*, irreducible quality of moral goodness by virtue of whose possession an entity/agent constitutes itself as a moral entity/agent. Now, as such, the formulation admittedly places the criterion for ethical evaluation/judgment in the ontological constitution of the entity/agent and indeed places it in an aspect of the ontological constitution that is primary and fundamental.[20] However, this aspect (i.e.., the quality of moral goodness) is not available to empirical/rational experience (i.e., it is not given in any of our sense-data nor can it be logically deduced from any other aspects in these sense-data, seeing that the quality of moral goodness is irreducible to any of these other aspects). Indeed, the only way available to this formulation by which to validate the criterion in terms of which the ethical evaluation/judgment is to be made, i.e., to validate the existence of the quality of moral goodness, is direct, unmediated intuition. But clearly, such intuition is not accessible to our empirical experience, seeing that it is safe to say that most of us do not possess this intuition. As such, notwithstanding the fact that the formulation places the criterion for its evaluation/judgment in the ontological constitution of the entity/agent, the formulation fails to provide us with an evaluation/judgment that is ethically viable.

Alternatively, Hume's formulation can exemplify for us a formulation that while satisfying the first pre-condition fails to satisfy the second pre-condition. For while Hume's formulation in placing the criterion for ethical evaluation/judgment in the sentiment of fellow-sympathy clearly places the criterion in an aspect of the ontological constitution of the prospective moral/entity agent and, indeed, in an aspect that is clearly validated in our empirical experience (there can be no denying that we are aware of possessing the sentiment in ourselves and of witnessing its manifestation in others), it is equally clear that Hume's formulation places the criterion in an aspect of the ontological constitution that is not primary and most fundamental but rather in an aspect that is merely secondary and derivative. For while there is no denying that the sentiment of fellow-sympathy does manifest, i.e., express, itself in individuals belonging to the human species, there is also no denying that this manifestation, i.e., expression, is not constant and universal but rather sporadic and selective—the same individual will at times manifest the sentiment while at other times it will not, and while some individuals will manifest the sentiment in a heightened form and/or frequently, other individuals will manifest the sentiment in a diminished form and/or infrequently (while still others may not even manifest the sentiment at all). But as we have seen above, manifestations, expressions, that are sporadic and selective (rather than constant and universal) cannot be manifestations, expressions, of aspects of the ontological constitution that are primary and fundamental; they can only be manifestations, expressions, of aspects that are secondary and derivative. Thus, with respect to Hume's formulation too, notwithstanding the fact that the formulation places the criterion for its evaluation/judgment in the ontological constitution of the entity/agent, the formulation fails to provide us with an evaluation/judgment that is ethically viable (except that here, in contra-distinction to the failure of Moore's formulation, the failure is due to its not being able to satisfy the second rather than the first pre-condition, which is to say, its not being able to satisfy the stipulations of universality and absoluteness rather than not being able to satisfy the stipulation of empirical/rational validation).

In light of the foregoing, it is clear that the crucial task that must confront us in this undertaking is to identify in our empirical experience the aspects (or aspect) that will truly prove themselves to be the primary and thus the most fundamental aspects in the ontological domain, namely, the aspects into which all other aspects can be reduced while they themselves remain irreducible to any other further aspects to any further aspects. For if this can be attained, then we would indeed have at our disposal a criterion (i.e., the criterion in terms of which the ethical evaluation/judgment is to be established) that is accessible to empirical validation (this by virtue of the fact that the aspect that is to serve as the criterion is, in the first place, located within our empirical experience) and that is truly universal in and absolute (this by virtue of the fact that it constitutes itself in terms of that which is ontologically most fundamental and therefore in terms of that which would inevitably be present in every entity and which would express itself in each one of them continuously) and, as such, we could finally establish evaluations/judgments that are ethically viable. And this being the case, our next step must clearly be to survey the ontological domain with an eye to identifying those aspects that are the primary, the most fundamental aspects, the aspects that are the ultimate "building-blocks" in the ontological domain.

11) But what do we mean by the ontological structure? We mean those features, aspects, of an entity that in the most fundamental sense constitute the entity and place it within the totality of entities making up the world. Thus, we certainly do not mean features that are merely accidental or particularistic to the individual entity; nor do we even mean features by which an entity can be arrogated to a species or even to a genus. We are looking for those features in terms of which the most fundamental and, indeed, the very primary division in the ontological domain occurs—the division that precedes and underlies not only the division into species and genus but even, more fundamentally, the division into minerals, vegetables and living entities. We are looking for the most essential, the ultimate, so to speak, bit or bits of reality in terms of which the ontological structure of any and all entities comprising the world given to us in our sense experience may be constituted.

And, in this connection, what we find, we would submit, are two bits of reality, i.e., two bits of reality into one or the other of which all the entities comprising the world can ultimately be reduced and which are themselves irreducible the one to the other. These two ultimate bits of reality are power and consciousness—blind power, on the one hand, and conscious awareness, on the other. Namely, we would submit, that all the entities, bar none, compromising the world given in our sense-experience reduce themselves to sub-atomic particles that, in turn, reduce themselves to power (i.e., energy).[21] At the same time, however, there are some entities (albeit, relative to the sum-total of entities, very few indeed) that in addition to the blind power to which their ontological structure ultimately reduces itself, manifest also conscious awareness. Thus far, it would seem to us, there can be no real contention regarding the claims made. But now (and this is the critical point that per force must brand us as ontological dualists), it is our further claim, all entities comprising the world given in our sense-claim, all entities comprising the world given in our sense-experience reduce themselves. And if this be so, then clearly we end up with two ultimate realities or, put somewhat differently, we end up with two ultimate principles by which reality divides itself, two dimensions into which it bifurcates itself—the reality, principle, or dimension of power and that of consciousness.

Now, this claim is certainly not incontestable or universally accepted. Indeed, under the impact of the positivist-scientific orientation the overwhelming trend is to deny such dualism and insist that ultimately consciousness too is reducible to power—consciousness is but an epiphenomenon emerging from certain transactions in power (that it is but a result of certain inter-neural transmissions). And certainly there is no denying that in our experience the only consciousness that is encountered is inescapably a consciousness that is linked to and dependent upon an entity that is ultimately reducible to power, i.e., that collection of molecules, neurons, that we call brain—without brain we do not encounter consciousness. Also, it would seem that full-fledged consciousness does not appear on the scene all of a sudden out of nowhere, but rather that it is possible to trace within the process of evolution an emergence of consciousness that is graded—from a mere reflexive response to an awareness of an other confined exclusively to the fleeting momentary present to an awareness that is preserved in memory to a conscious awareness (i.e., being aware of being aware of an other) to self-consciousness (i.e., being aware of oneself as the other)—and this would suggest that ultimately it should be possible to reduce it to power.

Still, notwithstanding these contra-indications, we find ourselves compelled to hang on to the dualistic view and this is so, because, try as hard as we may, we cannot possibly grasp, comprehend, how blind power (energy, pure and simple) can possibly give rise to conscious awareness; no matter how complex and intricate we make the transactions of power, the atomic or sub-atomic interactions, this cannot account for the emergence of conscious awareness—the difference between the two is qualitative and not merely quantitative, and consequently, no matter how complex or intricate the former may be, it could not possibly account for the emergence of the latter. So, we must insist that we are confronted with a reality that bifurcates itself into two qualitatively different realities, into two qualitatively different dimensions (the dimension-of-power and the dimension-of-consciousness) that are mutually irreducible to each other.

Indeed, another way of putting this is to say that we must insist that ultimately we are confronted with two qualitatively different and mutually irreducible kinds of beings, the being-of-power and the being-of-consciousness. For we take the category of being to be that which connotes the primary and most fundamental concrete expression of the ultimate reality and as such the category of being is commensurate with the kinds of reality or with the dimensions of reality that have been established. In our case, since we have established that the ultimate reality bifurcates itself into two dimensions, i.e., the dimension-of-power and the dimension-of-consciousness, we must commensurately accept two kinds of being, the being-of-power and the being-of-consciousness. But we should not confuse the category or the notion of being with that of entity. For while "being" is to connote the primary, most fundamental, concrete expression of the ultimate reality, "entity" connotes the thing, the object, that, when taken in its sum-total plurality, constitutes the world that is given in our concrete experience, i.e., that which in its sum-total plurality populates and thus constitutes the world given in the experience that remains within (i.e., that does not transcend) the mundane routines of ordinary life, the world of every-day experience. True, in every-day speech we are likely to use the two terms interchangeably, i.e., using "being" in the same connotation that "entity" possesses, and indeed in those cases where the entity is constituted in terms of one being only, there is a confluence of the two notions—the entity is identical with the being that constitutes it and as such it is understandable that "being" may be substituted for "entity" in referring to the thing, to the object. But inasmuch as not all entities are necessarily constituted exclusively in terms of one kind of being (there is no inherent necessity that compels a one-to-one relationship between "entity" and "being"), it would be confusing to use the two notions interchangeably (certainly, in those instances where the entity is constituted by more than one kind of being). In the last analysis, "entity" is really not identical with "being." Indeed, in theory, in principle, having two kinds of being, i.e., the being-of-power and the being-of-consciousness, gives us the possibility of having three different kinds of entities, i.e., the entity constituted exclusively by the being-of-power, the entity constituted exclusively by the being-of-consciousness, and the entity constituted by the combination of the being-of-power and the being-of-consciousness.[22]

Now, in view of our contention above that the criterion for ethically evaluating/judging an act/relation is to be provided by the ontological constitution of the agent, i.e., the entity that is the subject of the act, and inasmuch as there can be, as we have seen, three different kinds of ontological constitution, it follows that we have three possible criteria by which an ethical evaluation/judgment can be formed—the criterion provided by the attributes characterizing the dimension-of-power, the criterion provided by the attributes characterizing the dimension-of-consciousness, and the criterion provided by a mixture of the attributes characterizing the dimension-of-power and the attributes characterizing the dimension-of-consciousness. And only too clearly, these three criteria differ substantially from one another, seeing that the attributes characterizing the dimension-of-power are quite different from (indeed, diametrically opposed to) the attributes characterizing the dimension-of-consciousness, and a criterion constituted by mediating between the two sets of attributes would clearly differ from both.

Thus, the reality that constitutes itself within the dimension-of-power, which is to say, that constitutes itself in terms of power (i.e., in terms of energy, of movement, of force)[23] constitutes itself by its very essence as "imperialistic" in the sense of ever-striving to incorporate into itself (i.e., to engulf, to encompass, to "swallow" into itself) any and every power existing outside itself, knowing no point of saturation nor accepting any self-limitation. And this is so, because, by its very essence, what power signifies is nothing else but a striving to incur more power (or inversely—being, however, the expression of one and the same signification—it is but a persevering resistance to any diminution of its power).

But now, as one could readily anticipate, this, in turn, implicates with respect to the reality that constitutes itself in terms of power any number of further characterizations. In particular, there are three characterizations that impinge in a direct and a significant way on the point under discussion and that therefore need to be noted by us here. Thus first, the fact that the reality here constitutes itself in terms of power and as such, as we have seen, is fundamentally characterized as "imperialistic" implicates that this reality of necessity must constitute itself as a continuum, i.e., a continuous flow.[24] For inasmuch as power, as we have seen, is ultimately but the expression of movement, a reality that constitutes itself in its terms must be continuous, seeing that movement by its very nature cannot constitute itself as anything else except as a continuous flow; and likewise, inasmuch as power, by its very definition, has to be "imperialistic," a reality that constitutes itself in its terms must, again, be continuous, seeing that the capability to be "imperialistic" (i.e., to ever-strive to incorporate into oneself power that lies outside one's self) is contingent on the condition that the power lying outside one's self, i.e., the power to be incorporated, is to be contiguous with oneself (after all, incorporation, i.e., encompassing or engulfing, cannot be effected over a "gap").

Secondly, it also implicates that the reality here, i.e., the reality that constitutes itself in terms of power, must of necessity also constitute itself as a reality that is quantifiable. This is so, because this reality, as we have seen, is by its very nature characterized as "imperialistic" and the characterization of "imperialism" clearly cannot arise except in a quantifiable context (i.e., except with respect to a reality that constitutes itself as quantifiable), seeing that inasmuch as the very signification of the characterizations of "imperialism" implicates the notion of "increase" it must of necessity presuppose a context that is quantifiable, i.e., a context that allows for the notion of "more" (and, of course, also reversely for the notion of "less") to arise.[25] So, to the extent that the reality that constitutes itself in terms of power is necessarily "imperialistic" (and a continuous flow) it necessarily must also constitute itself as quantifiable.

Thirdly (and this is clearly the characterization that impinges most directly and pertinently on the point under discussion here, i.e., the way in which the criterion for ethical evaluations/judgments is to be determined by the ontological constitution of the subject/agent of the act/relation), it implicates that the reality that constitutes itself in terms of power and is thus characterized as "imperialistic" is of necessity further characterized by the fact that all acts/relations that arise within its context can only be acts/relations of utilization, namely, acts/relations where the other (any and every other) implicated in them can only be related to as a means—a means towards an increase in power.[26] And this is clearly inescapably so because of the fact that the reality that constitutes itself in terms of power is of necessity (as shown above) "imperialistic" and the characterization of "imperialism" denotes (again, in accordance with its definition put forth above) the striving on the part of such a reality to incorporate into itself any and every power external to itself. For this, in turn, clearly implicates that the relating of such a reality to any and every bearer of power lying externally to itself can of necessity only be a relating to that bearer as a means, a means towards the end of increasing its own power. So, to summarize, the reality that constitutes itself in terms of power constitutes itself of necessity as "imperialistic," as a continuum, as quantifiable and, finally, as a reality in which all acts/relations can only be acts/relations of utilization.

But now, this being the case, it follows that the criterion that can emerge from the ontological constitution of such a reality and that, as such, per our definition, would define the ethical evaluation/judgment of acts/relations of subjects that are thus ontologically constituated (i.e., subjects that constitute themselves exclusively as beings-of-power) is a criterion that would delineate itself in terms of the increase/decrease in the level of power possessed by the subject of the act—an increase in the level of power (or a warding-off of a diminution in the level of power) would implicate a positive ethical evaluation/judgment (the act would be evaluated as ethically good/right) while a decrease in the level of power (or a failure to increase the level of power) would implicate a negative ethical evaluation/judgment (the act would be evaluated evil/wrong).

Furthermore, it is a criterion that would allow (by virtue of the fact that it constitutes itself in terms of power and that power, in turn, is quantifiable) the introduction of gradations and thus a calculus leading to the establishment of a hierarchy with respect to the enterprise of ethical evaluation/judgment—the greater the increase in the level of power brought about by an act, the more positive will be its ethical evaluation/judgment (and commensurably with all the other alternative formulations that are possible here). Thus, for example, if act A brings about the greater increase in the level of power of its subject (or of the collectivity to which the subject belongs) than act B, then act A will be evaluated/judged as ethically better than act B. In other words, the ethical evaluation/judgment here is no longer restricted by the criterion to be carried out exclusively in terms of the single alternative between the ethically good and the ethically bad; rather, the criterion allows the ethical evaluation/judgment to be opened up and to be carried out in terms of a continuous succession of alternatives between the ethically better and the ethically worse.

Lastly, it is a criterion that would impinge (and this by virtue of the fact that the reality from which it emerges, i.e., a reality that constitutes itself in terms of power, constitutes itself as such, in turn, as a continuum) not on any intrinsic property that the act may possess but rather on the consequences that the act would bring about. Namely, the ethical evaluation/judgment of the act that would be carried out in the light of this criterion would be determined by the consequences that the act brings about rather than by any property or characteristic placed in the act itself—if the act leads to an increase in the power of its subject, it would be ethically evaluated/judged in a positive manner, i.e., it would be evaluated/judged as being an ethically right/good act, while if it leads to a diminution in the power of its subject, it would be ethically evaluated/judged in a negative manner, i.e., it would be evaluated/judged as being an ethically wrong/evil act (and, per the foregoing observation, we can add that the greater the increase in power, the more positive the ethical evaluation/judgment, while the greater the diminution, the more negative the ethical evaluation/judgment). Clearly, the ethical formulations that constitute themselves in terms of this kind of criterion will have to be consequentialist (rather than deontological) formulations.

As against this, the reality that constitutes itself within the context of the dimension-of-consciousness, i.e., in terms of consciousness (awareness), is by its very essence not only just "non-imperialistic," but actually, "anti-imperialistic." This is so because of the fact that, as has been widely noted (e.g., Brentano, Husserl), consciousness by its very essence is of necessity always a consciousness-of-something—consciousness by its very constitution is intentional. Thus, consciousness in the very act of constituting itself must implicate the existence of an other over-against its subject—in the absence of the existence of such an other, consciousness cannot arise. As such, an "imperialistic" orientation, i.e., the orientation whereby all acts are acts striving to incorporate any and every other into their respective subjects, is inescapably countermanding to the very possibility of the arising of consciousness. Not only can consciousness not arise if the other is eliminated, i.e., incorporated, "swallowed" into its subject, its very arising is predicated on its positing the existence of an other outside itself. Clearly, consciousness by the very essence of its constitution cannot arise in the context of an "imperialistic" orientation. And, conversely, it must follow that the very arising of consciousness must of necessity implicate the absence, i.e., the rejection, of the "imperialistic" orientation, which is tantamount to saying that a reality that constitutes itself in terms of consciousness is by its very constitution of necessity "anti-imperialistic." Indeed, commensurate with this is the further fact that a reality that constitutes itself in terms of consciousness does not constitute itself as a continuum. Each act of consciousness is a discrete, self-enclosed occurrence—it does not point beyond itself nor does it flow into or connect with another act of consciousness.[27] Indeed, this separation, discreteness, between acts of consciousness is but a reflection of the even more deeply-seated separation, "gap," that constitutes the internal make-up of the single, discrete act of consciousness itself. For the very act of consciousness is constituted by an inescapable over-againstness, a "gap" between the subject of the act, the subject who is conscious, and the other subject, which is being grasped in the act of consciousness. It is this over-againstness, the "gap," that in the most fundamental and primary sense constitutes the act of consciousness—in its absence the act cannot constitute itself.[28]

Furthermore, given this "anti-imperialistic" orientation that characterizes the very essence of the act of consciousness, it should be only too clear that the relating to the other implicated in the act of consciousness cannot, in principle, be a relating of utilization. For if it were, the act would inescapably have to be "imperialistic," seeing that utilization is but an expression, a manifestation, of the "imperialistic" orientation—an act cannot be "imperialistic" towards an other without at the same time, *ipso facto*, being an act of utilization towards that other. Indeed, the act of consciousness, taken in its own terms, cannot relate to the other as a means (a relating that is presupposed, implicated, by the relating of utilization), seeing that in its very essence it is an act of recognition, awareness, of an other that, as such, necessarily implicates the taking of the other in its own terms, the establishing of the other in its otherness, and this, in turn, is tantamount to saying that in the act of consciousness when taken in its own terms, the other, per force, can only be related to as an end-in-itself and not as a means to some other end.[29] The relating in an act of consciousness, taken in its own terms, far from being a relating that expresses itself in terms of utilization, is a relating that expresses itself solely in terms of affirmation—far from being utilized as a means towards some ulterior end, the other here can only be affirmed in its otherness, as an end-in-itself.

Lastly, in diametric opposition to an act of power, an act of consciousness, when taken in its own terms, does not lend itself to being quantified. The act of consciousness, like its signification in terms of the act of affirmation, cannot be fractionized or graded. These acts, like the state of pregnancy, are either/or, all or none. In the same way that one cannot be half or quarter pregnant, one cannot be half or quarter conscious or half or quarter affirming—one is either pregnant, conscious, affirming or one is not (it is a hundred percent or zero but not in-between).[30] Now, we can clearly surmise that the criterion that emerges from this context, from the context of the dimension-of-consciousness, i.e., the criterion that formulates itself in terms of consciousness, is a criterion that implicates that an act that affirms an other as an end-in-itself is to be evaluated/judged as ethically good/right while an act that fails so to affirm (i.e., an act that instead of affirming utilizes the other) is to be evaluated/judged as ethically blameworthy/wrong. Further, we can also conclude that the ethical evaluations/judgments that formulate themselves on the basis of this criterion would be evaluations/judgments that do not lend themselves to gradation; the evaluations/judgments that can arise here would, per force, be evaluations/judgments that are in terms of all or none and not in terms of more or less. Finally, we can conclude that the ethical evaluation/judgment here would formulate itself on the basis of the intrinsic character of the act itself (to wit, does it or does it not affirm the other as an end-in-itself) and not on the basis of consequences that it may or may not bring about. In other words, the formulation here of the ethical evaluation/judgment is not consequentialist but a deontological formulation.

Thus, given the way by which we proposed to delineate the enterprise of ethics above, to wit, its delineation as the enterprise that undertakes to evaluate/judge any and every act/relation (and secondarily and derivatively any every subject/agent of these acts/relations) in light of the criterion of whether or not it authentically expresses and conforms to the ontological constitution of its subject/agent, the bifurcation of the ontological domain into two ultimate "bits of reality" (i.e., two phenomena or principles or perspectives), that of power and that of consciousness, namely, the reduction of any and every entity within the ontological domain to one or the other of these two ultimate "bits of reality" (ultimate in that they themselves are not further reducible to anything else and, as such, of course, excluding also the possibility of either of them reducing itself to the other) gives rise to two alternative meanings as regards the signification of ethical evaluation—a positive ethical evaluation, i.e., the ethical good/right, can either mean expressing and being in conformity with the dictates of power or it can mean expressing and being in conformity with the dictates of consciousness and, conversely, a negative ethical evaluation, i.e., the ethical bad/wrong, can either mean failing to express and not being in conformity with the dictates of power, or it can mean failing to express and not being in conformity with the dictates of consciousness.[31] The justification for our identification of the It-being with the being-of-power and of the Thou-being with the being-of-consciousness is derived from the fact that a rationale for the characterizations that Buber attributes to the It-being and the Thou-being respectively (e.g., utilization as regards the It-being, address as regards the Thou-being; a means as regards the It-being, an end-in-itself as regards the Thou-being) can be established only on the basis of the It-being being identical with the being-of-power (i.e., constituting itself exclusively in terms of the being-of-power) and the Thou-being being identical with the being-of-consciousness (i.e., constituting itself exclusively in terms of the being-of-consciousness). For, indeed, as we have shown above, these characterizations arise quite clearly from the very nature and constitution of power and consciousness respectively—power being "imperialistic" of necessity implicates that its acting/relating can only be an acting/relating of utilization (and all other characterizations that necessarily follow from this) while consciousness being affirmation of necessity implicates that its acting/relating can only be an acting/relating of address (and all the other characterizations that necessarily follow from that). Indeed without this identification of the

It-being with the being-of-power and of the Thou-being with the being-of-consciousness Buber's characterizations of the I-It relation and of the I-Thou relation respectively would have to be judged as being completely arbitrary and capricious. Thus, we feel justified in claiming that the notion of the being-of-power and that of the It-being are fully interchangeable and likewise that the notion of the being-of-consciousness (or, on the basis of the identity established above, of the person) and that of the Thou-being are also fully interchangeable.

12) But while it seems to us that in terms of our delineation of the ethical enterprise the foregoing conclusions are perfectly valid and tenable (to wit, one is completely justified in holding them), we must also concede that they are really vacuous, i.e., that they are really devoid of any ethical "cash value." For the ethical judgment/evaluation does not tell us anything that we do not already know, seeing that no alternative ethical judgment/evaluation (e.g., an ethical judgment/evaluation that the act is wrong) is possible here. The evaluation/judgment is a foregone conclusion.

This is so, for, after all, the acts that are at the disposal of an entity, i.e., that an entity can perform, are determined completely and exclusively by the ontological structure that characterizes that entity; the ontological structure sets the parameters of the kind of acts that are available to an entity—which acts it cannot possibly perform and which acts it cannot possibly not perform (this is the sense of what is being said when we say that one cannot possibly jump out of one's skin). Namely, an entity can act only in conformity with and obedience to what its ontological structure imposes and, given our delineation of what makes an act ethically right, all such acts would be *ipso facto* ethically right. But now, if this be so, then when an entity in its totality constitutes itself exclusively in terms of one or the other of the two possible fundamental ontological structures, one can say *ab initio* and without a shadow of a doubt that any and every one of its acts, bar none, is ethically right. But this empties the ascription "ethically right" of any additional significant content that it may add to the situation—the most it can do is to pronounce something an x when that something is already *de facto* and *de jure* an x. In the absence of the possibility of judging/evaluating an act as unethical, judging/evaluating it as ethical, while not false or meaningless as such, does not really add anything significant to the judgment/evaluation.

Thus, while we can say meaningfully with respect to the acts of an entity that constitutes itself, in its totality, exclusively in terms of one kind of being (be it in terms of the being-of-power or in terms of the being-of-consciousness) that its acts/relations are ethical (i.e., that its acts/relations are evaluated/judged as being ethically right/good), we are not really saying very much, seeing that what we are saying is the case and could under no circumstances ever not be the case and as such the saying, while not untrue or invalid, is certainly not much of a saying.[32] Indeed, with respect to these entities there really can be no meaningful distinction between "ought" and "is." The distinction evaporates inasmuch as, on the one hand, the "ought" is reduced to the "is" (seeing that the "ought" here is defined by the "is") while, on the other hand, the "is" is identified with the "ought" (seeing that the "is" here is identical with the "ought"—the "is" can only be what ought to be). With respect to these entities, what they are doing is what they ought to do and what they ought to do is what they are doing. A meaningful distinction between "is" and "ought" can arise only with respect to entities that constitute themselves in terms of both the being-of-power and the being-of-consciousness, i.e., to entities that constitute themselves as beings-of-refracted consciousness (i.e., to humans). For here, with respect to these entities, the "is" actually encompasses three different "ises," seeing that these entities can express themselves in three distinct alternative ways—they can express themselves in terms of the being-of-power only or in terms of the being-of-consciousness only or in terms of both the being-of-power and the being-of-consciousness at the same time (i.e., in terms of the being-of-refracted consciousness). And as such, this of course is tantamount to saying that they can establish three distinct and different "ises." In such a context where alternative options are present and thus choice is available an "ought" can be applied meaningfully, namely, it is no longer reducible to or identical with the "is" (we shall have occasion to elaborate further on this in the following two sections when we come to deal with various possible ramifications in the evaluating/judging of the acts of an entity that constitutes itself in terms of the being-of-refracted consciousness). It would follow, therefore, that with respect to entities that constitute themselves exclusively either in terms of the being-of-power, i.e., in terms of the It-being, or in terms of the being-of-consciousness, i.e., in terms of the Thou-being (which is to say with respect either to the entities that constitute the realm of nature or to the entities that constitute the realm of the divine), the ethical enterprise can be applicable only in a very restricted, minimal sense, indeed, only in a sense that would not be of much significance or concern to us.

By the way, the vacuity or superfluousness of the ethical judgment/evaluation in these circumstances (i.e., when the entity constitutes itself exclusively in terms either of the being-of-consciousness or of the being-of-power) can be seen even more poignantly when we shift from considering the judging/evaluating of the act/relation itself to the judging/evaluating of its subject/agent. For while here, too, such an ethical evaluation/judgment is, in principle, feasible when the ethical evaluation/judgment is exclusively and wholly in terms of the subject's/agent's acts/relations (namely, that in judging/evaluating an agent/subject as being ethically good one is merely signifying that the agent/subject is an agent/subject of acts that have been judged/evaluated as ethically right/good), it is much more problematic to want to claim that such an ethical evaluation/judgment is applicable when it is directed not towards the acts/relations perpetrated by a subject/agent but towards the subject/agent itself. For it is very questionable whether a subject/agent can be subject to a *bona fide* ethical evaluation/judgment when it is deprived of the capacity, the possibility, of pursuing an alternative course of action. Can we really say that a subject/agent can be legitimately subjected to *ethical* evaluation/judgment when it does not have the option to have acted differently? After all, how can the subject/agent, in these circumstances, be held accountable and thus responsible for its acts/relations? But if it cannot, then it seems to us that it also cannot be legitimately subjected to ethical evaluations/judgments. For it would seem elementary to insist that only a subject/agent that can be held accountable and thus responsible for its acts/relations can be legitimately subjected to ethical evaluation/judgment and an entity that constitutes itself exclusively either in terms of the being-of-power or in terms of the being-of-consciousness is clearly not such a subject/agent.[33]

13) The ethical enterprise comes into its own, i.e., becomes applicable in its full sense, only when (with regard to the subject/agent of the acts/relations that are to be ethically evaluated/judged) we move away from entities whose ontological structure constitutes itself exclusively either in terms of the being-of-power or in terms of the being-of-consciousness to entities whose ontological structure constitutes itself in terms of both the being-of-power and the being-of-consciousness (namely, only when we move away from the entities that constitute themselves exclusively either in terms of the It-being or in terms of the Thou-being, i.e., from the entities that make up either the realm of nature or the realm of the divine, or to the entities that constitute themselves in terms of both the It-being and the Thou-being, i.e., to the entities that place themselves between these two realms and thus

partake in both, to wit, to the entities that place themselves in the realm of the human). For now, with respect to entities whose ontological structure constitutes itself in terms of both the being-of-power and the being-of-consciousness (i.e., in terms of both the It-being and the Thou-being), the option of alternative ways of acting/relating is clearly made available, seeing that such entities can act/relate either in accordance with their ontological constituent of the being-of-power (i.e., of the It-being) or in accordance with their ontological constituent of the being-of-consciousness (i.e., of the Thou-being) or, indeed, in accordance with both their ontological constituent of the being-of-power (i.e., of the It-being) and their ontological constituent of the being-of-consciousness (i.e., of the Thou-being). Thus, unlike the entities constituted exclusively as beings-of-power or exclusively as beings-of-consciousness, which, as such, are per force locked into only one possible way of acting/relating, the entities that constitute themselves in terms of both the being-of-power and the being-of-consciousness have three possible ways of acting available to them and in such a context a *bona fide* choice is clearly feasible.

Of course, in order for the choice to be actually carried out, the availability to a subject/agent of alternative ways of acting/relating, though necessary, is in itself not yet sufficient. One also requires that the subject/agent implicated here have the capacity, i.e., the freedom, to choose between the alternative ways of acting that are made available to it. Now, this capacity, this freedom, to choose between alternative ways of acting is indeed provided to the subject/agent implicated here (i.e., to the human entity, to the entity that constitutes itself in terms of the It/Thou-being) by virtue of the fact that it is constituted, albeit not in its totality but only in part, by the being-of-consciousness, for the being-of-consciousness by its very essence (and in stark contra-distinction to the being-of-power) possesses the capacity, the freedom, to choose. Thus, by virtue of constituting itself in terms of both the being-of-power and the being-of-consciousness, the human entity is presented with the possibility of making a choice between alternative ways of acting; and by virtue of the fact that one of its constituent beings is the being-of-consciousness, it has the capacity, the freedom, to effect such a choice. And if choice is available and can be effected by the subject/agent, then the ethical evaluation/judgment (with respect both to the act/relation and to its subject/agent) and the prescription that it necessarily implicates with respect to the act/relation (a favorable evaluation/judgment necessarily implicating an affirmative prescription and an unfavorable evaluation/judgment necessarily implicating a negative prescription) receive full and meaningful significance for us—the evaluation and the prescription are no longer an empty and superfluous exercise (establishing for us only what has already been established independently of it) as is the case with respect to entities whose ontological structure constitutes itself exclusively in terms of the being-of-power or exclusively in terms of the being-of-consciousness. And this being the case, a subject/agent that constitutes itself in terms of both the being-of-power and the being-of-consciousness, i.e., a subject/agent that constitutes itself in terms of a human entity (and this in stark contra-distinction to a subject/agent that constitutes itself either exclusively in terms of the being-of-power, i.e., an entity of nature, or exclusively in terms of the being-of-consciousness, i.e., a divine entity) is a subject-agent that lends itself to ethical evaluation/judgment in its full sense which, in turn, means that with such an entity as the subject/agent of the act/relation to be evaluated/judged the ethical enterprise can be carried out in its full significance.

But now, with respect to such a subject/agent, seeing that it has at its disposal three alternative modes of acting/relating towards an other (i.e., acting/relating towards an other in terms of its being-of-power ontological constituent, or in terms of its being-of-consciousness ontological constituent, or in terms of both of these ontological constituents, in terms of both the being-of-power and the being-of-consciousness), the question must inevitably arise as to when is any one of these three modes of acting/relating, rather than the remaining alternative two modes, the mode that would be applicable (i.e., the mode whose application would make sense) and thus the mode that could be validly subjected to ethical evaluation/judgment. Or, to put it more specifically and concretely, we must identify and establish the factor that would determine when the subject's/agent's acting/relating in terms of its ontological constituent of the being-of-power, when its acting/relating in terms of its ontological constituent of the being-of-consciousness and when its acting/relating in terms of both of these ontological constituents (rather than acting/relating in each of these instances in terms of the available alternative modes) is the acting/relating that would be applicable and thus the acting/relating that could be validly subjected to ethical evaluation/judgment.[34] Thus, the criterion of justice, in combining the utilization and affirmation of the other (i.e., in relating to the other as a means and as and end), does indeed constitute itself as a combination of the criterion of power (emanating from the being-of-power) and the criterion of consciousness (emanating from the being-of-consciousness) and as such it can be applied most fittingly and authentically to entities (and, of course, first and foremost to their acts/relations) that constitute themselves in terms of both the being-of-power and the being-of-consciousness when these entities are taken in the totality of their ontological constitution.

So, where can we locate in the context confronting us here the factor that would determine which of the three possible modes of acting/relating is the mode that would be applicable (i.e., the mode whose application would make sense) and thus the mode that could be validly subjected to ethical evaluation/judgment? We would submit that this factor is located in the ontological constitution of the other towards which the act/relation (i.e., the act/relation that is to be ethically evaluated/judged) is directed. For it is the ontological constitution of the entity towards which the act/relation is directed that would clearly determine whether or not the act/relation directed towards it is applicable. The situation here, we would suggest, is analogous to the situation that obtains in the opening up of a lock—the key being analogous to the act/relation and the lock being analogous to the entity towards which the act/relation is directed; and in the same way that the question of which key among the different possible keys is to be applicable, i.e., is to unlock the lock, would be determined by the form of the lock (the key whose form corresponds to the form of the lock is clearly the key that would be applicable) so would the question of which mode of acting/relating among the different possible modes of acting/relating is to be applicable would be determined by the kind of ontological constitution that characterizes the entity towards which the act/relation is directed (the acting/relating whose ontological mode of acting/relating, i.e., whether the acting/relating is in terms of the dimension-of-power or in terms of the dimension-of-consciousness or in terms of the combination of both dimensions, corresponds to the ontological constitution of the entity towards which it is directed is the acting/relating that is applicable).

Thus, we would submit, that if the other is an entity that constitutes itself exclusively in terms of the being-of-power, then the only mode of acting/relating that would be applicable is the mode that formulates itself in terms of the dimension-of-power (i.e., the mode of acting/relating that expresses itself in terms of utilization); and clearly such a mode could be validly subjected to ethical evaluation only if the ethical evaluation is to be carried out solely in the light of the criterion that formulates itself in terms of the same dimension in which the acting/relating formulates itself, which is to say that in the circumstances here it is the criterion of power (i.e., whereby the accruing of power is evaluated positively while the diminution in power is evaluated negatively). The available alternative mode of acting/relating, i.e., the mode that formulates itself in terms of the dimension-of-consciousness (i.e., the mode of acting/relating that expresses itself in terms of address, affirmation) cannot be applicable here. For while it must be granted that in actuality the applicability of this mode of acting/relating is feasible, it is at the same time also inescapably true that in the circumstances here such a mode of acting/relating could not possibly make any sense (namely, while it is certainly feasible for an entity constituting itself in terms of both the being-of-power and the being-of-consciousness, e.g., a human entity, to actually address, affirm, an entity that constitutes itself exclusively in terms of the being-of-power, e.g., a wall, an automobile, such a mode of acting/relating towards such an entity would simply not make any sense).

On the other hand, if the other is an entity that constitutes itself exclusively in terms of the being-of-consciousness, then the only mode of acting/relating towards it that would be applicable is the mode that formulates itself in terms of the dimension-of-consciousness (i.e., the mode of acting/relating that expresses itself in terms of address, affirmation); and here too, of course, this mode can be validly subjected to ethical evaluation only if the ethical evaluation is to be carried out solely in light of the criterion that formulates itself in terms of the same dimension in which the acting/relating formulates itself, which is to say that in the circumstances here it is the criterion of consciousness (i.e., whereby the addressing, the affirming, of an other is evaluated positively while the withholding of such addressing, affirming, of an other is evaluated negatively and whereby the evaluation, be it positive or negative, does not lend itself to gradation but is all or none). Lastly, here too the available alternative mode of acting/relating, i.e., the mode of acting/relating that formulates itself in terms of the dimension-of-power (i.e., the mode of acting/relating that expresses itself in terms of utilization) cannot be applicable but this time not because it does not make sense but because it is simply not feasible, seeing that utilization can be feasible only with respect to an other which is an entity that constitutes itself (at least in part) as a material substance which a being-of-power can effect but which a being-of-consciousness cannot and consequently an other which is an entity that constitutes itself exclusively in terms of the being-of-consciousness cannot lend itself to utilization.[35] Now, in the instance before us here we encounter such a situation—both the other and the subject/agent constitute themselves in terms of the being-of-consciousness (and it does not matter that the subject/agent constitutes itself in terms of the being-of-consciousness only in part, for what matters is the mere presence, i.e., availability, of the being-of-consciousness, not the extent of its presence) and this being the case, the other has an ethically justifiable claim on the subject/agent to act/relate towards it in the mode that formulates itself in terms of the dimension-of-consciousness (i.e., act/relate towards it in terms of address, affirmation) and the failure of the subject/agent to so act/relate (which evidently is the case when the subject/agent acts/relates in terms of the dimension-of-power, i.e., in terms of utilization) validly invites an ethical evaluation/judgment that is negative. True, the negative ethical evaluation/judgment here is not because of the act itself, i.e., because the act taken in its own terms is evaluated/judged negatively, but rather because the perpetrating of such an act/relation must of necessity preclude the perpetrating of the alternative act/relation, i.e., the act/relation that formulates itself in terms of the dimension-of-consciousness, and it is this preclusion, i.e., the failure to act/relate in the mode that formulates itself in terms of the dimension-of-consciousness, that precipitates an ethical evaluation/judgment that is negative. Still, this does not change the fact that, in the last analysis, the ethical evaluation/judgment that obtains here is negative rather than neutral.

Thus, with respect to an other that constitutes itself exclusively in terms of the being-of-power, the only tenable mode of acting/relating towards it is the mode that formulates itself in terms of the dimension-of-power, while with respect to an other that constitutes itself exclusively in terms of the being-of-consciousness the only tenable mode of acting/relating towards it is the mode that formulates itself in terms of the dimension-of-consciousness.

14) But now, what clearly emerges from the foregoing analysis is the fact that in order to have an ethical evaluation/judgment that is not vacuous, empty, but carries content and is thus meaningful (an ethical evaluation/judgment that has "the beef") it is not enough that the subject/agent of the act/relation to be ethically evaluated/judged be an entity that constitutes itself in terms of both the being-of-power and the being-of-consciousness (i.e., a human entity)—it is indeed a necessary condition but not a sufficient one. For, as we have seen, when the other towards which the act/relation is directed is an entity that constitutes itself exclusively either in terms of the being-of-power (i.e., as an entity of nature), or in terms of the being-of-consciousness (i.e., as a divine entity), a subject/agent that is an entity that constitutes itself in terms of both the being-of-power and the being-of-consciousness (i.e., as a

human entity), even though it has at its disposal three alternative modes of acting/relating (and as such is, in principle, a *bona-fide* subject/agent for a content-full, meaningful, ethical evaluation/judgment), it has in actuality, for all intents and purposes, only one mode of acting/relating that can be applicable and is ethically viable (i.e., can be validly subjected to ethical evaluation/judgment). Thus, when the other towards which the act/relation is directed is an entity that constitutes itself exclusively either in terms of the being-of-power or in terms of the being-of-consciousness, the subject/agent that is an entity that constitutes itself in terms of both the being-of-power and the being-of-consciousness is, from the ethical vantage point, reduced to the same status in which subjects/agents that are entities that constitute themselves exclusively either in terms of the being-of-power or in terms of the being-of-consciousness find themselves—a subject/agent whose acts/relations are from the ethical vantage point without "cash value."

To have acts/relations that lend themselves to ethical evaluation/judgment in its full signification, to ethical evaluation/judgment that is meaningful (i.e., that has "the beef" in the sense that its approvals are not merely *pro forma* inasmuch as the acts could not be otherwise, seeing that no alternative acts can be applicable), requires not only that their subjects/agents be entities that constitute themselves in terms of both the being-of-power and the being-of-consciousness (i.e., human entities) but that their objects too, i.e., the others towards which they are directed, be likewise entities that constitute themselves in terms of both the being-of-power and the being-of consciousness (i.e., human entities). For only with regard to an other that is an entity that constitutes itself in terms of both the being-of-power and the being-of-consciousness is a subject/agent that is likewise an entity that constitutes itself in terms of both the being-of-power and the being-of-consciousness in a position to act/relate in a way that is applicable and that indeed can be validly subjected to ethical evaluation in all three modes of acting/relating that are at its disposal. The three possible modes of acting/relating here are not only at the disposal of the subject/agent but the subject/agent can now actually act/relate through them in a way that is ethically viable inasmuch as all three modes can be applicable and can be validly subjected to ethical evaluation.

Thus, the subject/agent has now a *bona fide* option, choice, among three alternative modes of acting/relating. It has the option, choice, of acting/relating towards the other in terms of its being-of-power constituent in which case the applicable mode of acting/relating would be the mode that formulates itself in terms of the dimension-of-power, i.e., the mode that expresses itself in terms of utilization (and this mode would, of course, validly subject itself only to the ethical evaluation/judgment that is carried out in the light of the criterion of power); the alternative mode of acting/relating that is, in principle, also available here, i.e., the mode that formulates itself in terms of the dimension-of-consciousness, would clearly be inapplicable and if, in these circumstances, it were nonetheless applied, then its ethical evaluation/judgment could be, we would want to claim, in the negative.[36]

Alternatively, it has also the option, choice, of acting/relating toward the other in terms of its being-of-consciousness constituent in which case the applicable mode of acting/relating would be the mode that formulates itself in terms of the dimension-of-consciousness, i.e., the mode that expresses itself in terms of address, affirmation (and this mode would, of course, validly subject itself only to the ethical evaluation/judgment that is carried out in the light of the criterion of consciousness); and as in the preceding option, the alternative mode of acting/relating that is, in principle, available here, i.e., the mode that formulates itself in terms of the dimension-of-power, would likewise be inapplicable and if, in these circumstances, it were nonetheless applied, then its ethical evaluation/judgment would be, we would submit, in the negative.[37] Thus, while in the above instance the rationale, justification, for the negative evaluation/judgment of the acting/relating lies in the fact that it preempts the alternative available mode of acting/relating (i.e., the mode that formulates itself in terms of the dimension-of-consciousness) and that it is precisely this mode of acting/relating that is called for by the context of the situation there, in the instance before us the rationale/justification for the negative evaluation/judgment lies in the fact that there is a mismatch between the mode of the acting/relating and the specific constituent within the other towards which the acting/relating is directed.

Lastly, it has the option, choice, of acting/relating towards the other in terms of its wholeness, i.e., in terms of both its being-of-power constituent and its being-of-consciousness constituent, in which case the applicable mode of acting/relating would be the mode that formulates itself in terms of both the dimension-of-power and the dimension-of-consciousness, i.e., the mode that expresses itself in terms of both utilization and affirmation (and this mode would, of course, validly subject itself only to the ethical evaluation/judgment that is carried out in the light of the criterion of justice); and in similar fashion to the foregoing two options, choices, here too an acting/relating in any one of the two available modes of acting/relating, to the exclusion of the other mode, would be inapplicable. And if it were nonetheless applied, the ethical evaluation/judgment would have to be in the negative or, alternatively, the application would have to be viewed as changing the very make-up of the situation that obtains here in that the other is no longer acted upon/related to in terms of its wholeness but rather either exclusively in terms of its being-of-power constituent or exclusively in terms of its being-of-consciousness constituent and in which case a mismatch between the ontological constitution of the other and the mode of acting/relating that is directed towards it (as, for example, an other that is constituted in terms of the being-of-consciousness and an acting/relating directed towards it in a mode that formulates itself in terms of the dimension-of-power) would dictate an evaluation/judgment of the acting/relating that is negative while a correspondence between the ontological constitution of the other and the mode of acting/relating that is directed towards it (as, for example, an other that is constituted in terms of the being-of-consciousness and an acting/relating directed towards it in a mode that formulates itself in terms of the dimension-of-consciousness) would dictate an evaluation/judgment of the acting/relating that is positive.

Thus, we can conclude that only when the other is an entity that constitutes itself in terms of both the being-of-power and the being-of-consciousness (i.e., as a human entity) can the ethical evaluation be applied in its fullest range—if the other is an entity that constitutes itself exclusively in terms of either the being-of-power (i.e., as an entity of nature) or the being-of-consciousness (i.e., as a divine entity), the range of applicability of the ethical evaluation is per force limited. And since we have already established that only when the subject/agent of the acting/relating is an entity that constitutes itself in terms of both the being-of-power and the being-of-consciousness (i.e., a human entity) can the ethical evaluation of the acting/relating possess full "cash value" (which the subject/agent is an entity that constitutes itself exclusively in terms of either the being-of-power, i.e., in terms of an entity of nature, or the being-of-consciousness, i.e., in terms of a divine entity, the ethical evaluation of its acting/relating, while in principle feasible, is inescapably devoid of any "cash value"), it follows that the ethical evaluation can apply in its full range and "cash value" only to the acting/relating that obtains between a *human* subject/agent and a *human* other, which is to say that the ethical enterprise, when taken in its full range and relevancy, is an enterprise that impinges on acts/relations that obtain between humans and not really on acts/relations that obtain between humans and nature or between humans and the divine.

15) In light of the discussion in the foregoing section, we would want to suggest that what many people would take to be the three principal formulations of the ethical enterprise that arose within the history of philosophy, namely, the utilitarian formulation, the deontological formulation (in particular in its classical, i.e., Kantian, expression) and the formulation in terms of the notion of justice, are formulations that reflect respectively the three alternative modes of evaluating/judging that can arise with regard to the acts/relations that obtain between a subject/agent and an other, both of which are entities that constitute themselves in terms of both the being-of-power and the being-of-consciousness (i.e., both of which are human entities), to wit, the mode that formulates itself in terms of the dimension-of-power (and where the criterion is in terms of the increase/decrease in the power of the subject/agent), the mode that formulates itself in terms of the dimension-of-consciousness (and where the criterion is in terms of the affirmation of the other), and the mode that formulates itself in terms of both the dimension-of-power and the dimension-of-consciousness (and where the criterion is in terms of the notion of justice, i.e., in terms of balancing the requirements implicated in both of these dimensions).

Thus, we would submit that a good case can be made that inasmuch as the utilitarian formulation formulates itself in terms of happiness or pleasure (i.e., the ethical good being constituted in terms of happiness or pleasure), it really, in the last analysis, formulates itself on the basis of the criterion of power, seeing that the notions of happiness and of pleasure ultimately reduce themselves to that of power—they are but the emotional, dispositional, expressions of power in the sense that the possession or presence of power elicits the emotional state of happiness or pleasure and, reversely, that the lack or absence of power elicits the emotional state of anguish and pain (and, of course, the more power is present the greater the happiness or pleasure and, reversely, the less power is present, the greater the anguish and pain). And indeed, as such, it should not be surprising in the least (keeping in mind our analysis above) to find that this formulation, by its very essence, implicates a consequentialist approach, i.e., the act is evaluated/judged not in its own terms but in terms of its consequences (and this, of course, implicates, in turn, that the other is related to not as an end-in-itself but as a means to a further end) and that its evaluations/judgments lend themselves to being quantified (i.e., the ethical good is defined as the greatest happiness or as the greatest pleasure for the greatest number of people.) Clearly, all these characteristics, which are essential to the utilitarian approach, can arise only in the context of the dimension-of-power, namely, only with regard to entities that constitute themselves as beings-of-power.[38]

By the way, it may not be amiss to note in this connection that these two contexts are represented respectively by Buddhism and Christianity—Buddhism pursuing the total rejection of power exclusively within the context of the dimension-of-power and Christianity pursuing the same by transcending the dimension-of-power into the dimension-of-consciousness. As such, it should not be surprising that some people see a kinship between these two religions and, indeed, if one focuses exclusively on the question of the presence of power (is it present or absent) in the salvific formulations of these two religions then there is no denying that there is close similarity between these two religions. But the very point of our analysis here is to show that this kinship is really superficial and that underlying the similarity there is a basic difference between these two religions. And between these two alternative orientations, that of Buddhism and that of Christianity, Schopenhauer clearly takes his stance in the context of the Buddhist orientation. Even so, even though he rejects power totally, Schopenhauer, like Nietzsche, formulates his position completely within the context of the dimension-of-power (indeed, here lies ultimately the impact of Schopenhauer on Nietzsche) except that he places himself at the diametrically opposite pole to that of Nietzsche—while Nietzsche affirms power unreservedly, Schopenhauer rejects power totally.

Likewise, a good case can be made that inasmuch as the deontological formulation (clearly in its classical Kantian expression) formulates itself in terms of the respect for the other as an end-in-itself and never as a means (i.e., the ethically good/right being constituted in terms of the relating to the other as an end-in-itself), it formulates itself on the basis of the criterion of consciousness. And as such, it should also not be in the least surprising to find that this formulation by its very essence rejects the consequentialist approach, insisting on evaluating/judging the act in its own terms, and totally irrespective of any consequences that it may or may not implicate; also, that it rejects in no uncertain terms the possibility of its evaluations/judgments lending themselves to being quantified, seeing that its prescriptions express themselves as categorical, i.e., as unconditional, unquantified commands, which, as such, per force implicate evaluations/judgments and prescriptions being, as we have argued above, but the two sides of one and the same coin and therefore, per force, identical in their characterizations). And clearly, just as the characteristics of the utilitarian approach could arise only in the context of the dimension-of-power, i.e., only with respect to entities that constitute themselves as beings-of-power and to acts/relations between such entities thus establishing that the utilitarian formulation grounds itself in the criterion of power, so the characteristics of the deontological approach can arise only in the context of the dimension-of-consciousness, i.e., only with respect to entities that constitute themselves as beings-of-consciousness and to acts/relations between such entities, thus establishing that the deontological formulation is a formulation that grounds itself in the criterion of consciousness.

Finally, it should be only too clear that the formulation of justice in endeavoring to establish a balance between the dictates that emanate from the dimension-of-power and those that emanate from the dimension-of-consciousness can arise only in a context that combines these two dimensions (i.e., in the context of the dimension of a consciousness that is “refracted” through power) and thus with respect only to entities that constitute themselves as a combination of the being-of-power and the being-of-consciousness, which is to say that it can arise only with respect to human entities.

Thus, it would seem that these three formulations have indeed much to recommend them. Certainly, between them they do cover the whole range of the ethical enterprise in that between them they implicate and utilize every possible ethical criterion; taken together they cover the whole gamut of possible evaluations/judgments that constitute the ethical enterprise. Indeed, as such, there is no denying that all of these three formulations are from the perspective of our delineation of the ethical enterprise *bona fide,* valid ethical formulations. There is, however, a serious flaw with these formulations and it is that each of them as it formulates itself in the philosophical tradition commits the sin of *hubris.* Namely, each of them claims that its formulation preempts the ethically valid evaluations/judgments, that its formulation captures and represents the ethically valid evaluations/judgments in their totality (and that, therefore, it and it alone represents the valid ethical formulation). Thus, the utilitarian formulation formulates itself as if all the acts/relations of the human are in the dimension of power (i.e., that the acts/relations between humans can only be acts/relations between entities that constitute themselves exclusively in terms of the being-of-power); the deontological formulation formulates itself as if all the acts/relations of the human are in the dimension-of-consciousness (i.e., that the acts/relations between humans can only be acts/relations between entities that constitute themselves exclusively in terms of the being-of-consciousness); and the formulation of justice formulates itself as if all the acts/relations of the human belong inextricably to both the dimension-of-power and the dimension-of-consciousness (i.e., that acts/relations between humans can only be acts/relations that subsist between entities that constitute themselves in terms of both the being-of-power and the being-of-consciousness).

Now, clearly, both the reduction by the utilitarian formulation and that by the deontological formulation of the *totality* of the human activity to one dimension exclusively, either to the dimension-of-power or to the dimension-of-consciousness respectively, is manifestly invalid. For while it is true that the acts of the human can and do belong to either of these two dimensions, it is not true that they are locked in their totality exclusively in one or the other of these dimensions. The human as always has the possibility and capacity to act in the alternative dimension. And as to the formulation of justice, it is true that the human constitutes itself as an inextricable combination of the being-of-power and the being-of-consciousness. But this does not mean that as such all its acts/relations must inescapably belong at one and the same time to both the dimension-of-power and the dimension-of-consciousness, i.e., that all of them must be a mixture of the dimension-of-power and the dimension-of-consciousness. Rather, it means that the human constituting itself as an inextricable combination of the being-of-power and the being-of-consciousness can indeed act/relate as a combination of the being-of-power and the being-of-consciousness and that such acts/relations would indeed, at one and the same time, belong to both the dimension-of-power and the dimension of consciousness (and where as such the criterion of justice would indeed be applicable, seeing that a proportion between the two dimensions has to be determined) but it does not mean that this is the only way the human thus constituted can act. The human constituting itself as an inextricable combination of the being-of-power and the being-of-consciousness can also act exclusively as a being-of-power or exclusively as a being-of-consciousness. For as we have seen, there are instances where the applicable acts would be acts belonging to the dimension-of-power (and here not only as regards entities that constitute themselves exclusively as beings-of-power, i.e., entities of nature, but also as regards entities that constitute themselves as a combination of the being-of-power and the being-of-consciousness, i.e., entities that are human, but where the act is with regard to the being-of-power constituent of the entity, e.g., the human in terms of his/her body) and also instances where the applicable acts would be acts belonging to the dimension-of-consciousness (and here again not only as regards entities that constitute themselves exclusively as beings-of-consciousness, i.e., divine or angelic entities, but also as regards entities that constitute themselves as a combination of the being-of-power and the being-of-consciousness, i.e., entities that are human, but this time where the act is with regard to the being-of-consciousness constituent of the entity, e.g., the human in terms of its consciousness, spirit) and in these instances, seeing that the human is capable of carrying out these acts, the human could be acting and could be ethically evaluated/judged either as a being-of-power (in the former instances) or as a being-of-consciousness (in the latter instances).

Thus, as regards the acts of an entity that constitutes itself as a combination of the being-of-power and the being-of-consciousness, i.e., as regards the human entity (the only entity, as we have seen, that can be taken as an ethical agent/subject in the fullest sense, namely, the only entity that lends itself to the ethical evaluation/judgment in its fullest extent), they can be evaluated/judged from the perspective of all three possible criteria; in other words, all three possible criteria, that of power, that of consciousness, and that of justice, are applicable. Any ethical formulation, therefore, that settles on only one of these criteria to the exclusion of the other two (like the utilitarian or the deontological formulation or, indeed, the formulation of justice) is, per force, falling short of covering the whole range of the ethical enterprise. It is not that they are totally invalid or irrelevant; it is that their validity and relevancy is only partial.

16) Now, given the delineation of the ethical enterprise as presented here, one can make a good case that this delineation gives us an ethical enterprise that is non-cognitivist and as such, of course, also non-descriptivist. For clearly, in the delineation presented here the ethical enterprise is involved in evaluating and judging acts and relations and not in gaining and communicating knowledge (thus implicating also a description) of entities. Indeed, we would want to argue that being non-cognitivist and non-descriptivist lends our delineation a distinct advantage, seeing that as such it is spared the necessity of postulating or claiming that there are certain kinds of realities, i.e., certain properties, qualities or attributes, distinguished from the other kinds of realities in being ethical, that confront us and which as such we can get to know and describe. For clearly, such a claim is most dubious.

Certainly, our normal, ordinary sense perception can provide no support for the existence of such properties/attributes in things; nor can their existence be deduced from any valid premises. Indeed, no wonder that proponents of the cognitivist/descriptivist delineation of the ethical enterprise are all too often forced, in the last analysis, to posit a special kind of perception, intuition, by which to establish their claim. But this is really spurious since the vast majority of people (indeed, one suspects that, objectively speaking, all people) do not possess such intuitive power.

Furthermore, how is one to define, in this context (i.e., in the context where the "morally good" denotes a property/attribute that characterizes an entity), the ethical dimension? What would make a property/attribute moral rather than non-moral? One alternative, that of defining "ethical good" by identifying it with one or another naturalistic property/attribute (e.g., pleasure, happiness), is undermined by Moore's naturalistic fallacy charge as it bases itself on the "open question" argument, namely, on the argument that such a naturalistic definition (i.e., a definition whereby the "ethical good" is reduced to one or another naturalistic property/attribute) would necessarily lead to an infinite regress in as much as with respect to any naturalistic property/attribute that is to serve as the defining factor one can raise the further question as to what makes it ethically good, thus forcing one to reduce it into yet another naturalistic property/attribute. The other alternative (and in view of the rejection of the former alternative, the only remaining alternative) is to claim that the "ethical good" is a property/attribute that by its very constitution is undefinable, a position that Moore does indeed adopt.[39] But being undefinable is tantamount to being erased. A term or a notion that is totally undefinable is meaningless (a mere emission of sound) and as such might just as well be cancelled out. For, if the notion of the "ethical good" is to denote a special property/attribute of an entity, yet the notion being by its very essence undefinable, the denotation implicated here would be vacuous, namely, there could be no difference between asserting and denying its existence and this is tantamount to conceding bankruptcy.

Thus, the cognitivist formulation is caught in an insoluble difficulty in that the two approaches available to it with respect to the notion of the "ethical good," namely, defining it in terms of some naturalistic property/attribute or declaring it to be undefinable, are untenable—the former by reason of the "open question" argument and the latter by reason of being vacuous. In contrast to this, in the context of non-cognitivist formulations (the context to which the formulation presented here belongs) these difficulties do not arise. For, in the context of the non-cognitivist formulation, one is playing in a totally different ball park. One is now no longer involved with identifying the existence of a property/attribute but rather with the passing of an evaluation/judgment and consequently the focus of the ethical enterprise is no longer on the presence of a property/attribute but rather on the availability of a criterion.

And indeed, in these circumstances, neither the problematic connected with the undefinable term nor the problematic connected with the "open question" argument can arise here. For, to begin with, one cannot have the option here of establishing the ethical enterprise on the basis of something that, by its very essence, must remain undefinable, seeing that this something is the criterion in the light of which the ethical evaluation/judgment is to be carried out and that to have a criterion that is, by its very essence, undefinable is a contradiction in terms. Similarly, the problematic connected with the "open question" argument, to wit, the problematic of infinite regress (i.e., the problematic arising from the ever-present possibility of challenging any and all naturalistic properties/attributes as to why they are to be taken as "morally good") cannot arise here, seeing that the issue of regressing cannot arise vis-à-vis the delineation of a criterion as it can arise vis-à-vis the entities, e.g., properties/attributes, that are to be evaluated/judged in its light.[40]

What can arise vis-à-vis the delineation of a criterion is the issue of justification, namely, the question of why take x and not y as the criterion. But here, we would want to argue, the issue of infinite regress does not really arise. For once a proposed justification is accepted, this is it; there is no inbuilt propulsion towards a further justification for the given justification. The issue here is rather what consideration or considerations should determine the acceptability or unacceptability of the proposed criterion. And here, we would submit that, in the last analysis, it is a question of persuasion, namely, it is a question of whether or not the proposed criterion succeeds in persuading one of its applicability and this, in turn, would depend, to a great extent, on how one conceives of the ethical enterprise. Thus, for example, given our conception of the ethical enterprise as delineated above, the criterion that formulates itself in terms of the ontological constitution of the subject/agent of the act/relation proved to be most persuasive; but no doubt, there are others who possess a different conception of the ethical enterprise (as we will have occasion to mention below) and for them, as is to be expected, a criterion that formulates itself differently will, in all likelihood, prove most persuasive.

By the way, in this connection we may note that Toulmin's most perceptive thesis regarding the different degrees and kinds of evidence that different contexts call for (as, for example, the passing of a sentence by a Court of Law or the acceptance of a hypothesis by the community of scientists) would not apply to our conception of the ethical enterprise (though for Toulmin it clearly does apply to the ethical enterprise). The reason for this, it would seem to us, lies in the fact that this differentiation in the kind and degree of evidence called for by the different enterprises is confined exclusively to enterprises that are concerned with the establishment of facts. Here, different categories of facts, in order to be established, may well call for different kinds and degrees of evidence (and for Toulmin the ethical enterprise is included here precisely because he takes the ethical enterprise to be concerned with the establishment of certain kinds of facts, i.e., with the establishment of moral facts). But in our delineation of the ethical enterprise, the enterprise is not concerned with the establishment of facts (i.e., moral facts) but rather with their evaluation/judgment (the "facts" here being primarily acts/relations and secondarily their subjects/agents) and consequently it is not the right kind and degree of evidence that is called for, but rather the selection of the right kind of criteria, which is to say, the selection of criteria that would be applicable to the kind of evaluation/judgment that the ethical enterprise implicates. Or, to put the matter slightly differently, criteria are not established on the basis of evidence but on the basis of persuasion that, in turn, is determined by the applicability of the criteria to the kind of evaluation/judgment implicated in the enterprise that, in our case, happens to be the ethical enterprise.

We may also note, in this connection, that the problematic of deriving an "ought" from an "is" does not apply to our formulation and, this is so, even though, at first sight, it might well have appeared that the case here is just the opposite, namely, that the problematic of deriving an "ought" from an "is" would only too readily arise in the context of our formulation. For, after all, the ethical "ought" is derived here from the "is" of the ontological structure of the subject/agent of the act/relation (an "is," by the way, that is quite clearly naturalistic). But, on more careful examination, we can see that this is not really so, seeing that the "is" here from which the "ought" is derived is the "is" of a criterion, i.e., the "is" of the entity from which the "ought" is to be derived, but not also, at one and the same time, the entity to which the "ought" is to be referred. For, in these circumstances, we would submit, there should really be no problem with the derivation of an "ought" from an "is."

Namely, we would want to argue that the problematic arises only when the "is" from which the "ought" is derived is, at one and the same time, also the "is" to which the "ought" is referred. In such circumstances, there is really no justification for the derivation of the "ought" from the "is"—just because A is something it does not mean that A ought to be that something. But when the "ought" refers to a different "is," then there should be no problem in deriving the "ought" from the "is." For, to begin with, it is only too clear that in not being a cognitivist kind of formulation our formulation is not a formulation that conceives of the ethical enterprise in terms of the ascertainment/description of a particular kind of property/attribute (i.e., the kind that is ethical), seeing that what defines a formulation as cognitivist is precisely its conception of the ethical enterprise in terms of ascertainment/description. But this means, in turn, that our formulation, in being a non-cognitivist kind of formulation, is a formulation that conceives of the ethical enterprise in terms of the evaluation/judgment of acts/relations, indeed, in principle, of any and all acts/relations (and, secondarily, of their subjects/agents) from a particular vantage point, a particular perspective. This is so because the conception of the ethical enterprise in terms of the evaluation/judgment of acts/relations is the only alternative conception of the ethical enterprise that suggests itself. Namely, we would submit, that there are only two possible delineations in terms of which the ethical enterprise can be conceived—it can be conceived either in terms of the ascertainment/description of a particular class of properties/attributes or in terms of the evaluation/judgment of acts/relations from the vantage point of a particular criterion; no other kind of delineation suggests itself. And as such, this means that if the delineation of the ethical enterprise in terms of the ascertainment/description of properties/attributes is preempted by the cognitivist formulation, the only delineation available to the non-cognitivist formulation is the delineation in terms of the evaluation/judgment of acts/relations (and, secondarily, of their subjects/agents).

But if this be the case, as indeed it is (i.e., that in the context of the non-cognitivist formulation the ethical enterprise is delineated in terms of the evaluation/judgment of acts/relations and, secondarily, of their subjects/agents), then it further follows that in the case of the non-cognitivist formulation, and this in clear contra-distinction to the case of the cognitivist formulation, the "is" from which the "ought" is derived is not the same "is" towards which the "ought" is to be directed. Namely, while in the context of the cognitivist formulation the "is" from which the "ought" can be derived is the "is" of the ethical property/attribute and it is precisely towards this very same ethical property/attribute that the "ought" is to be directed (by being a property/attribute that is ethical its existence implicates that it ought to exist, seeing that *qua* ethical its existence is clearly to be commended and desired), in the context of the non-cognitivist formulation the "is" from which the "ought" is derived is the "is" of the criterion and the "ought" is clearly not directed towards it, i.e., towards the criterion, but rather towards the acts/relations that are to be evaluated/judged.

Thus, as we have indeed already stated, this difference between the context of the cognitivist and that of the non-cognitivist formulation (i.e., the difference whereby in the context of the cognitivist formulation the "is" and the "ought" impinge on one and the same entity while in the context of the non-cognitivist formulation they impinge on two distinct entities) makes all the difference in the world as far as the problematic of deriving an "ought" from an "is" is concerned. For the problematic is precipitated only when the "is" towards which the "ought" is to be directed is, at one and the same time, also the "is" from which the "ought" is derived. Here, indeed, one "cannot get an 'ought' out of an 'is'." But when the "ought" is directed towards a different "is" from that from which it was derived, there should be, as already argued, no problem in its derivation from such an "is." Indeed, a good case can be made that the very meaning of the notion of a criterion is precisely to be that "is" from which an "ought" that is to be directed towards another "is" can be derived, that its very function is to provide such a derivation of an "ought" from an "is." Thus, in contra-distinction to an "is" that is an "is" of a property/attribute and with respect to which the problematic of the derivation of an "ought" from an "is" clearly arises, with respect to an "is" that is an "is" of a criterion, the problematic of the derivation of an "ought" from an "is" does not really arise. And this, in turn, means of course that while the problematic of the derivation of an "ought" from an "is" can arise in the context of a cognitivist formulation, it cannot arise in the context of a non-cognitivist formulation (which is to say that it cannot arise in the context of our formulation).

As an aside, it should be noted, however, that in actuality the problematic of deriving an "ought" from an "is" does not really arise also in the context of a cognitivist formulation. But here this is so not because the context does not allow the problematic of deriving an "ought" from an "is" to arise but rather because in this context there is no "ought" to begin with. And this is so because unlike the "is" of a criterion, the "is" of an ethical property/attribute implicates commendation and appreciation but not prescription. And this, in turn, is so because unlike the "is" of a criterion that implicates the activity of the ethical enterprise in terms of evaluation/judgment, the "is" of a property/attribute implicates the activity of the ethical enterprise not in terms of evaluation/judgment but rather in terms of ascertainment/description and while, as we have seen, the activity of evaluation/judgment does indeed implicate prescription, i.e., an "ought," the activity of ascertainment/description may well implicate commendation/appreciation but not prescription. Thus, the non-cognitivist formulation in implicating the ethical activity in terms of evaluation/judgment does implicate an "ought" but at the same time does not precipitate the problematic of deriving an "ought" from an "is." In contra-distinction, the cognitivist formulation does precipitate the problematic of deriving an "ought" from an "is" but in implicating the ethical activity in terms of ascertainment/description does not provide the "ought" whose availability is obviously required for the problematic to be precipitated in actuality. In the last analysis, therefore, in both formulations the problematic is not actually precipitated, except that in the context of the non-cognitivist formulation it is not precipitated because there is no problematic to be precipitated (the derivation of an "ought" from an "is" does not present a problematic), while in the context of the cognitivist formulation it is not precipitated because even though the derivation of an "ought" from an "is" does present a problematic, the unavailability of one of its necessary ingredients, i.e., the unavailability of the "ought," precludes its precipitation in actuality.

Finally, it would behoove us in this connection to also address the problematic of what has been referred to as the naturalistic fallacy, namely, the contention that one cannot reduce an ethical term in its totality to naturalist terms or, to make the same point from a somewhat different angle, that one cannot define an ethical term exclusively in naturalist terms and that any undertaking to do so (such as an undertaking being the defining characteristic of the naturalistic stance) is bound to be fallacious. For after all, the problematic of the naturalistic fallacy is clearly linked with the problematic of deriving an "ought" from an "is," the two problematics being, in the last analysis, but mirror images of each other, two sides of one and the same coin. As has been remarked, "'you cannot get an ought from an is' is the motto of non-naturalism." Indeed, it should not be too difficult to see the close association that obtains between these two problematics. For if I cannot derive an "ought" from the "is" (which as such would clearly allow us to conclude that there is nothing in the "is" that would yield, produce, for us an "ought"), then clearly no "ought" could have been reduced to the "is" in the first place, seeing that if an "ought" were reduced to the "is," then the "is" would have contained within itself that "ought" and thus could have yielded, produced, it. These two relationships, however, that obtain between the "ought" and the "is" (i.e., deriving an "ought" from an "is" and reducing an "ought" to an "is") should readily lend themselves to being translated into relationships that obtain between ethical and naturalistic entities on the basis of identifying the "ought" with the ethical entity and the "is" with the naturalistic entity thus allowing us to conclude (in a fashion parallel to what has just been established with respect to an "ought" and an "is") that a naturalistic entity cannot, by its mere existence, implicate an ethical prescription nor can an ethical entity be exclusively defined by, i.e., be totally reduced to, a naturalistic entity.

But now, using the same line of argument presented above, one can apply with equal force the conclusion reached there with respect to the derivation of an "ought" from an "is" to the challenge of the naturalistic fallacy. Namely, the reduction of the ethical entity in its totality exclusively into naturalistic terms would precipitate a problematic for the ethical enterprise only when the entity is taken as an ethical property/attribute and the ethical activity is delineated in terms of the ascertainment/description of that property/attribute but not when the entity is taken as a criterion and the ethical activity is delineated in terms of the evaluation/judgment that emanates from such a criterion. But, of course, this means that in contra-distinction to ethical formulations that formulate themselves in a cognitivist context, ethical formulations that formulate themselves in a non-cognitivist context (as is the case with our formulation) do not have to contend with this twin-problematic, i.e., the problematic of deriving an "ought" from an "is" and the problematic of reducing the "is" in its totality exclusively to naturalistic terms, seeing that in their formulation the "is" is not the "is" of an ethical property/attribute but rather the "is" of some other entity—in the case of our formulation it being the "is" of a criterion (and thus constituting the ethical activity in terms of evaluating/judging) while, for example, in the case of an emotivist formulation it being the "is" of feelings (and thus constituting the ethical activity in terms of expressing/evoking). Thus, the fact that in our formulation the "ought" is derived from an "is" and the "is" is reduced in its totality to naturalistic terms (the "is" in the latter instance being constituted exclusively by the fundamental ontological structure of the subject/agent and the "ought" in the former instance being derived from the dictates of the fundamental ontological structure of the subject/agent) should present no problem whatsoever inasmuch as the "is" involved here is not the "is" of an ethical property/attribute.

But to return to the main thrust of our observations here, an equally good case can be made that the delineation of the ethical enterprise presented here also gives us an ethical enterprise that is (in addition to being non-cognitivist and descriptivist) objectivist and empirical. For in grounding the criterion in the ontological structure of the subject/agent the formulation clearly gives us a criterion (and, of course, also the evaluation/judgment that emanates from it) that is both objective and empirical. It is objective, seeing that it places the criterion beyond the subjectivity of the individual subject/agent in aspects that are shared by all other members of the species (thus in aspects that essentially characterize the species of which the individual subject/agent is a member). The criterion (and as such also the evaluation/judgment that follows from it) thus transcends the particular interests and preferences of an individual subject/agent to be determined by the dictates and requirements of aspects that are grounded in the species and that as such lie beyond the individual—rather than being the expression of the individual in its subjectivity, i.e., its expression in terms of such aspects as its feelings, wishes or desires, they are the expression of the individual in its objectivity, i.e., its expression in terms of those aspects that constitute it as that which it is. At the same time, it is also empirical, seeing that in grounding the criterion (and thus also the evaluation/judgment that emanates from it) in the ontological structure of the subject/agent of the acts/relations that are to be ethically evaluated/judged one is grounding the criterion (and thus also the evaluation/judgment that emanates from it) in a context that is open to empirical examination and validation.[41] Indeed, this state of affairs may be analogous to the state of affairs that obtains in the context of science. For in the context of science too the existence, the reality, of entities, which in their own terms do not lend themselves to being directly sense-perceived, is nonetheless established as empirically valid on the basis that they implicate the existence, the reality, of other entities that, in contra-distinction to themselves, do lend themselves to being directly sense-perceived; namely, the existence, the reality, of entities that in their own terms is not available to sense-perception is nonetheless empirically validated on the basis of the "traces," the "footprints," that these entities leave behind and that are available to sense-perception. Thus, for example, the existence, the reality, of sub-atomic particles that in their own terms are not available to sense-perception is nonetheless accepted by science as empirically validated when the existence, the reality, of occurrences that it implicates can be established on the basis of being sense-perceived. Indeed, such a state of affairs must inevitably arise whenever we push towards the very limits that circumscribe the context delineated by sense-perception, whenever we deal with entities that are posited on the very boundary (or perhaps already beyond the boundary) of the domain available to sense-perception as, for example, the sub-atomic particles in the context of science or the power and consciousness constituents in the context of our own formulation—the existence, the reality, of such entities cannot be empirically validated by direct sense-perception but only by the sense-perception of that which they implicate. And this being the case, it gives our formulation, by virtue of its being objectivist, the all-important advantage of being a formulation that escapes the charge of relativism, a charge that, given our conception of the ethical enterprise, is clearly fatal to the very validity of the ethical enterprise.

Indeed, as such, our formulation has a most telling advantage over all alternative formulations that remain imprisoned within the subjectivist orientation (and consequently are inescapably relativistic) such as, for example, the emotivist formulation (as formulated by C. L. Stevenson or A. J. Ayer) or the prescriptivist formulation (as formulated by R. M. Hare). For while there can be no denying that these formulations point to aspects (i.e., the emotive and prescriptive aspect respectively) that validly and, indeed, inextricably characterize ethical utterances,[42] in making these aspects (rather than the aspect of evaluation as in our formulation) the aspects that primarily and most fundamentally define the ethical utterance, these formulations inevitably fall into a subjectivist and consequently also into a relativistic orientation.

Thus, the emotivist formulation is subjectivist (and consequently also inescapably relativistic) inasmuch as it identifies the ethical with (i.e., reduces it to) the feelings or attitudes of the subject of the ethical utterance, more specifically and precisely, with the subject's feelings or attitudes that obtain at the moment of its articulating the ethical utterance and as such identifying the ethical with feelings or attitudes that are not permanent or constant but rather ever-changing and, indeed, most significantly, where the change involved can readily be arbitrary and capricious. Clearly, such a formulation of the ethical can only give us an ethical that is inescapably relativistic.

Similarly, the prescriptivist formulation (à la Hare) is likewise a subjectivist, and thus also a relativistic, formulation, seeing that it identifies the ethical with any prescriptivist utterance as long as the applicability of such an utterance is universalizable; namely, an utterance that is both prescriptive and universalizable is ethical. The formulation here is clearly subjectivist, seeing that it is here the subject who by himself/herself chooses and decides (i.e., there is no other factor outside the subject that plays any role in the choice or the decision), and chooses and decides in a completely unfettered, i.e., arbitrary, fashion which utterance or, more precisely, the content of which utterance is to be made prescriptive. Any utterance, irrespective of its content, can be made prescriptive by the subject; the choice, the decision, is completely at the discretion of the subject. And being subjectivist, it, in turn, implicates its being also relativistic. For clearly, different subjects may well choose to prescribe different utterances; indeed, the one and the same subject may well choose, at different times, to prescribe different utterances. And as such, of course, one could readily encounter a state of affairs where two utterances diametrically opposed to each other are deemed to be ethical, or where one and the same utterance is deemed to be at one time ethical and at another time unethical. And the fact that this formulation (i.e., the prescriptivist formulation à la Hare) adds the further stipulation (and, indeed, adds it as an essential stipulation) whereby an utterance can be taken as ethical only if in addition to being prescriptive it is also universalizable, does not change the picture here, seeing that the universalizability of the utterance is made to depend exclusively on its being posited by the subject who, in turn, is completely free of all constraints from any external factor in its decision of whether or not to posit the utterance as universalizable. For as such, any utterance can qualify for such positing, the positing being dependent exclusively on the subject's free choice—the subject can claim any utterance as being universal in its applicability.[43] Thus, in being objective our formulation, unlike current, widely held alternative formulations, has a significant advantage in clearly avoiding the problematic of relativism.

At the same time, in being empirical our formulation has an equally significant advantage over all non-empirical formulations such as, for example, the religious or the intuitive type of formulation of being, in principle, available for assessment and validation by all normal humans, i.e., by all humans endowed with the capacity to sense-perceive and to reason. Indeed, this advantage has been already alluded to in the critical evaluation we had occasion to undertake above with respect to the religious formulation (i.e., the formulation that grounds the criterion for the ethical evaluation/judgment in a divine revelation or in a *suis generis* experience of the sacred). And, *mutatis mutandis,* the same critical evaluation can be raised and consequently the same advantage established with respect to the intuitivist formulation. Namely, with respect to both kinds of formulations, the essential (and, indeed, fatal) weakness lies in the fact that, in principle, these formulations are not open, accessible, for validation to any and all normal humans. Thus, not withstanding what other advantages these formulations may or may not have in comparison with our formulation, the advantage that our formulation possesses, namely, that it is accessible for validation to any and all normal humans, is the decisive advantage. Thus, for example, although the religious formulation may indeed have the advantage over our formulation with respect to the aspect of absoluteness (i.e., it being more rigorously absolute, seeing that its criterion is grounded in the divine), it is nonetheless, unlike our formulation, unacceptable because it cannot lend itself for validation to all humans but only to a particular sub-group of humans.[44]

Thus, so far we have tried to show that our formulation, in being objectivist and empirical, has a clear advantage over alternative formulations that are subjectivist and/or non-empirical. But, of course, there are also alternative formulations to ours that at the same time, however, claim to be, similarly to the claim of our formulation, both objectivist and empirical and with respect to them the question must naturally arise as to what advantage, if any at all, our formulation may have. Clearly, if we are going to make a case for an advantage on behalf of our formulation over such alternative formulations (as, indeed, we would like to), the case cannot be made on the grounds that these alternative formulations are either relativistic or not accessible to any and all humans—being objectivist and empirical, these alternative formulations are not afflicted with these weaknesses. And this being so, the case would have to be established, we would submit, on the grounds that the empirical validation that can be offered on behalf of such alternative formulations is, in the last analysis, not persuasive as is the empirical validation that can be offered on behalf of our formulation.

Let us exemplify this point by turning to a rather prominent alternative formulation (prominent in the sense of being fairly widely accepted and certainly of having a very long and impressive tradition) on whose behalf the objectivist and empirical claims can be readily advanced, to wit, the natural law formulation in its assertion that "there is an unchanging normative order that is part of the natural world," that there are eternal laws directing the actions of all rational beings and built into the very structure of the universe (in other words, that we can attribute to the natural world not only necessary descriptive laws, i.e., scientific laws, but also necessary prescriptive laws, i.e., moral laws). Now, we can readily grant the claim that the natural law formulation is objectivist, seeing that it formulates itself in terms of a reality that lies outside the individual subject/agent, and as such, indeed, that it succeeds in escaping the problematic of relativism that arises in conjunction with formulations that are subjectivist. But we cannot grant the further claim that the assertions of the natural law formulation are in fact empirically validated as, we would argue, are the assertions of our formulation.[45] There is no encounter in our experience (and for that matter, we dare say, in the experience of the overwhelming majority, if not, indeed, of all, humans) with any laws pertaining to conduct that are built into the very structure of the world—we do not encounter in the world moral laws built into the very structure of reality in the same array that we do encounter scientific laws.

We must concede, however, that when the natural law formulation is formulated in a more restrictive way, namely, when it is formulated not in terms of the nature of the world as such but rather more restrictively in terms of *human* nature (as is the case, for example, in the Ciceronian or Thomistic formulation), the foregoing criticism does not apply. For a good case can be made that while we cannot encounter empirically traits in the nature of the world as such that determine the conduct of its entities, we can encounter empirically traits in the nature of human entities that determine their conduct. Indeed, as such, our formulation (which, true, recognizes such determining traits not just in the nature of human entities but in the nature of all the various kinds of entities and yet, nonetheless, clearly recognizes at the same time that, as regards dealing with the ethical enterprise in its fullest expression, it is, indeed, specifically the nature of the human entity that enters the picture) is very close to the restrictive model of the natural law formulation (i.e., the Ciceronian model) and consequently it is, indeed, very sympathetic and accepting of many of its features.[46]

Still, notwithstanding the closeness, a substantive and significant difference between the restrictive natural law formulation and our formulation remains, a difference that pertains to the way in which the ontological constitution of the human entity is perceived in the two formulations (the human entity being for all serious intents and purposes the subject/agent of acts/relations that can be submitted to ethical evaluation/judgment in its full sense). Thus, while in our formulation the ontological constitution of the human is essentially perceived in terms of power and consciousness (and the inter-action between them), in the restrictive natural law formulation (certainly, in its main expression, i.e., the stoic/Ciceronian expression) it is essentially perceived in terms of reason—the distinctive and defining aspect, element, of the human ontological constitution is reason; the human is perceived as essentially a bearer of reason, an entity that is rational, and thus it is reason (and not power or consciousness as in our formulation) that determines the patterns of conduct that the natural law formulation would dictate. But this being the case, our formulation, we would want to argue, possesses a clear advantage over the restrictive natural law formulation. For in perceiving the ontological constitution of the human (in the context of grounding the natural law in it) in terms of reason—leave alone in terms of such other factors as upright posture, speech, expressive features as indeed Cicero has suggested (*Laws* I, vii-xiii, as quoted in Singer 1991, 164)—the ontological constitution of the human, we would submit, is not captured in terms of its most fundamental elements. Clearly, the elements of power and consciousness, the elements in terms of which the ontological constitution of the human is perceived in our formulation, are more fundamental than the element of reason (in fact, a good case can be made that they are indeed the most fundamental elements) and therein lies a significant advantage for our formulation over the restrictive natural law formulation. Still, it must be admitted that as regards the essential question that is before us here (i.e., the question of where the ultimate criterion for ethical evaluation/judgment is to be located) our formulation is actually at one with the restrictive natural law formulation. For both locate the criterion in which the ethical evaluation/judgment is to be grounded in the ontological constitution of the subject/agent of the act/relation that is to be ethically evaluated/judged (which, for all intents and purposes, is to say in the ontological constitution of the human subject/agent). Where the difference between them enters the picture is with regard to the way by which they respectively perceive the ontological constitution of the human—while for the restrictive natural law formulation the distinctive constitution lies ultimately in a unitary factor, i.e., the factor of reason, for our formulation it lies in the dual factors of power and consciousness and, consequently, also in the proper balance between them, and thus also in a third factor, i.e., the factor of justice.[47]

Lastly, it should also be clear that the delineation of the ethical enterprise presented here gives us an ethical enterprise that grounds itself in an egotistical rather than in an altruistic vantage point. This is so not only because in our formulation the criterion in the light of which the ethical evaluation/judgment is to be carried out is placed in the subject/agent of the act/relation that is to be ethically evaluated/judged rather than in the object/recipient of the act/relation or in a third kind of entity that is outside both the subject/agent and the object/recipient (such as an abstract universal maxim or law or a divine being), but because, and this is much more significant and to the point, the criterion here is formulated in terms of the interests of the self, i.e., of the subject/agent, and not in terms of the interests of the other, i.e., of the object/recipient. We should hasten to note, however, that notwithstanding the fact that the criterion is placed here in the subject/agent, our formulation escapes the problematics of subjectivism, seeing that it insists, as was made clear above, that the ethical criterion be placed in the most fundamental ontological factors that can be identified in the ontological constitution of the human and not in any secondary, contingent or derivative, factor and certainly not in any passing or arbitrary whim or desire. For as such, although our formulation is clearly egotistical (one cannot help but act in conformity with one's ontological constitution and as such always act in one's own interest), it is not at the same time reduced to being subjectivist. And this is so because in formulating the criterion here in terms of the fundamental, the permanent, factors in the ontological constitution of the human, the criterion is being formulated in terms of something that transcends the *individual* human and locates itself in the *species* of the human, thus reflecting the vantage point of the species rather than of the individual.[48] But while this argument may well be, in principle, valid, it nonetheless clearly misses the mark as far as the issue before us here is concerned. For as we have had occasion to argue above, the ethical enterprise is not viable (indeed, it cannot arise) in any other context except the human context and, this being the case, it means that the absoluteness that the ethical enterprise requires in order to be viable is only an absoluteness that would be commensurate with the existence of the human species. As long as the human species exists the ethical criterion must indeed be applicable at all times and with regard to all members for the ethical enterprise to be viable. But before the human species arose or, for that matter, after it disappears, the ethical criterion need not be applicable (indeed, by the very nature of things, it cannot be applicable), seeing that in these circumstances the ethical enterprise as such is no longer available. Thus, the "absoluteness" (both in its temporal dimension of eternity and in its spatial dimension of encompassing all members) that in our conception of the ethical enterprise must be taken as a condition *sine qua non* is only an "absoluteness" that must be available with respect to the human species but not beyond it, and such an "absoluteness" is fully safeguarded by the fact that in our formulation the ethical criterion is placed within the ontological constitution of the human species.

Still, overcoming the problematic of relativism implicated in a subjectivist formulation, though certainly important, is not in itself sufficient to establish in a conclusive manner the acceptability of our egotistical formulation—though it is certainly a necessary condition, it is not, as such, a sufficient condition. To establish the acceptability of our formulation more convincingly we need in addition to show that our formulation has a telling advantage over possible competing alternative formulations, which, given the circumstances before us here, is to say that we need to show that it has a telling advantage over alternative formulations that equal it in satisfying our fundamental conception of the ethical enterprise formulated above (namely, that they too place the criterion for evaluations/judgments that are to be ethical in the ontological constitution of the subject/agent, i.e., in the ontological constitution of the human species),[49] but which, at the same time, differ from it in not being egotistic, which is tantamount to saying that they are altruistic. Three such altruistic formulations come to mind and it is, therefore, incumbent upon us to examine them briefly in order to establish the advantage of our formulation over them.

To begin with, there is Hume's formulation in which all humans are seen as being endowed with a sense of sympathy towards their fellow-humans, and this sense of sympathy, in turn, is being taken as the ground on which morality is established (thus, indeed, transforming the sense of sympathy to the "moral sense")—acts/relations that conform to this sense (they being acts/relations that give pleasure/satisfaction to their human subjects/agents) are ethically evaluated/judged as right/good while those that do not are ethically evaluated/judged as wrong/bad. Now, this formulation clearly formulates morality in altruistic terms (it is, after all, the advantage, the welfare, of the other, rather than the self-interest of the subject/agent, which is to define an act/relation as moral);[50] at the same time it grounds morality in the ontological constitution of the human (after all, the ethical criterion is lodged here in the sentiment of sympathy, a sentiment that is supposedly an inextricable aspect of being human), which, as such, satisfies our fundamental stipulation regarding the ethical enterprise, to wit, the stipulation that the ethical criterion is to be grounded in the ontological constitution of the subject/agent or, more precisely, of the human subject/agent. It would seem, therefore, that we may well have here a formulation that is altruistic and yet just as viable as our egotistic formulation.

On a closer, more critical, examination, however, one would have to conclude that this is not really the case. For it is not valid to claim (insinuate?) that a sense of sympathy for fellow-humans is present *universally* in all humans. True, there is no denying that there are humans, even a great many humans, that are characterized by this sense of sympathy for fellow-humans (and, indeed, even for animals). However, at the same time, it is equally undeniable that there are also humans that are devoid of this characterization, humans that are characterized not by a sense of sympathy but rather by a sense of sadism towards their fellow-humans. But if this be the case, then the claim that a sense of sympathy is an inextricable aspect of the ontological constitution of the human is clearly undermined, seeing that for such a claim to be valid the sense of sympathy must express itself universally in all humans. Furthermore, this undermining of the claim that a sense of sympathy is an inextricable aspect of the ontological constitution of the human is further buttressed by the fact that the expression of the sense of sympathy in the human is not constant but rather sporadic (at one time it may well express itself while at a different time, even though the circumstances be the same, it may not). For as such, the sense of sympathy clearly cannot be a foundational, inextricable aspect of the ontological constitution of the human, seeing that to be such the sense of sympathy has to express itself not only universally but also constantly in all humans. Lastly, there are good grounds to doubt whether, granting that a sense of sympathy is present in the human, such a presence would overcome the egotistical tendencies in the human subject/agent and lead it to act altruistically towards the other. For a good case can be made that as regards the overwhelming majority of humans, notwithstanding the presence of a sense of sympathy in them, acting altruistically towards an other would not be effected if such acting would entail any appreciable cost on their part. Most humans would act on their sense of sympathy only if there is no cost to them or the cost is minimal. But this is tantamount to conceding that for most humans their acts are guided, in the last analysis, not by altruistic but by egotistic motivation.[51] Thus, we would want to contend that the relatively few cases of authentic self-sacrifice (of the self authentically sacrificing itself in favor of an other), to wit, the cases of saintly acting, do not undermine our claim that, in the last analysis, human acting (as, indeed, the acting of all other worldly entities) is guided by egoistic and not by altruistic motivation. On this point we are clearly at one with the Nietzschean position—in the last analysis all human acting is determined by egoistic considerations.

Thus, we may well conclude that the formulation of the ethical enterprise in terms of a sense of sympathy (namely, a formulation that formulates itself in altruistic terms) fails to prove itself as a viable alternative to our formulation (namely, to a formulation that formulates itself in egotistic terms), let alone, prove itself as an alternative that possesses an advantage over such a formulation. And this is so, seeing that 1) the purportedly altruistic acts are, on closer examination, really acts that, in the last analysis, are not altruistic but egotistic and 2) even if one were to concede that the acts emanating from the sense of sympathy are, after all, altruistic, the sense of sympathy (and consequently the acts emanating from it, acts that are purportedly altruistic) is nonetheless clearly not a primary, foundational element in the ontological constitution of the human, inasmuch as it is neither permanent nor universal in its expression within the human.

The second formulation is the formulation put forth by Schopenhauer. This formulation appears to be in its basic orientation rather similar to the foregoing formulation, i.e., to Hume's formulation, except that it formulates itself in terms of a feeling of compassion, of pity, rather than in terms of a sense of sympathy. Namely, in Schopenhauer's formulation the ethically good/right act/relation is the act/relation that expresses a feeling of compassion, of pity, towards the other. But, of course, as such, the criticism raised earlier against Hume's formulation would, *mutatis mutandis,* apply also here. Thus, one can argue with equal persuasion that as with the sense of sympathy, here too, the feeling of compassion, of pity, is neither universal nor permanent in the human (i.e., it does not characterize all humans without exception nor, in most humans, is its expression consistent) and, this being the case, it does not constitute itself as a foundational element in the ontological constitution of the human and consequently, given our delineation of the ethical enterprise, it cannot be taken as the ethical criterion, i.e., as the criterion by which the ethical evaluation/judgment is to be carried out.

But even more so, it would seem to us, that one may well go beyond the criticism raised against Hume's formulation and mount an even more radical criticism against Schopenhauer's formulation by challenging the very claim that it is altruistic and arguing that, in the last analysis, it is really an egotistic formulation.[52] True, at first sight, the state of affairs might well appear to be just the opposite, namely, that Schopenhauer's formulation, far from being egotistic, is clearly altruistic and, indeed, radically so. For its ethical criterion implicates not only a clear shift to being other-centered (after all, other-centeredness is an inextricable implication of the signification of the notions of compassion and pity) and thus altruistic in its formulation. But inasmuch as the subject/agent in the context of Schopenhauer's formulation is perceived exclusively in terms of the dimension-of-power (namely, it is perceived as being constituted exclusively in terms of the being-of-power), the shift from subject/agent-centeredness to other-centeredness implicates not merely the loss of centeredness for the subject/agent but its very abrogation (i.e., the undermining of its ontological constitution). For, as we had occasion to point out above, power is, by its very essence, "imperialistic" (i.e., ever-striving to accrue more power to itself), which, as such, means that any entity that constitutes itself in terms of power (as is the case here with regard to the subject/agent) must, per force, be self-centered (its very existence being the expression of power, it must, per force, implicate self-centeredness) and, consequently, the undermining of such self-centeredness (as is clearly the case with the shift from the subject/agent-centeredness to other-centeredness that the notion of compassion or of pity implicates) must, per force, be tantamount to the abrogation of the existence of the bearer of this self-centeredness—it would be a contradiction in terms to have an entity constitute itself in terms of power and at the same time not be "imperialistic," i.e., self-centered, but other-centered; an entity that constitutes itself in terms of power and is at the same time other-centered is an oxymoron. As such, it would indeed appear that Schopenhauer presents us with a formulation of the ethical enterprise that is altruistic in a radical way—it not only shifts the ethical act from constituting itself in terms of self-centeredness to constituting itself in terms of other-centeredness but it implicates the very elimination of the self altogether.

And yet one may well argue that this estimation of Schopenhauer's formulation is not really valid; that, in the last analysis, Schopenhauer presents us with a formulation that is not really altruistic but egotistical after all. What brings about this about face is the additional factor, left out of consideration thus far, that in Schopenhauer's formulation power is evaluated negatively. Namely, power is seen as the source of human suffering.[53] Indeed, being constituted in terms of power constitutes the fundamental predicament of the human self and correspondingly the goal must be to escape the grip of power—the salvation for the human self lies in abrogating its power. Now, it is precisely in view of this that acts of compassion or pity are ethically evaluated/judged as right/good. For these acts, inasmuch as they redirect the concern of the self from itself to the other, i.e., from being self-centered to being other-centered, are salvific acts for the self (seeing that they undermine the "imperialistic" aspect and this, as we have seen, is tantamount to their abrogation of the very power in terms of which the self constitutes itself) and salvific acts clearly implicate their being ethically evaluated/judged as right/good. But this being the case, the positive ethical evaluation/judgment here is not because of the acts being altruistic, but rather, just the opposite, because of their being egotistic—it is the advantage to the self and not to the other that ensues from acts of compassion and pity that makes the ethical evaluation/judgment of these acts as right/good. Thus, we would want to claim that Schopenhauer's formulation does not really present us with an authentic altruistic alternative to the egotistic orientation of our formulation; in the last analysis, it too is egotistic in its orientation.

But whether we take Schopenhauer's formulation as being altruistic or as being egotistic, it is, we would submit, at a clear disadvantage in comparison with our formulation. Thus, if we take the formulation to be altruistic, it would suffer from the same weakness that characterized Hume's formulation in terms of the sense of sympathy, namely, that the feeling of compassion or of pity is neither a universal nor a permanent feature of human nature (not all humans manifest these feelings nor would any individual human manifest these feelings consistently at all times) and as such they cannot be taken as foundational constituents in the ontological constituency of the human. On the other hand, if we take the formulation to be egotistic, it would suffer from the weakness that its perception of the ontological constitution of the human, being a perception that is exclusively in terms of power (i.e., a perception of the human as exclusively an it-entity), is an invalid perception; the valid perception is, we would submit, the perception put forth by our formulation, namely a perception that is in terms of both power and consciousness (i.e., a perception of the human as an It/Thou-entity).[54] But, of course the involvement in such implication is only possible but not necessary—there can be expressions of the religious enterprise that would identify the predicament in some other aspect than the way the ontological constitution of the human is made up and as such may well overlap with the ethical enterprise (prophetic Judaism being a good example of this). But if this be so, then a good case can be made that Schopenhauer's formulation, unlike our formulation, is a formulation that, in the last analysis, does not really belong to the ethical enterprise but rather to the religious enterprise and it is, indeed, in this context that its kinship to the Buddhist and Christian formulations is to be seen (in contra-distinction to this, the kinship between our formulation and that of Judaism is to be seen in the context of the ethical enterprise, namely, in light of the fact that both belong to the ethical enterprise, the Judaism implicated here being prophetic Judaism, which is, as pointed out above, an expression of the religious enterprise that overlaps into the ethical enterprise so that it partakes not only in the expression of the religious enterprise but also in the expression of the ethical enterprise thus enabling it to be linked in kinship with a variant formulation in the domain of the ethical enterprise, e.g., our formulation).

Thirdly and lastly, there is Levinas' formulation. This formulation is clearly altruistic, seeing that for it the ethical enterprise is to be constituted in terms of the responsibility that a self bears towards its other—an act/relation assuming responsibility towards an other is an act/relation that is ethical, namely, an act/relation that is evaluated/judged as ethically right/good. For as such, the ethical act/relation is, in terms of this formulation, by its very essence other-directed and not self-directed and this is tantamount to establishing that the formulation here is altruistic and not egotistic in its orientation. Indeed, it is perhaps the most radical expression of the altruistic orientation, seeing that Levinas goes so far as to claim that the self bears responsibility for the acts of the other even when these acts are acts of persecution directed against itself; the self is responsible for the other even when the other is its persecutor—"I am responsible for the persecutions that I undergo" (Levinas 1985, 99).[55] But it should be noted that the bifurcation that the notion of justice is to resolve is established here, strictly speaking, not in terms of two separate entities, i.e., the entity of the persecuted and the entity of the persecutor, but rather in terms of a sole entity, i.e., the entity of the self. Namely, the bifurcation is established here in terms of two roles that one and the same entity, i.e., the entity of the self, can assume, to wit, the role of assuming responsibility for the entity that is the persecutor and the role of assuming responsibility for the entity that is the persecuted. The self must assume responsibility for the other (but apparently not for itself) and since both the entity that is persecutor and the entity that is persecuted are others to the self, the self must assume responsibility for both. In this connection, it is interesting to note that in our formulation too the bifurcation that the notion of justice is to resolve is established in terms of the self but in our formulation it is established not in terms of the kinds of responsibility that the self may assume but rather in terms of the kinds of ontological dimensions that may enter into its constitution. This difference suggests some further interesting contrasts to which we will have occasion to refer below.

Now, we would submit that the rationale for such a delineation of the ethical enterprise can be established only in terms of a context in which the entities involved are entities that implicate a Thou-being in their ontological constitution. Namely, the rationale for claiming responsibility on behalf of the self for an other can be established only if the self and the other are entities that implicate a Thou-being in their ontological constitution. For clearly, the only alternative being available (certainly in terms of our delineation of the ontological domain) in terms of which an entity can constitute itself, i.e., the It-being, is a being that cannot assume responsibility toward an other. Indeed, inasmuch as Levinas (following Buber, it would seem) delineates the notion of responsibility in terms of that of responding, namely, responsibility for an other constitutes itself in terms of responding to that other (the responsibility that a self bears for an other is the responsibility to respond), it is clear that an It-being cannot relate to an other in terms of its response. For after all, the act of responding to an other of necessity implicates an affirmation of that other in its otherness while an It-being by its very make-up can relate to an other only in terms of utilization and manipulation but not affirmation (it can relate to an other only as a means but not as an end-in-itself). Thus, it can make sense to attribute responding and consequently responsibility only to an entity that implicates a Thou-being in its ontological constitution.

And this indeed is the case not only with regard to the entity that is the subject but equally so with regard to the entity that is the object, the recipient, of the responding/responsibility. By the same token that it would not make sense to have a response from an It-being, it would also not make sense to have a response directed towards an It-being. For the act of responding is by its very essence re-active and not pro-active—it does not initiate, it answers. And this, in turn, means that for an act of response to take place it must be instigated, triggered, by its recipient and this being so a good case can be made that only a recipient that implicates a Thou-being in its ontological constitution can instigate, trigger, a response, seeing that only a thou-being can address or challenge thus bringing about the possibility of a response—an It-being cannot.[56] Indeed, Levinas' formulation, while it is true that it does not explicitly state it, would nonetheless clearly seem to intimate that the responsibility that it established between the self and its other is established between the self and the other *qua* entities that implicate a Thou-being in their ontological constitution. For as regards the self, it is clearly a human self with which Levinas' formulation is concerned and as such there can be no question that it is an entity that implicates a Thou-being in its constitution. Where a question may well arise is with regard to the other that is encountered and here in referring to that other as an other that looks at the self, e.g., "since the other looks at me, I am responsible for him" (Levinas 1985, 96), indeed, in referring to it as a "face," e.g., "before the face I don't simply remain there contemplating it, I respond to it" (p. 88), Levinas' formulation, it would seem to us, clearly intimates that the other encountered is likewise an entity that implicates a Thou-being in its ontological constitution. An It-being could not be encountered as a "face" that elicits response. Thus, it would seem to us, that the intimation in Levinas' formulation is quite clear that the entities involved in the ethical enterprise are entities that implicate a Thou-being in their respective ontological constitutions. Certainly, given the way the formulation delineates the ethical enterprise, the rationale and justification for such a delineation can be established only on the basis that the entities involved are entities that implicate a Thou-being in their respective ontological constitutions.[57]

Indeed, even more, a persuasive case can be made that as regards the subject of the ethical act/relation Levinas' formulation intimates not only that it has to be an entity that implicates in its ontological constitution a Thou-being but that it has to be an entity that ontologically constitutes itself *exclusively* in terms of the Thou-being, which is to say, that it intimates that the subject of an act/relation that is to be taken as ethical has to be a pure, absolute Thou-entity (and not just, for example, an It/Thou-entity). This is so, seeing that the responsibility towards the other that Levinas' formulation arrogates to the subject (and as a subject of an act/relation that is to be taken as ethical the arrogation of a responsibility towards the other, i.e., towards the object of the act/relation, is of necessity implicated) is delineated as a responsibility that is in no way limited, circumscribed or compromised (the subject, the self, assumes responsibility for the other even to the point of assuming responsibility for its being persecuted by the other), and such a delineation can be arrogated only to a subject that is an absolute, pure Thou-entity, namely, the rationale and justification for the arrogation of a responsibility that is unlimited and uncircumscribed can be established only on the grounds of the subject being an absolute, pure Thou-entity. For, as was established above, the very arrogation of a responsibility towards an other (irrespective of the extent of such arrogation) is feasible only with respect to a Thou-being, seeing that it is the Thou-being that by its very essence constitutes itself as a being-for-another; the alternative kind of being that is available in our scheme of things, i.e., the It-being, cannot be a recipient of such arrogation of responsibility, seeing that, in contra-distinction to the

Thou-being, it, by its very essence, constitutes itself as a being-for-itself (when active) or as a being-in-itself (when passive). It follows, therefore, that it is feasible to arrogate to an entity responsibility for an other only if the entity in question implicates in its ontological constitution a Thou-being and that to the extent, however, that the entity in question also implicates in its ontological constitution an It-being, namely, to the extent that it constitutes itself as an It/Thou-being, the responsibility for an other arrogated to it cannot be unlimited—it is, per force, circumscribed and limited by its It-being constituent. The responsibility for an other can be unlimited only if the entity in question here, i.e., the entity to which such responsibility is being arrogated, constitutes itself exclusively in terms of the Thou-being, i.e., constitutes itself as a pure, absolute Thou-entity. Thus, Levinas' formulation in arrogating to the self a responsibility for an other that is unlimited (after all, the self in this formulation is to assume responsibility even for the acts of persecution perpetrated by the other against itself) per force implies that in its context the self is an entity that constitutes itself as a pure, absolute Thou-entity.[58]

But now it is precisely this implication in Levinas' formulation, i.e., the implication that the self involved in the ethical enterprise is an entity that constitutes itself as a pure, absolute Thou-entity, that exposes, in our judgment, a serious weakness in this formulation. For this implication of the self as being constituted as a pure, absolute Thou-entity includes in Levinas' formulation the further implication that this self exists, i.e., is available to one and all, in the present, namely, that it exists in the world as it is presently constituted and not merely in the world as it might have been constituted in a remote past (i.e., in some paradisaic context) or as it may be constituted in some distant future (i.e., in some eschatological context). This is so because the self that is implicated in Levinas' formulation is a self that is clearly being situated in the context of the ethical enterprise (i.e., it is a self that is to be the subject/agent of the act/relation that is to be ethically evaluated/judged), and as such it is indeed a self that, per force, is located in the world as it exists in the present, seeing that the ethical enterprise can address itself meaningfully to its task only in the context of the world as it is presently constituted—it is the self as it is presently constituted in the given world and not as it may have been constituted in a paradisaic past or may be constituted in an eschatological future that can be meaningfully subjected to ethical evaluation/judgment.

But if this be the case, then implicating the human self as an entity that constitutes itself exclusively in terms of the Thou-being, as Levinas' formulation seems to be doing, clearly flies in the face of reality as we perceive it. For the human entity, when taken in the context of the world as presently constituted, is manifestly not an entity that constitutes itself as a pure, absolute Thou-entity; the overwhelming and indubitable evidence of our sense-perception clearly implicates the presence of the It-being in the ontological constitution of the human entity when taken as it exists in the context of the world as presently constituted thus implicating it as an entity that constitutes itself as an It/Thou-entity.[59] Levinas' formulation, therefore, in implicating within its delineation of the ethical enterprise the human entity as being constituted as a pure, absolute Thou-entity clearly undermines its validity—it, so to speak, shoots itself in the head. In the world as presently constituted there is no human entity that constitutes itself as a pure, absolute Thou-entity.[60] Namely, in a religious context it is quite valid to resort to the ontological constitution of the human entity as it would be constituted in the context of the eschaton rather than as it is presently constituted (i.e., as it would be constituted in its state of salvation rather than as it is constituted in its state of Fallenness) as the criterion by which the ethical evaluation/judgment is to be determined. Of course, the ethical guideline that would obtain in these circumstances would, per force, reflect an idealistic, perfectionist rather than a realistic orientation (as is, indeed, clearly the case in Christianity). Still, it is a formulation of an ethical guideline (ethical at least in the sense of being a guideline for acting and relating towards others, though to the extent that the ontological constitution of the human entity implicated here is not the ontological constitution that it possesses in the present but only that which it will come to possess in the remote future, it is certainly questionable whether we can really claim the guideline here to be ethical in the full sense of the notion) and as such it shows that it is possible to have an ethical guideline that implicates the human entity as a pure, absolute Thou-entity if the guideline is formulated in a religious context. But, it is possible only in a religious, and not in a secularist, context. Thus, while implicating the human entity as a pure, absolute Thou-entity does undermine Levinas' formulation, seeing that it formulates itself in a secularist context, it does not undermine Christianity's formulation, seeing that it formulates itself in a religious context. Indeed, it is precisely at this point that the disadvantage of Levinas' formulation and the advantage of our own formulation can be appreciated. For while in Levinas' formulation the self is not a self that can function in the context of the ethical enterprise, in our formulation the self, in being constituted as an It/Thou-entity (and, as such, as a self that is clearly available in the present), is manifestly a self that can function fully and unambiguously in the context of the ethical enterprise.

17) In the preceding section our comparison with alternative formulations of the ethical enterprise was with respect to formulations that shared with our formulation the same fundamental context, namely, the context whereby the ethical enterprise is to be ultimately grounded in the ontological constitution of the human subject/agent—they all, in common with our formulation, locate the criterion by which the act/relation is to be ethically evaluated/judged in one or another aspect or feature of the ontological constitution of the human entity.[61] Indeed, we may say that they all share with our formulation the common denominator of being ontological formulations of the ethical enterprise.

But now, what about the comparison between our formulation and formulations that do not share this common denominator, i.e., the common denominator of locating the criterion for the ethical evaluation/judgment in one or another aspect of the ontological constitution of the human subject/agent (formulations which may be referred to as the "ontological formulations" of the ethical enterprise), such formulations as those which locate the criterion for the ethical evaluation/judgment in the values, ideals or interests of the collectivity (e.g. the society, the class) to which the individual human subject/agent belongs (formulations which may be referred to as the "societal formulations" of the ethical enterprise) or those which locate the criterion in the prescriptions of a divine revelation (formulations which may be referred to as the "religious formulations" of the ethical enterprise)? These two kinds of formulation, the "societal" and the "religious," certainly present us with a difference that goes to the very heart of how the ethical enterprise is to be grasped.

Now, as will be recalled, we did already have occasion above to address the difference between our formulation and these two alternative formulations. But our concern there was focused exclusively on our attempt to establish their disadvantage (indeed, their invalidity) in comparison with our formulation on the basis either of their relativism (this with respect to the "societal formulation") or of their lack of universal acceptability (this with respect to the "religious formulation")—the "societal formulation" being relativistic in as much as different societies possess different sets of values and ideals (not to mention that the same society may well change its values and ideals with the passage of time) and the "religious formulation" being limited in the scope of its adoption in as much as the revelation in which it grounds itself is not universally available. We did not, however, undertake there to address the underlying question of whether relativism and lack of universal acceptability are indeed aspects that would undermine the credibility of the ethical enterprise—it was taken for granted by us that this would be the case. But from the vantage point of the "societal formulation" or the "religious formulation" this is by no means granted. Indeed, if anything, if in terms of the "social formulation" the ethical enterprise is really nothing else but the articulation of the ethos and mores of a society (as indeed is the case in such a formulation), then clearly ethics and morality cannot be but relative, seeing that every society has its own peculiar ethos and mores and that the ethos and mores of any particular society is most likely to change with the passage of time. And if, regarding the "religious formulation," the scope of acceptability is limited (as indeed is the case in this kind of formulation), this does not present an insurmountable problem for the "religious formulation," seeing that it is inherent within this formulation to expect that eventually, at some point in the future, acceptability will indeed become universal.[62]

How is one to respond to such alternative conceptions of the ethical enterprise? Let us start by readily conceding that, in principle, one can delineate the ethical enterprise as one chooses, and as long as the delineation is not self-contradictory it would be, at least theoretically, viable. Now, the two alternative delineations under consideration here, namely, the "societal formulation" and the "religious formulation," are clearly not self-contradictory and consequently they must be taken as being, at least theoretically, valid. But even more so, in as much as these two alternative formulations utilize as the criteria that are to underpin their evaluation/judgment of acts/relations (and the prescriptions emanating from such evaluation/judgment) situations or events that are accessible to us, they are not only theoretically but also practically viable.[63] And the fact that their evaluations/judgments are, in the last analysis, inescapably relativistic may well not be problematic when the ethical enterprise is perceived from a vantage point that is different from ours. Who says that the ethical enterprise must be, by the very essence of its constitution, absolute and universal in its evaluations/judgments? After all, it cannot be established that an implication of the aspect of the absolute and of the universal is inherent to the very signification of the notion of the ethical. Whether or not these aspects are to be implicated by the notion of the ethical would depend on how, in the first place, one would wish to grasp the notion of the ethical—from what vantage point one would choose to perceive the ethical enterprise.

Thus, it is not really tenable to reject either of these two alternative formulations as invalid and we would readily concede this—we certainly would recognize that an ethical enterprise that formulates itself in terms of the "societal formulation" or in terms of the "religious formulation" is a valid enterprise and that people can adopt it and adhere to it with full legitimacy. What we can, however, maintain (and this in contra-distinction to the stance implicated by the alternative formulations) is that not *all* evaluations/judgments are inescapably relativistic (either in the sense of not applying to all humans at all times and at all places, or in the sense of not being accessible to being appropriated by all humans). Indeed, we would want to claim that there are evaluations/judgments that are absolute and universally accessible to all humans. Thus, for example, murder, exploitation, enslavement are acts, we would submit, that must always and everywhere be evaluated/judged negatively; and commensurately, acting/relating toward other humans according to the dictates of justice must always and everywhere be evaluated/judged positively. With respect to such acts/relations the evaluation/judgment has to be absolute and universal.[64]

But if this be valid, as we believe it to be, then we do indeed have at our disposal beside the "societal formulation" and the "religious formulation" a third kind of delineation of the ethical enterprise, the one presented in the "ontological formulation." At the same time, however, if, as we have clearly intimated, all three kinds of formulation can claim validity (each, of course, from its own vantage point), then the issue confronting us here is really not the issue of validity but rather that of appellation, namely, which of the three formulations has the best claim to appropriate the appellation "ethical."

Now here, with respect to this issue, it may well appear, at first sight, that it is the "societal formulation" that would have the best claim on appropriating the appellation of "ethics" and "morality," seeing that it formulates itself in terms of ethos and mores and that etymologically "ethics" and "morality" derive themselves respectively from "ethos" and "mores." But this argument may not be really valid. For one may well argue that this derivation should lead one to expect precisely the opposite, namely, it should lead one to expect a change in signification between the original terms and the new, derived terms. For after all, the derivation implicates a phonic transformation of the original terms to new ones (e.g., from "ethos" to "ethics" or from "mores" to "morality"). And such a transformation, in turn, by virtue of introducing a difference, a distinction, in the phonetic expression between the original terms and the derived ones (and no matter how minimal this difference may be) is indeed to be taken as implicating a parallel difference, distinction, between the signification borne by the original terms and that borne by the derived terms. Otherwise, if no such difference, distinction, ensues, we would end with having two different words (i.e., two different phonetic sounds) that signify one and the same thing, and what is the point of this? It stands to reason, therefore, that we should expect that the change from "ethos" to "ethics" implicates a change not only in phonetics but also in signification. Thus, from the vantage point of this argument, it is the formulation that perceives the enterprise of ethics as being different from the enterprise of ethos, the formulation that does not equate "ethics" with "ethos," that is the formulation that possesses the stronger claim on the appellation of the "ethical." And this, of course, is tantamount to saying that it is our formulation (precisely in not reducing ethics to ethos, which is to say, in not accepting that ethical evaluations/ judgments can be relativistic, insisting that they must be absolute and universal) rather than the "societal formulation" (the formulation that does reduce ethics to ethos and does accept the relativism of ethical evaluations/judgments) that is the formulation that is to be taken as the formulation in which the ethical enterprise is validly depicted.

But now, what about the "religious formulation"? As will be recalled, we have observed above that the "religious formulation," namely, the formulation that grounds itself in an act of divine revelation, can present itself in two forms depending on which one of two aspects connected with the act of revelation is to be emphasized—is it the act as such taken in its own terms or is it the act as it is mediated and thus refracted by a religious tradition. Now, our assessment here would greatly depend on which one of these two aspects is to be emphasized. For clearly in the former case, i.e., the case where the emphasis is placed on the act itself (the act of direct divine communication to the human), the "religious formulation" places itself on the side of our formulation (or, to put it more generally, on the side of the "ontological formulation"), seeing that for it the evaluations/judgments that constitute the ethical enterprise are also absolute and universal (indeed, in an even more radical sense than is the case with the "ontological formulation"), and consequently that for it, it is also the case that the signification of "ethics" is different from and irreducible to the signification of "ethos." On the other hand, in the latter case, i.e., the case where the emphasis is placed on the religious tradition that mediates and refracts the act of revelation, the "religious formulation" places itself on the side of the "societal formulation," seeing that in its context (indeed, just as in the context of the "societal formulation") "ethics" is reduced to and identified with the signification of "ethos" and that consequently the evaluations/judgments that are to constitute the ethical enterprise cannot be really absolute and universal, but must remain, in the last analysis, relativistic. Now, given our argument above against identifying the signification of "ethics" with that of "ethos," it would follow that the "religious formulation," when it is taken in terms of the latter case, i.e., in terms of emphasizing the religious tradition (and, indeed, like the "societal formulation"), has a weaker claim to appropriate the designation of being the formulation that authentically depicts the ethical enterprise than does our formulation (or, for that matter, other "ontological formulations"). This assessment, however, would not apply when the "religious formulation" is taken in terms of the former case, i.e., in terms of emphasizing the act of revelation as such. For clearly here there is no reduction of "ethics" to "ethos" and, indeed, the evaluations/judgments that are to constitute the ethical enterprise are as absolute and universal as can be.[65]

Is this, then, to mean that the claim to the appellation of the "ethical" by the "religious formulation," when its emphasis is on the act of divine revelation as such (rather than on its mediation and refraction through a religious tradition), is equal in strength to the claim of our formulation (a formulation that constitutes itself in terms of the "ontological formulation")? While at first sight this may indeed appear to be the case, a more careful consideration, we would submit, would lead us to question the validity of such an implication. For while it is true, as we have just observed above, that the "religious formulation" when its emphasis is on the act of divine revelation succeeds every bit as well as, if indeed not better than, our formulation in safeguarding against the identification of "ethics" with "ethos" and in bestowing absoluteness and universality (indeed, in the most radical sense conceivable) upon the evaluations/judgments and prescriptions of the ethical enterprise, it nonetheless falters in inescapably having to implicate the supernatural dimension in order to provide such safeguarding and bestowal (after all, it can provide such safeguarding and bestowal only because it grounds itself in the act of divine revelation). It is our claim that in doing this, the "religious formulation" falters because, as argued above, the ethical enterprise is an enterprise that formulates itself exclusively within the parameters of the natural world—namely, its justification, which is to say, the justification of its evaluations/judgments (and thus of its prescriptions) has to be established on an empirical basis and in terms of considerations that are acceptable to human reason. Divine revelation, however, is an act that clearly implicates a transcending of the parameters of the natural world. Consequently, the "religious formulation," when it grounds itself in the act of divine revelation as such, must abdicate its claim to the appellation of the ethical.

Thus, although the "religious formulation" that grounds itself in the act of divine revelation taken in itself as such, is at one with our formulation in blocking the identification of "ethics" with "ethos" and in safeguarding the absoluteness and universality of the evaluations/judgments (and thus also of the prescriptions) that are to be taken as ethical (having in both of these respects a clear advantage over the "societal formulation" and, indeed, also over the "religious formulation" that grounds itself in the act of divine revelation taken not in itself as such but as it is mediated and refracted by a religious tradition), it nonetheless is not a viable alternative to our formulation, seeing that, in the last analysis, it cannot pass muster as an *ethical* formulation in as much as the justification it can offer for its evaluations/judgments and prescriptions is not a justification that grounds itself within the parameters of the natural world.

To sum up, therefore, our comparative examination of the three leading kinds of formulation that offer us a depiction of the ethical enterprise, to wit, the "societal formulation," the "religious formulation" and the "ontological formulation," has led us to the conclusion that the advantage in claiming the appellation of "ethical" goes to the "ontological formulation" (more specifically, to the particular ontological formulation that we have put forth here) rather than to the "societal formulation" or the "religious formulation."[66] Of course, we should be clear that this advantage could be gained only on the basis of defining "ethics" in a certain way (to wit, as an enterprise that is constituted by evaluations/judgments of acts/relations, and thus also by prescriptions directed towards the latter, that are absolute and universal and whose justification is grounded within the parameters of the natural world). At the same time, however, we should also be equally clear that, in the last analysis, this definition is, so to speak, arbitrary in the sense that one could opt to adopt a different definition (as indeed we saw the alternative formulations do). True, one may well endeavor to advance considerations and arguments in support of one's chosen definition (as indeed we did above), but if others do not find them persuasive, there is really nothing else that one can do—in the last analysis, a term can be defined as one chooses to define it. In such a context, the one thing we can and, indeed, must insist upon is that it is incumbent upon the various proponents of the different definitions of the term "ethics" to state their respective definitions as fully and clearly as possible so that there can be no ambiguity or fudging in the way the term is being applied. Indeed, this is what we have tried to do here.

18) Lastly, we should briefly address one further issue (an issue that, if not sorted out, can muddle our understanding of the ethical enterprise) before bringing this chapter to a close. The issue in question here is the relationship that may obtain between the enterprise of ethics and yet another enterprise, to wit, the enterprise of political philosophy. What is the relationship between these two enterprises? Clearly, there is a division of opinion among philosophers with regard to this question. Thus, for some the two enterprises coalesce into a continuous single enterprise either (as in antiquity) by seeing the enterprise of political philosophy as encompassing the enterprise of ethics, or (as in some contemporary formulations as, for example, that of Richard Popkin) by seeing the enterprise of political philosophy as a kind of "applied ethics" or as being "continuous with morality." As against this, for others (and we would certainly place ourselves in this group), while there is no denying that the enterprises are in some ways rather close to each other, the two enterprises remain, in the last analysis, distinct from each other. How is one to account for this discrepancy in the viewing of the relationship between the ethical enterprise and the enterprise of political philosophy, and which one of the two views is, after all, the valid one? Namely, can we sort out the dividing-line between the ethical enterprise and the enterprise of political philosophy or must we resign ourselves to the fact that it must be left blurred and ambiguous?[67]

It would seem to us that the crux of the problem that faces us here revolves around the question of what role and status is being arrogated respectively to the notion of the collectivity and to that of the individual. Thus, we would want to argue that the view that sees the two enterprises as coalescing grounds itself in (i.e. derives its rationale and justification from) the claim that both the enterprise of political philosophy and that of ethics focus on the collectivity, namely, that the collectivity is the primary and main object of concern for the enterprise, the principal object to which the enterprise directs itself. In contradistinction to this, the view that sees the two enterprises as distinct grounds itself in the claim that while the enterprise of political philosophy does indeed focus on the collectivity, the ethical enterprise does not likewise focus on the collectivity but rather on the individual. Now, if these claims are tenable, then our argument here should be persuasive. For clearly in having both the enterprise of political philosophy and that of ethics share the same kind of entity as the object of their concern, of their focusing, a "bridging," a continuity, between the two enterprises is established, thus effecting their coalescence. As against this, if the object of the concern, of the focusing, in the two enterprises is constituted by the two different kinds of entity (i.e. the enterprise of political philosophy focusing on the collectivity while the ethical enterprise focuses on the individual), no "bridging" and thus no coalescing between the two enterprises is feasible, which is to say, a distinction between the two enterprises must be retained. But if this is the case, then it follows that our argument here must, per force, be reduced to the question of whether it is indeed the case that the enterprise of political philosophy focuses on the collectivity while the ethical enterprise focuses on the individual, or is it rather that both the enterprise of political philosophy and that of ethics focus on the collectivity. Determining the relation between the enterprise of political philosophy and that of ethics would thus depend on how this question is answered. So, how is the foregoing question to be answered? Turning first to the enterprise of political philosophy, it would seem to us that there can be no question that the primary object upon which the core concern of the enterprise focuses is the collectivity and not the individual. For however one wishes to delineate the enterprise there can be little doubt that the delineation would have to implicate (and implicate in an essential way) a concern with such issues as how a national entity comes to be constituted in the first place,[68] how best to regulate and order the various networks of relations and functions within such an entity (i.e., what political arrangement would best express the entity's sovereignty), what institutions would best safeguard and promote the interests of the entity; and in all of these issues, their substance clearly impinges upon a collectivity and not upon an individual. A delineation, therefore, which by its very essence cannot not encompass these issues, will have to have as its object of primary concern a collectivity and not an individual.

When we turn, however, to the ethical enterprise, the matter is not so clear-cut. For, on the one hand, one could argue that, in the last analysis, the ethical enterprise too implicates a collectivity, seeing that, after all, we have delineated the ethical enterprise as constituting itself primarily in terms of the evaluation/judgment of acts/relations and that acts/ relations, in turn, per force implicate an other which, as such, means that the evaluation/judgment constituting the ethical enterprise, per force, implicates a twosome and a twosome is already a collectivity (true, a collectivity in the most minimal sense, but a collectivity nonetheless).[69] And if the ethical enterprise too implicates a collectivity (as the enterprise of political philosophy clearly does), then a coalescence between the two enterprises can clearly be established.

On the other hand, however, one can argue that while a collectivity may well be implicated in the ethical enterprise, such a collectivity does not, however, constitute itself within the ethical enterprise as the primary object of concern and it is after all not the implication of the collectivity as such but rather the implication of the collectivity specifically as the primary object of concern for the enterprise (and which as such constitutes itself as the factor that defines the very nature of the enterprise) that is at issue here. Indeed, an implication of a collectivity as such, certainly of a collectivity in the minimal sense of a twosome, is to be encountered in most enterprises. For after all, most enterprises would implicate the presence of acts/relations, and acts/relations, in turn, of necessity implicate not only a subject/agent but also an object/recipient, thus of necessity implicating a twosome, which is to say that they of necessity implicate a collectivity. It is the implication of a collectivity in this sense that one encounters in the ethical enterprise. But, as said, such an implication of the collectivity is not to the point, given our concern here. What is to the point is whether we can have an implication of the collectivity that constitutes itself as the primary concern for the ethical enterprise. And here, a good case can be made that in contrast to the enterprise of political philosophy where an implication of the collectivity as the prime object of concern for the enterprise can be established, with respect to the ethical enterprise such an implication of the collectivity as the prime object of concern for the enterprise cannot be established. With respect to the ethical enterprise, the object of primary concern for the enterprise is the individual and not the collectivity. The ethical enterprise, in its essential structure, constitutes itself in terms of the evaluation/judgment of individual acts/relations between individual subjects/agents and individual objects/recipients. But if this be the case, then there is after all no common denominator between the ethical enterprise and the enterprise of political philosophy in both implicating the collectivity as their primary object of concern and consequently the feasibility of the two enterprises coalescing is undermined. The two enterprises remain distinct.

But is the foregoing claim with regard to the way by which the domain of political philosophy can be distinguished from the domain of ethics (i.e., the claim that the former formulates its object of primary concern in terms of the collectivity while the latter formulates it in terms of the individual) really valid? Namely, is it really universally applicable within the domain of ethics? Could not one undermine the validity of this claim, for example, by the instance of the "societal formulation," a formulation that, as its appellation intimates, seems to formulate the ethical enterprise in terms of the collectivity and not of the individual?

At first sight this may indeed seem to present a serious challenge to our claim here. For there is no denying that the "societal formulation" is seen by many as a valid delineation of the ethical enterprise and that the formulation clearly implicates the collectivity and not the individual. Of course, we could respond by saying that those who see the "societal formulation" as a valid delineation of the ethical enterprise are mistaken and that the "societal formulation," precisely because it implicates the collectivity and not the individual, really belongs in the domain of political philosophy and not in the domain of ethics. But this may appear rather high-handed and arbitrary, seeing that the view that the "societal formulation" impinges upon the ethical enterprise is held not by a few, scattered individuals but by a good many people.

Indeed, we too can readily accede to the claim that the "societal formulation" impinges on the ethical enterprise and still, notwithstanding this and the fact that the societal formulation clearly implicates the collectivity, hold on to our claim that the determination of whether a formulation belongs to the domain of political philosophy or to the domain of ethics can be established by whether the formulation in question implicates the collectivity or the individual. For a more careful examination of our claim will clearly show that it is not all that open (i.e., lacking in further qualifications) and sweeping in its assertion, namely, it will show that our claim does not assert that any implication of the collectivity by a formulation would arrogate that formulation to the domain of political philosophy while any implication of the individual by a formulation would arrogate that formulation to the domain of ethics. Rather, our claim clearly limits the use of the implication of the collectivity or of the individual in arrogating a formulation either to the domain of political philosophy or to the domain of ethics exclusively only to those instances where this implication is to impinge specifically on the object of primary concern for the formulation in question and not on any other aspect that may be involved in the formulation. But if this be the case, then clearly the "societal formulation" as such (i.e., without any further elaboration) does not necessarily have to be seen as undermining our criterion for distinguishing between those formulations that belong to the domain of political philosophy and those that belong to the domain of ethics (implicating the collectivity being the condition for the former and implicating the individual being the condition for the latter). For as long as the collectivity implicated in the "societal formulation" does not impinge on the object of primary concern but rather on some other object operating within the enterprise, our proposed criterion for arrogating a formulation to the domain of political philosophy or to the domain of ethics remains unaffected, which is to say, it is not undermined.

And indeed, in the various ethical formulations that can be ascribed to the "societal formulation," i.e., in the various ethical formulations that implicate a collectivity, the collectivity is implicated not with respect to the object of primary concern, i.e., with respect to that which is to be ethically evaluated/judged, but rather with respect to that which is to provide the criterion in the light of which the ethical evaluation/judgment is to be carried out (and very significantly for the case we are making here, the recipient, i.e., the object, of the ethical evaluation/judgment, thus the object of primary concern, always remains here the individual).[70] Thus, for example, this can be seen, we would submit, in Aristotle's ethical formulation, a formulation that exemplifies as best as any the "societal formulation" type.[71] For, in the Aristotelian formulation, the collectivity does indeed enter the picture not as the object of the ethical evaluation/judgment, thus as the object of primary concern for the enterprise, but rather as the source that provides the criterion by which the formulation/judgment is to be carried out and, as such, it is valid to view the formulation here, notwithstanding the fact that it clearly implicates the collectivity, as belonging to the ethical domain rather than to the enterprise of political philosophy.[72] At the same time, however, when the collectivity implicated in a formulation belonging to the "societal formulation" class of formulations[73] seems to go beyond implicating itself exclusively as the provider of the criterion for the ethical evaluation/judgment and seems to lend itself to being implicated also as the object of the evaluation/judgment, i.e., as the object of the primary concern of the enterprise, there would be, in all likelihood, an openness to consider the possibility of (and, indeed, in many instances the actual tendency towards) arrogating such a formulation not to the domain of ethics but rather to the domain of political philosophy.

The above point can be exemplified, we would suggest, by Hegel's *Sittlichkeit* formulation. For, on the one hand, one can indeed see that within the formulation of *Sittlichkeit* the society to which the individual belongs (thus the collectivity) functions (through its instrument of the state) as the source providing the criterion for the evaluation/judgment that constitutes the essence of the enterprise. This is so in as much as in terms of this formulation the norms by which the evaluation/judgment is to be carried out are provided by the institutions of the social life—the family, civil society and, above all, the state. The grounds for the ethical enterprise are the values of a person's society—ethics is social ethics. Indeed, the values embodied in the state constitute, in the last analysis, the only morality a person can have—there is no higher authority above the state. And as such, of course, given our view of the differentiation between the domain of ethics and that of political philosophy, the formulation may well be arrogated to the domain of ethics and not to that of political philosophy.

On the other hand, however, it is clear that the formulation here takes an "organicistic" view in that for it full, true being is vested only in entities that constitute themselves as organic wholes, and that the being of any entity that constitutes itself as a part of such a whole is derived from that whole. The applicable analogy here is that of an organism (the whole) and its cells (the parts)—the individual human person is the "cell" and the society (i.e., the collectivity) to which he/she belongs is the "organism." Thus, in the formulation here the individual person finds his/her essence only in the state (the state being the institutional expression *par excellence* of a collectivity)—he/she is made for the state, everything that he/she is, he/she owes to the state. The will of the state (of the collectivity), what Rousseau called the "general will," is the real will of the individual. Any rights or liberties an individual person may possess, he/she comes to possess them by virtue of their being given to him/her by the state (i.e., the collectivity). Indeed, it is the supreme duty of the individual person to be a member of the state, to identify himself/herself with the state appropriating its values and customs. For only by immersing himself/herself in the society (the collectivity) to which he/she belongs, can the individual person gain consciousness of his/her selfhood. As such, in the context of this formulation, even when the object of evaluation/judgment (and thus the object of primary concern) is the individual human person, the real object is, in the last analysis, the society, i.e., the collectivity, to which the individual human person belongs.

This comes to the fore even more emphatically, seeing that the formulation here expresses itself even more radically in taking the collectivity as the individual. Thus, it proclaims explicitly that the state, i.e., the collectivity, is the 'true individual.' The society to which the individual belongs is not a mere conglomerate of individuals. Rather, it is taken as an entity that possesses its own reality—it is a spiritual reality. Indeed, the state (i.e., the institutional expression of the collectivity) is taken here as being a 'person' having a life of its own. But this being the case, our proposed criterion for distinguishing between the domain of ethics and that of political philosophy would clearly arrogate the *Sittlichkeit* formulation not to the ethical domain but to the domain of political philosophy and, as such, we would have to conclude that in formulating the *Sittlichkeit* formulation, Hegel, so to speak, shifts gears and moves from the domain of ethics to that of political philosophy.

It should be noted, however, that Hegel seems to consider his *Sittlichkeit* formulation as continuing to belong to the domain of ethics. Indeed, he presents the *Sittlichkeit* formulation as the ethical formulation that overcomes what he now perceives to be the weakness of his ethical formulation of *Moralität* (and, for that matter, equally so, of Kant's ethical formulation).[74] Namely, the *Sittlichkeit* formulation, being objective, outwardly-oriented and contentful, overcomes the weakness of the *Moralität* formulation and of Kant's ethical formulation of being subjective, inwardly-oriented (in the sense of seeing the ethical enterprise as evaluating/judging acts/relations exclusively in terms of their intentions and not in terms of their concrete consequences) and, most significantly for Hegel, of being purely formal, i.e., devoid of any concrete content.[75] Indeed, the *Sittlichkeit* formulation is presented as being encompassed within the dialectic that is operative within the ethical domain, a dialectic that is seen to proceed from the *Moralität* formulation (as thesis) through the formulation in terms of objective rights (as antithesis) to its culmination in the *Sittlichkeit* formulation (as synthesis).

But not only does it appear that Hegel's stance regarding the arrogation of the *Sittlichkeit* formulation does not conform to the stance that is implicated by our proposed criterion (i.e., the criterion by which the domain of ethics is a domain that is delineated in terms of the individual, while the domain of political philosophy is a domain that is delineated in terms of the collectivity), even more fundamentally, Hegel, in the last analysis, could most probably not accept (leave alone appreciate) the very distinction between the individual and the collectivity as the primary object of concern, the distinction that underlies our proposed criterion—in all probability such a distinction would not have made sense to him. For it would seem that Hegel cannot conceive of an individual human who exists in isolation and is not lodged in some kind of collectivity. The individual human is, per force, always situated in one or another kind of collectivity, be it the collectivity of the family or of civil society or of the state.[76]

Indeed, one would have to concede that this view has a great deal to commend itself—the individual human, if it is to retain its humanity and, indeed, become human in the first place, must lodge itself in some kind of collectivity. But if this be the case, then we do have after all in some sense a closeness, a coalescence, between the ethical enterprise and the enterprise of political philosophy. We would not (and, indeed, could not) deny this.[77] After all, there is in some sense a closeness that the domain of political philosophy has to the domain of ethics, which it does not have to other domains, as for example to those of aesthetics, epistemology or metaphysics. Still, we would want to maintain that our proposed criterion retains its validity. For, we would submit that notwithstanding the coalescence between the domain of ethics and that of political philosophy, a distinction and thus a differentiation can be introduced on the basis of where the primary concern of the enterprise is to focus itself—is it to focus itself on the individual *qua* individual or on the individual *qua* part of a collectivity (the former defining the ethical enterprise while the latter would define the enterprise of political philosophy).[78]

Notes

1. As such, our delineation differs substantially from some alternative delineations of the ethical enterprise (for example, G. E. Moore's delineation) for which there exists an objective moral realm, a set of moral entities, "facts" (e.g., certain attributes that by their very constitution are ethically good or, alternatively, a specific attribute of ethical goodness) and for which, accordingly, the delineation of the ethical enterprise is in terms of capturing and describing these ethical "facts" rather than in terms of evaluating facts that in themselves are ethically neutral (thus facts that do not carry the ethical value in themselves but rather receive it through the process of our evaluations). Such an alternative delineation clearly presents the ethical enterprise in a way that parallels the presentation of the scientific enterprise—they both are in the business of identifying and describing facts, i.e., states of affairs that constitute reality. The ethical enterprise distinguishes itself from the scientific enterprise (as indeed the various particular sciences distinguish themselves from each other) not by the nature of its activity but only by the kind of object it undertakes to describe (though, true, the object of the ethical enterprise differs

from the object of the scientific enterprise qualitatively and not only quantitatively as is the case in distinguishing the particular sciences from each other). In contra-distinction to this, in our delineation the ethical enterprise distinguishes itself from the scientific enterprise in terms of the very nature of its activity (and not merely in terms of the kind of object that it is concerned with)—it does not undertake to identify and describe states of affairs that constitute reality but to evaluate them. One may say that in our delineation the ethical enterprise belongs to the realm of axiology and not to the realm of epistemology or metaphysics.

2. The validity of this last claim can be readily seen if the signification of the notion of truth is established, as in our view it should be, in terms of the correspondence theory. For correspondence (i.e., correspondence with the data of our sense-perception) can be established only with respect to assertions and assertions articulate themselves only in propositional statements and certainly not in commands. Thus, wherever assertions are made (which is to say, propositional statements are articulated) as, for example, in the scientific enterprise, raising the question of truth (i.e., the question of whether what is being asserted does or does not correspond to the data of our sense-perception, this data constituting reality for us) will in principle always be relevant and meaningful. By the same token, however, wherever commands are articulated (as, for example, in the ethical enterprise), raising the question of truth (i.e., truth in terms of correspondence) cannot in principle be relevant or meaningful.

3. But, as we shall see below, this sweeping delineation of the parameters of the ethical enterprise, a delineation that proposes to incorporate every conceivable act (which is to say, acts of all conceivable entities) under the legitimate jurisdiction of the ethical enterprise, will have to be considerably modified in our final delineation of the parameters of the ethical enterprise.

4. True, to be more accurate, the kind of relation that is implicated here by the act that does lend itself to ethical evaluation/judgment (i.e., the act that can be encompassed within the ethical enterprise) can only be a relation that is a one-way relation, a relation that moves exclusively in one direction, to wit, from the subject to the object, and this would mean, of course, that relations of authentic mutuality (i.e., relations whose mutuality is not attained by the mere imposition of two one-way relations on each other so that the mutuality is but the result of the simultaneous occurrence of two opposite one-way relations but rather is attained, so to speak, by the oscillations of a single relation between its two end-points, both end-points being subjects at one and the same time rather than alternating between subject and object) would be excluded from being encompassed within the ethical enterprise. Now, although the occurrence of relations of authentic mutuality may indeed be relatively infrequent, they are relations that, from our perspective, may well occupy a significant place within the ethical domain and consequently it would be important to ascertain that it is feasible for such relations to be also encompassed within the ethical enterprise.

5. As such, our approach must be distinguished from alternative approaches that formulate the essential and primary ethical evaluation/judgment in terms of the agent/subject and derive the ethical

evaluation/judgment of the act/relation from this preceding ethical evaluation/judgment of the agent/subject (an example that readily comes to mind is the approach taken by virtue theory). We would attempt to argue below that our approach of placing the primary and essential ethical evaluation/judgment with respect to the act/relation rather than with respect to its agent/subject has the clear advantage that in such an approach a persuasive rationale and justification for carrying out an ethical evaluation/judgment can be provided while in the alternative approach, which places the primary and essential ethical evaluation/judgment with respect to the agent/subject rather than with respect to the act/relation, it could not.

6. True, to be precise, this is not completely the case. There is still one way in which the agent/subject can express its capacity to choose freely (and its possession of rationality) and that is in freely choosing not to perpetrate/establish the one act/relation that is available to it. Just because it is available to the agent/subject, in no way implies that the agent/subject has to perpetrate/establish it. Thus, the capacity to choose freely can be expressed though only, so to speak, in a negative way, i.e., in the agent/subject freely choosing not to express itself, or rather (to put it more precisely) freely choosing not to avail itself of the only way of expression available to it. This possibility can manifest itself, as we shall see below, with respect to entities belonging to the domain of the divine.

7. And clearly, all of these three conditions must be satisfied not only if the ethical evaluation/judgment of the agent/subject (in its own term and in the fullest sense) is to be possible but equally so if prescribing to the agent/subject is to make sense to begin with. Namely, it should be quite clear that in the absence of any one of these three conditions it simply would not make sense to prescribe to the agent/subject—it simply does not make sense to prescribe to an entity that does not possess rationality or is not endowed with the capacity to choose freely or is not presented with the option of alternative acts/relations.

8. But this implicates that the ethical enterprise, when taken in its fullest and most extensive sense (i.e., when the agent/subject is to be ethically evaluated/judged in its own terms and in the fullest sense), can be carried out only with respect to the agent/subject that belongs to the human domain. For, as we will enlarge upon below, it is only entities that constitute themselves in terms of the human domain, i.e., human beings (and not entities that constitute themselves in the other domains, to wit, the domain of nature or the domain of the divine), that can satisfy all three conditions, to wit, the possession of rationality, the capacity to freely choose and being presented with the option of alternative acts/relations.

9. It is important to underline the fact that the evaluation/judgment with which we are concerned here is the *ethical* evaluation/judgment. For clearly there are evaluations/judgments that are not ethical as, for example, aesthetic or technical evaluations/judgments. And indeed, in the last analysis, these different evaluations/judgments distinguish themselves from each other not so much in terms of the kinds of ends that they are to pursue or in terms of the kinds of objects to which they are to relate but rather in terms of the criteria to

which they are to conform (though it is true that in the aesthetic, but not in the technological, evaluation/judgment we have also the further distinction whereby, in contrast to the ethical evaluation as presented by us here, the evaluation/judgment impinges primarily on the entity involved and not on the act/relation—indeed the entity involved in the aesthetic evaluation/judgment is passive and all acts/relations are directed towards it rather than from it—but this distinction is secondary to the distinction in terms of the kind of criteria involved and is derived from it). Thus, it may be suggested that an evaluation/judgment would be characterized as aesthetic if the criterion in the light of which it is carried out is to be that of harmony and it would be characterized as technical if the criterion is to be that of efficiency. And, of course, in this context the fundamental issue that we must, in turn, address will be the issue of how to characterize the criterion by which evaluations/judgments carried out in its light are to be taken as evaluations/judgments that are ethical.

10. Assuming that the act/relation and the circumstances in which it takes place remain the same, the very meaning of what constitutes for us an evaluation/judgment that is moral would not permit its evaluation/judgment today as morally right/good and at the same time allow to stand as valid its evaluation/judgment of yesterday or of tomorrow as being morally wrong/bad nor would it permit its evaluation/judgment as morally right/good in, let us say, the United States and at the same time allow to stand as valid its evaluation/judgment in China as morally bad/wrong. Such relativity with respect to time and place may certainly characterize acts/relations that belong to the domain of mores but not to the domain of morality. Mores can certainly vary from place to place and from time to time but the very essence of morality is that it transcends the relativity of time and place—what applies here must also apply in any other place in the universe and what applies today must have applied from time immemorial and will continue to apply for eternity. True, it is easy to confuse morality with mores but this should in no way validate such confusion.

11. Rationality by itself will not do for rationality can impinge only on the process of argumentation that leads from a starting-point, a grounding, to a conclusion. It itself cannot provide the starting-point, the grounding—it can provide only the guidance by which to move from the starting-point, whatever it may be, to the conclusion; the starting-point, the grounding, must be provided by some source other than reason. Thus, on this point we follow Hume's position except that he articulates it in terms of means and ends (i.e., reason can serve only as the means by which to attain, to realize, ends that have been provided, established by another source, that other source being for him the sentiments) while we articulate it in terms of a starting-point, a grounding, and a conclusion (i.e., reason being able only to guide us from a starting-point to a conclusion, the starting-point being provided by another source, that source being for us the data of sense-perception).

By the way, it may also bear pointing out that while the preceding two stipulations are called for because they define what for us are the essential and thus inextricable characterizations of an *ethical* evaluation/judgment (to wit, that all other things being equal, if it is to be applicable, for example, in India then per force it must also be applicable in England, Japan and all other places in the universe and if it is applicable today then per force it must also be applicable yesterday, the day before yesterday, tomorrow, the day after tomorrow, and at all other points in time as far as the past and future may stretch, and finally, that if it is applicable with regard to Tom then, per force, it must also be applicable with regard to Dick, Harry and every other moral agent), this third stipulation is called for because only on its basis can we establish that not only must ethical evaluations/judgments claim to be applicable to all members of the group, i.e., to all prospective moral entities (or, to use Kant's phrasing, to all members of the "kingdom of ends"), but they actually must also be universally adopted as ethically valid evaluations/judgments by all prospective moral entities.

Now, the significance of the first two stipulations is quite clear—it is to ensure and safeguard the essential characteristics that delineate an evaluation/judgment as being ethical rather than some other kind of evaluation/judgment. But what possibly can the significance of the third stipulation be? It certainly cannot be the same significance that we encountered in the preceding two stipulations. After all, this stipulation does not impinge upon the issue of the delineation of ethical evaluations/judgments (i.e., upon the issue of what delineation is called for an evaluation/judgment to be rendered an *ethical* evaluation/judgment). Rather, we would submit, that in stipulating that the justification of the evaluation/judgment must be grounded in rationality the stipulation impinges upon the extent of the adoptability of the ethical evaluations/judgments by the members of the class of moral entities (i.e., by the members of the "kingdom of ends"). Indeed, we would submit that it stipulates that the ethical evaluations/judgments will ultimately (and at least, in principle) be adoptable by *all* members of the class of moral entities. For in stipulating that the justification be grounded in rationality, it grounds the justification in an aspect that is possessed by all members of the class of moral entities, namely, it grounds the justification in that which serves as a common denominator in all moral entities (see our observations in section 8 above where we have tried to show that for an entity to be moral, i.e., a moral agent, it has to be endowed with reason) and as such it makes it feasible that (at least, in principle) all moral entities would ultimately be persuaded of the justification and consequently compelled to adopt the ethical evaluations/judgments so justified.

12. Clearly, therefore, our delineation here of what we take to be a subjectivist formulation does not encompass within its confines the formulations belonging to what has been referred by some as "extended subjectivism," i.e., where the criterion is placed in an aspect or property shared by a collectivity of individual moral entities/agents(such a delineation being "subjectivist" by virtue of the fact that the aspect or property in which the criterion is placed remains internal within the moral entity/agent while at the same time this subjectivism is being "extended" by virtue of the fact that the aspect or property is not confined to a single individual moral entity/agent but

rather is placed in a multiplicity of moral entities/agents). In our judgment, and certainly for our purposes here, such "extended subjectivist" formulations really belong, in the last analysis, to the domain of objectivist formulations.

13. This can be claimed because in all the alternative formulations (excluding, of course, the religious formulation where the single individual is the divine being, indeed, the monotheistic divine being, who as such is clearly not finite in the duration of its existence) the moral entity/agent is taken to be exclusively the human being and this being the case, the claim of a finite duration of existence is clearly perfectly valid. And while we have not as yet addressed this issue and are therefore, indeed, talking in terms of the general concept of a moral entity/agent without ascribing it more specifically to the kinds of entities that may qualify for that role, it is in our judgment, as we will try to argue below, perfectly valid to confine the concept of a moral entity/agent exclusively to the human being and not to any other being (though again, as we shall also see below, the exclusion of the divine being from being a moral entity/agent is not all that clear and definite).

14. It should be noted, however, that while the determination focused upon here whereby the ethical evaluation/judgment is to be determined by whether or not the act is performed in total freedom from any constraints, outward or inward (i.e., by whether or not the prospective moral entity/agent acts authentically), is certainly central to the existentialist formulation, it is not the only determination that the existentialist formulation offers. The existentialist formulation also offers a different determination (indeed, a determination that would seem to be in contradiction with the determination focused upon here, i.e., the determination in terms of authenticity), namely, a determination in terms of whether or not the prospective moral entity/agent escapes the pitfall of "bad faith," to wit, whether or not it escapes the illusion of seeing itself either exclusively as a "being-in-itself" or exclusively as a "being-for-itself" and thus failing to harmonize the two (the morally positive act being the act that takes into consideration and harmonizes the two aspects of being that characterize the prospective moral entity/agent, i.e., the human entity/agent—its being a consciousness that makes it free and its being located in a situation that proscribes this freedom). And while the determination in terms of authenticity certainly lends itself to the criticism that it is subjectivist and thus invalid, this is not the case with regard to the determination in terms of "bad faith." Indeed, as we will try to show below, this latter determination may well correspond to a determination that the formulation that we will try to present will put forth.

15. The nation-state, i.e., the nation possessing full sovereignty as expressed through the institution of statehood being the fullest, maximal expression of these interests and/or values, seeing that in its context alone are all possible dimensions of collective existence, i.e., the political, social, economic and cultural, covered

16. True, the duration of its existence is very likely to be considerably longer than that of any prospective individual moral entity/agent. Still, the difference is only quantitative and relative. In essence, the duration of its existence is also finite and thus its existence is also contingent and not absolute.

17. Indeed, if morality is to be defined in terms of correspondence to the interests and/or values of a community/society, it is difficult to see how one can distinguish and differentiate between morality and legality. And although it is true that one would certainly desire that there be no conflict between ethics and law (that, indeed, the law should express, reflect, morality), a distinction and differentiation between the two is certainly called for. For not only must one allow for the possibility of the law being in conflict with morality (thus being subject to being criticized and, indeed, opposed by morality) but there can be no denying that a good deal of the law has nothing to do with morality but rather with the regulation (i.e., with the ordering and the facilitating) of the various economic, social, and political interactions and transactions that constitute the very existence of a community/society.

18. It should be noted, however, that such a formulation does not slip back into the problematical subjectivist context that we had to reject above as being incompatible with a viable ethical enterprise but remains fully within the objectivist context. True, the criterion is placed here within the subject of the act and not in some entity or factor outside it such as the divine being or the community/society. As such, it is indeed placed in a subjectivist context but in a subjectivist context that is taken in its broad sense. The problematic for the viability of the ethical enterprise does not arise, however, in such a context of subjectivism taken in its broad sense. It arises only in the context of subjectivism when it is taken in its narrow sense, i.e., when the criterion is placed not just in some aspect or property of the subject of the act as such (thus covering all individuals that would qualify as the subject of the act) but rather in some aspect or property that specifically belongs to an *individual* subject to the exclusion of all other possible individuals that can be subjects of the act. But clearly a formulation that would place the criterion in the ontological constitution that characterizes the prospective moral entity/agent is not placing it in a context that is subjectivist in the narrow sense, seeing that the criterion is placed in that which belongs to all individuals of the class of prospective moral entities/agents. As such, for our purposes here, such a formulation, for all intents and purposes, belongs to an objectivist context, seeing that it places the criterion in a context in which the ethical enterprise can be viable. Indeed, when we characterize a context as subjectivist here we use subjectivism only in its narrow and not in its broad connotation. A formulation that belongs to a context that is subjectivist in the broad connotation we relegate to the objectivist context.

19. The reason for including the second pre-condition is that only by satisfying it can the satisfaction of the first two stipulations put forth above, i.e., the stipulation of universality and that of absoluteness, be safeguarded, thus, in turn, safeguarding the possibility of having an evaluation/judgment that is ethically viable. This is so for only with respect to aspects of the ontological constitution that are primary and most fundamental is it the case that they have to express themselves universally and absolutely (i.e., all entities/agents characterized by this ontological constitution would have to express these aspects and express them at all times). Aspects of the ontological constitution

that are secondary and derivative do not have to express themselves universally and absolutely; they can express themselves selectively and sporadically—indeed, this is what marks them off as being secondary and derivative and not primary and fundamental.

20. As an aside, however, it should be noted that, in contra-distinction to our approach here, in Moore's formulation the primary object of the ethical evaluation/judgment is not the act/relation but rather the entity/agent. The ethical evaluation/judgment of the act/relation is deduced from the ethical evaluation/judgment of the entity/agent that is its subject, namely, if the entity/agent is evaluated/judged to be morally good (which is to say, is evaluated/judged to possess the quality of moral goodness), then it will, per force, follow that its acts/relations will reflect this moral goodness and will, therefore, have to be evaluated/judged as being morally good rather than (as in our approach) where the ethical evaluation/judgment of the entity/agent is deduced from the ethical evaluation/judgment of its acts/relations, namely, if the acts/relations of an entity/agent are, by and large, evaluated/judged to be morally good, then it will per force follow that we would also want to evaluate/judge the entity/agent that is the subject of these acts/relations as being morally good.

21. As such, of course, the dimension-of-power i.e., the reality that is constituted by power and thus being the manifestation, the expression, of power, is all-pervasive in the world that is graspable in our sense-experience.

22. But, of course, in the concrete world given in our sense-experience we can encounter only the entities that are constituted exclusively in terms of the being-of-power or in terms of both the being-of-power and the being-of-consciousness. We do not encounter the entities that are constituted exclusively in terms of the being-of-consciousness; indeed, we cannot, seeing that for an entity to be graspable by our sense-experience the being-of-power must be implicated, if not exclusively then, at least, in part, in its ontological constitution. Thus, the existence of an entity constituted exclusively in terms of the being-of-consciousness must, per force, be relegated to a realm other than, i.e., transcending, the realm of the natural world—it must, per force, be relegated to the realm of the supernatural. Correspondingly, the existence of such an entity can be established not on the basis of our sense-experience but only on the basis of our projecting from our sense-experience. Thus, the existence of an entity constituted exclusively in terms of the being-of-consciousness is established by projecting from the existence (the existence being established by our sense-perception) of the entity constituted by the combination of a being-of-power and a being-of-consciousness—the projection being effected by proceeding from the partial implication of the being-of-consciousness in ontologically constituting the entity to its exclusive, all-encompassing, implication. Of course, the question of whether one can establish that such an entity has an existence independent of us (i.e., independent of the projectors) is a central question for the philosophy of religion but it need not concern us here.

23. Force being but the application, the impingement, of movement with

respect to an other bringing about in that other further movement.

24. True, in this state of continuous flow power is not directly graspable by our sense perception. It becomes manifest to our sense perception only when, through its diminution (i.e., diminution of its movement), it, so to speak, "sediments" itself and thus constitutes itself as a discrete entity (it can be sense-perceived only when it "sediments" itself into discrete entities). Still, inasmuch as these entities are, in the last analysis, constituted by power (they are but manifestations of various levels of power), they remain embedded within, and are part of, the continuum of power (and as such, indeed, they are also, in the last analysis, inescapably interlinked with every other manifestation of power).

25. But as such, of course, a necessary connection of implication is also established between a reality that constitutes itself as quantifiable and a reality that constitutes itself as a continuum. This is so, first, because the characterization of "imperialism" (the characterization that implicates a reality that is quantifiable) can arise only in the context of a reality that constitutes itself as a continuum. But also, and more directly, a reality that constitutes itself as quantifiable can arise only in terms of a reality that constitutes itself as a continuum, seeing that the notions of "more" and "less" (i.e., the notions that enable a reality to constitute itself as quantifiable) cannot arise except in a context of a reality that constitutes itself as a continuum. As such, a reality that constitutes itself as quantifiable presupposes in a direct manner a reality that constitutes itself as a continuum in addition to its presupposing this reality indirectly through the characterization of "imperialism."

26. Fundamentally, of course, the increase in power is to be applied here to the subject/agent of the act, namely, it is to be confined within the parameters of the individual subject/agent. But it is also possible, so to speak, to "stretch out" the application (i.e., such "stretching out" should be rationally appreciated, which is to say, grasped and accepted by reason) and place it within the more extended parameters of the collectivity of which the individual subject/agent is a member, seeing that by virtue of such membership the impingement of the increase in power of the individual subject/agent is not canceled out (indeed, one might say that the impingement of the increase in power continues to be upon the individual subject/agent, except that the individual subject/agent is now no longer defined exclusively in its own terms but rather in the more encompassing terms of the collectivity of which it is a part).

27. We get a stream of consciousness by the rapid succession of discrete, disparate, individual self-enclosed acts of consciousness. The situation here (i.e., the set-up, the mechanism) is analogous to that which obtains with regard to a movie-picture—the succession of individual still pictures, when sufficiently rapid, presents itself as an uninterrupted, continuously-moving, single picture.

28. By the way, in light of the above, it should not be surprising that the primary and the most fundamental expression of the dimension-of-consciousness, what we have defined as the being-of-consciousness (the category of being being the category that captures and represents the primary

and most fundamental manifestation, expression, of the dimension in question), is constituted by a relation, i.e., by an "in between"; in contra-distinction to the being-of-power, which constitutes itself in terms of a material substance, it being the entity constituted by the most minimal quantity of power (i.e., the quark and the lepton), the being-of-consciousness constitutes itself in terms of an "in-between," it being the entity constituted by a relation—the being-of-consciousness in its primary expression is a relation. It is only in its secondary expression, namely, when it expresses itself not in terms of the "in-between," but rather in terms of the poles that are the end-points, the boundaries, delimiting the "in-between," (a relation *qua* "in-between"—either as "gap," i.e., differentiation, or as linkage, i.e., bonding—cannot arise without simultaneously setting boundaries to itself at either end, these boundaries being the poles of the relation) that the being-of-consciousness manifests itself, expresses itself, as a discrete entity (like a material substance), seeing that it locates itself at a specific point in space, to wit, the spatial point occupied by the pole. Indeed, this expression of the being-of-consciousness at the pole, i.e., its expression as a discrete entity, constitutes what may be referred to as a person (or, to use Buberian terminology, as a Thou)—a person, a Thou, is but a being-of consciousness that expresses itself in terms of the pole of the relation rather than in terms of its "in between."

Now, it is here, at this juncture, with respect to the constituting of a person, a Thou, that one gets a first intimation, a minimal glimpse, of the "refraction" of the being-of-consciousness through the dimension-of-power in the sense of the being-of-consciousness expressing itself through the mediation (and thus in terms) of the dimension-of-power (a phenomenon that ultimately remains a profound mystery). For in placing itself at the pole, in contradistinction to placing itself in the "in-between," the being-of-consciousness places itself at a determinable point in space and as such presents itself in terms of an aspect (i.e., the aspect of space) that belongs to the dimension-of-power—indeed, it makes itself available as a discrete, identifiable (i.e., subject to a specific location in space) and thus concrete entity very much in the same manner as a material substance, i.e., as a being-of-power. So, while ontologically (and, indeed, temporally) the being-of-consciousness at the pole arises identically and simultaneously with the being-of-consciousness at the "in-between," logically (and, indeed, perspectively) it arises secondarily and derivatively, seeing that in the context of the dimension-of-consciousness it is the relation *qua* "in-between" which is the entity that arises primarily (and this is so in as much as it is the relation *qua* "in between" which primarily captures and thus expresses the very essence of the phenomenon of consciousness, seeing that by its very essence, consciousness must inescapably always constitute itself as a consciousness of something and therefore inescapably always constitute itself as a relation *qua* "in-between"). But now, for this entity to constitute itself it clearly must delimit itself on either side (without such delimitation there can be no "in-between"), such delimitation being nothing else but the constituting of the two poles, and this, in turn, would clearly imply that from a logical vantage point the poles are constituted secondarily and derivatively in as much as their constitution is called for and implicated by the constitution of the relation *qua* "in-between."

This, by the way, is in stark contrast to the situation that arises in the context of the dimension-of-power where the primary expression of the phenomenon of power is in terms of the constituting of discrete material substances (they, in their discreteness, being equivalent to the expression of the phenomenon of consciousness that takes place at the poles of the relation), which then may or may not relate to each other, so that here in the context of the dimension-of-power it is the discrete entity, i.e., the discrete material substance, that is primary and the relation is secondary. Indeed, unlike the context of the dimension-of-consciousness where the distinction between primary and secondary is only from the logical but, most significantly, not from the ontological vantage point, here in the context of the dimension-of-power the distinction is not just from the logical but also fully from the ontological vantage point. The relation is in no way an ontological expression of power; with respect to power, the ontological expression is solely in terms of the discrete material substance. Thus, the fundamental distinction between the being-of-consciousness and the being-of-power with regard to their respective ontological constitution and expression is that the former constitutes (and thus expresses) itself in terms of a relation while the latter constitutes (and thus expresses) itself in terms of a material substance.

Now, this distinction would be valid only to the extent that it could be derived from a comparison in which the two parties (i.e., the being-of-power and the being-of-consciousness) are placed on an equal footing, to wit, that they are both taken as primary ontological expressions. Indeed, we would submit that the comparison here (and, for that matter, any other comparison) can be valid and meaningful only in as much as the parties are fully placed on an equal footing.

But if this be so, then we must further specify in connection with the comparison between the being-of-power and the being-of-consciousness that the being-of-consciousness implicated in this comparison cannot be the being-of-consciousness *qua* "in-between" but must be the being-of-consciousness *qua* pole (namely, it cannot be the being-of-consciousness whose ontological expression is in terms of the relation *qua* "in-between" but must be the being-of-consciousness whose ontological expression is in terms of the relation *qua* pole). This is so because the ontological expression of the being-of-power (the other party in the comparison) is not only of necessity, per our definition, primary but it is inescapably also always concrete. Namely, the being-of-power (seeing that it constitutes itself as a discrete material substance) cannot ontologically express itself (not even if the expression is the primary and thus the most minimal expression) except in terms of concreteness, i.e., in terms that place it at a specific point in space and thus making it available to being sense-perceived. But as such, this means that if we are to have a fully valid comparison between the being-of-power and the being-of-consciousness, the being-of-consciousness that is to be implicated must be the being whose ontological expression is not only primary but also, commensurate with the being-of-power implicated in the comparison, concrete; and this, in turn, means that the being-of-consciousness that is to be implicated in the comparison has to be the being-of-consciousness whose ontological expression is not in terms of the relation *qua* "in-between" but rather in terms of the relation qua pole. For, as we have tried to establish above, it is only when the ontological expression is in terms of the relation *qua* pole (and not *qua* "in-between") that one gets an intimation of the "refraction" of the being-of-consciousness in the dimension-of-power, a refraction that, per force, bestows concreteness on the ontological expression of the being-of-consciousness.

Thus, a comparison that is fully meaningful will have to be a comparison between a material substance (i.e., the being-of-power) and a person (i.e., the being-of-consciousness as it ontologically expresses itself in terms of the relation *qua* pole). Such a comparison would yield any number of interesting distinctions. Thus, for example, we get the distinction whereby while with respect to the being-of-power the category of the relation is, ontologically speaking, external (namely, the ontological constitution of the being-of-power is independent and irrespective of the category of the relation—the relation subsists outside the fully established being-of-power that may or may not enter it with respect to other beings-of power), with respect to the being-of-consciousness the category of the relation is, ontologically speaking, internal (namely, the being-of-consciousness ontologically continues itself in terms of the category of the relation—the relation subsists inside the being-of-consciousness either in the sense of being identical with its ontological constitution or in the sense of the being-of-consciousness rising from within it in ontologically constituting itself). Another distinction that we get, and it is indeed this distinction that we need to note in particular (seeing that it plays an all-important role in the case we would present below on behalf of the claim for an ethical right to life), is the distinction whereby while the being-of-power in its ontological constitution constitutes itself (as a material substance) singly, as an individual, the being-of-consciousness in its ontological constitution constitutes itself (as a person) in twos, as a twosome—personhood can arise only as twosome, seeing that it constitutes itself in terms of the relation *qua* pole and that the pole of a relation, per force, can arise only as a twosome (a single pole is not a pole; a pole is a pole only if there is another pole at the other end of the relation). So, as regards personhood, and in stark contrast to a material substance, the adage "it takes two to tango" is to the point.

29. Of course, one can object that there are many acts of consciousness in which the other is cognized (i.e., related to) not as an end-in-itself but as a means to some further end (an example that comes readily to mind, but which is by no means the only kind of example that is available, is that of the animal of prey recognizing the other as a potential prey and thus as a means to satisfying its hunger). But it should not be difficult to see that in all these instances the consciousness that is implicated is not a "pure consciousness" but a "refracted consciousness" (namely, a consciousness that arises not in the context of the dimension-of-consciousness but in the context of the dimension-of-power, which is to say a consciousness that is, so to speak, bent by the

medium of power) that, as such, is a consciousness that places itself at the service of the dimension-of-power; it lends itself as a tool to serve the needs of power and to do this it clearly has to lend itself to the requirements and standards of power and not of its own. It is solely because of the consideration of power that the other is related to in "refracted" consciousness as a means. In "pure consciousness," i.e., in a consciousness that arises exclusively within the context of the dimension-of-consciousness, which is to say, in a consciousness taken in its own terms, this is not possible—here, the other can only be related to as an end-in-itself. In light of this, our repeated application in the discussion above of the qualification "in its own terms" to the act of consciousness may be excused perhaps.

30. Still, one can and does claim at times to be "barely conscious (half conscious, half unconscious or ten percent conscious, ninety percent unconscious) or that the affirmation received is dubious and questionable. This, however, does not refute our claim that the act of consciousness or of affirmation is all or none. For the statements implying the partialization or fractionalization of consciousness and affirmation can arise and, indeed, can be valid only with respect to a "stream of consciousness," i.e., to a string of successive acts, or to a sustained flow of affirmation. Here, indeed, one can enter consciousness in one act and exit in another or give affirmation at one instance but not at another and this clearly opens the door to gradation—depending on how frequently or infrequently consciousness comes into existence or affirmation is extended would determine the fullness, the "strength," of consciousness and the certainty of affirmation (the more acts in the "stream of consciousness" in which consciousness arises, the fuller or stronger is the experience of consciousness and the more instances in which affirmation is extended, the more convincing is the affirmation to the recipient). But our claim is made specifically with respect to the individual act (and not with respect to a collectivity of acts) of consciousness or of affirmation and with respect to the individual act the claim of all or none remains valid—in terms of the individual act there can be no gradation, no more or less, of consciousness or of affirmation; it is all or none.

31. No doubt it would not have escaped notice that the characterizations that we are attributing to actions/relations associated with the being-of-power (e.g., they being actions/relations of utilization, of acting/relating towards the other as a means, of being subject to quantification) parallel and, indeed, are identified with the characterizations that Buber attributes to I-It relations and correspondingly that the characterizations that we are attributing to actions/relations associated with the being-of-consciousness (e.g., they being actions/relation of address, of acting/relating towards the other as an end-in-itself of being all or none) parallel and are identical with the characterizations that Buber attributes to I-Thou relations. But this should not be all that surprising, seeing that the "I" in the I-It relation is an It-being (i.e., the I-It relation is a relation between two It-beings) and the "I" in the I-Thou relation is a Thou-being (i.e., the I-Thou relation is a relation between two Thou-beings) and that we would want to strongly claim that in the last analysis the It-being is

nothing else but an entity that constitutes itself exclusively in terms of the being-of-power and the Thou-being is nothing else but an entity that constitutes itself exclusively in terms of the being-of-consciousness.

32. And correspondingly, it is clearly also the case that applying here the act of prescription (an act whose application, as we have seen, is fundamental and essential to the ethical enterprise) would simply not make sense. There is no point in prescribing that one ought to do this and not that when one cannot but do what one does, i.e., when one cannot but do this and not that. Thus, with respect to entities that constitute themselves exclusively either in terms of the being-of-power or in terms of the being-of-consciousness prescription, just like evaluation/judgment, is devoid of any "cash-value."

33. But while it is clearly true that both an entity constituting itself exclusively in terms of the being-of-power and an entity constituting itself exclusively in terms of the being-of-consciousness share in common the characteristic of not having at their disposal alternative ways of expressing themselves (thus not having at their disposal alternative ways of acting/relating) and in consequence of which neither kind of entity can be subjected to ethical evaluation/judgment, these two kinds of entities (i.e., the entity that constitutes itself exclusively in terms of the being-of-power and the entity that constitutes itself exclusively in terms of the being-of-consciousness) do differ with respect to yet another characteristic that impinges in a significant sense on the issue before us here, namely, on the issue of whether or not the entity can be subjected to ethical evaluation/judgment. This characteristic consists in the entity being a *free* subject/agent, i.e., in its possession of the capacity to decide and thus to choose freely. For if the entity does not possess this characteristic, i.e., the capacity to decide and choose freely between alternative ways of expressing itself, which is to say, between alternative ways of acting, it would clearly not be valid to subject the entity to ethical evaluation/judgment—an entity that cannot choose and act freely (i.e., choose and act without being pre-determined by any factor outside itself) cannot be held accountable and thus responsible for its choices and acts and consequently cannot be subjected to ethical evaluation/judgment. Thus, to be subjected validly to ethical evaluation/judgment, an entity must not only be presented with alternative ways of acting but also be endowed with the capacity to choose *freely* among them.

But now, a persuasive case can be made that the capacity to choose freely can be attributed only to a being-of-consciousness and not to a being-of-power. For it is only the being-of-consciousness that, in being by its very constitution an expression of consciousness (i.e., awareness), can come into existence uncaused, i.e., spontaneously, and thus free in its acts and endowed with the capacity to decide (consciousness cannot be caused—it arises spontaneously and as such, *qua* awareness, its expressions, its acts, are per force not automatic and mechanical as reflexive or instinctive acts would be but the result of decision). The being-of-power, in contra-distinction, in being by its very constitution an expression of power, is totally "blind" in the sense that it can come into existence only by virtue of its being encompassed within an ongoing network of causation and that its expressions, its acts, are commensurately completely mechanical and automatic, being brought about and determined exclusively by the expressions, the acts, of the beings-of-power that precede it.

But if this be the case, then clearly regarding entities that constitute themselves exclusively in terms of the being-of-power (i.e., entities that constitute themselves as material substances) there can be no question that they would not lend themselves to ethical evaluation/judgment, seeing that such entities have neither alternative options from which to choose nor, indeed, the capacity to make a free choice between alternative options. But is the situation not different with respect to entities that constitute themselves exclusively in terms of the being-of-consciousness such as, for example, the God of biblical faith? For while it is true that such an entity is also devoid of alternative options of expressing itself (it being constituted in terms of a single kind of being), the fact that the single kind of being in terms of which it constitutes itself is the being of consciousness (and not the being-of-power) safeguards its capacity (unlike in the case of an entity where the single kind of being implicated in its constitution is the being-of-power) to freely choose and decide. Thus, could not one argue here that notwithstanding the absence of alternative options of expressing itself, such an entity can still exercise its capacity to make a free choice (due to its being constituted in terms of the being-of-consciousness) and thus be validly subjected to ethical evaluation/judgment in that it always has the option of either expressing itself in terms of the being-of-consciousness or not expressing itself at all, i.e., withholding its expression. Indeed, the God encountered in Judaism (and, for that matter, also in the other biblical faiths), the God that constitutes Himself exclusively in terms of the being-of-consciousness (i.e., as a pure Thou, a pure person), would seem to be a God that exercises this option—it is a God who at times reveals Himself and is accessible to the human while at other times hides Himself and is withdrawn from the human; a God who at times addresses, affirms, the human while at other times remains silent and unresponsive. In short, it seems to be a God who at times freely decides and chooses to express Himself in accordance with His ontological constitution while at other times freely decides and chooses to withhold such expression of Himself, thus a God who exercises His capacity to freely decide and choose, albeit not between alternative ways of expressing Himself but between expressing Himself in the only way available to Him and not expressing Himself at all. And of course, this being the case, such a God could be validly subjected to ethical evaluation/judgment.

Still, in the last analysis, one would have to concede that, notwithstanding its resourcefulness and its surface persuasiveness, the analysis contained in the preceding argument with respect to the kind of entity that constitutes itself exclusively in terms of the being-of-consciousness, i.e., with respect to the God of biblical faith, is not really valid. This is so inasmuch as the option of not expressing itself is not really available to any entity. It is certainly not available to an entity that constitutes itself exclusively in terms of the being-of-power, seeing that such an entity does not have at its disposal any capacity to freely decide and choose. But an even more fundamental consideration, and this consideration impinges equally on the entity that constitutes itself exclusively in terms of the being-of-consciousness (i.e., the kind of entity with which we are concerned here), is the consideration that the very existence of an entity, any and every entity, consists in its self-expression. For an entity to exist means to express itself in accordance with its ontological constitution, which is to say, to express its ontological constitution—for it to withhold, to abrogate, the expression of its ontological constitution is tantamount to its ceasing to exist, to its, so to speak, committing suicide. But it is precisely this latter alternative that, by the very nature of reality, is not feasible, seeing that the most fundamental and essential act of any and every entity is to strive and sustain its own ontological identity, which is tantamount to saying that it is to strive and sustain the expression of its ontological constitution.

But if our claim here is valid, how is one to account for the fact that acts of suicide can and do occur? Does not this fact undermine and refute the validity of our claim here? Not really, as can be shown, we believe, by a more detailed analysis of the phenomenon of suicide. Thus, first, it should be noted that the act of suicide takes place only with respect to humans and not with respect to any other kind of entity—not to the kind of entities that constitute the material, natural domain (e.g., the entities constituting the animal kingdom) nor the kind of entity or entities that may constitute the immaterial, supernatural domain (e.g., God or the angels). Now, with respect to the human entity, a good case can be made that the act of suicide does not really undermine our claim, to wit, the claim that it is not possible for the expression of the ontological constitution of an entity to be abrogated by that entity *in toto*. For while the human entity constitutes itself ontologically in terms of two kinds of being, i.e., the being-of-power and the being-of-consciousness, its act of suicide actually implicates the abrogation of expression of only one of these two kinds of being, namely, it implicates the abrogation of expression of only the being-of-consciousness (the dead body of the human who committed suicide continues to express its ontological constitution as a being-of-power, albeit on a different level than when it was the bearer of a being-of-retracted consciousness). As such, this means, of course, that the act of suicide by the human entity abrogates the expression of its ontological constitution only partially but not *in toto* and this, in turn, clearly means that it does not undermine our claim, seeing that our claim addresses itself only to an abrogation of expression that is *in toto* and not to an abrogation of expression that is partial. Indeed, our claim is not only not undermined but is actually substantiated by the further fact that the act of suicide does not manifest itself in all the other entities that are not human (i.e., in all the entities that comprise respectively the natural and the super-natural domains). For all these other than human entities constitute themselves in terms of a single kind of being (the entities comprising the natural domain, e.g., many of the entities constituting the animal kingdom, constituting themselves exclusively in terms of the being-of-power while the entities constituting the supernatural domain, e.g., the biblical God, constituting themselves exclusively in terms of the being-of-consciousness) and as such this means, of course, that the act of suicide, in being the act that abrogates the being in terms of which the entity committing suicide constitutes itself, must of necessity implicate here the abrogation *in toto* of the expression of the ontological constitution of the entity in question (after the abrogation of the being in terms of which the entity here constitutes itself, an abrogation that signifies the very essence of the act of suicide, there is no other kind of being left that can go on being expressed). But according to our claim such an abrogation *in toto* by an entity of the expression of its ontological constitution should not be possible and consequently the fact that indeed the act of suicide does not take place with respect to these entities must be taken as a clear corroboration of our claim. Applying now this conclusion to the issue before us, we would have to conclude that the God of biblical faith (i.e., the God whose ontological constitution is constituted exclusively in terms of a single kind of being, the being-of-consciousness) cannot commit, so to speak, suicide, which is to say that it cannot not express its ontological constitution (indeed, Buber, in presenting his notion of the eclipse of God, seems to be sensitive—whether consciously or unconsciously—to this point, seeing that he suggests that the eclipse is effected not so much by the God of biblical faith falling into silence as by the human erecting a partition, i.e., its technological civilization, between itself and this God thus blocking the voice of this God from reaching it). And this being the case, such a divinity cannot be subjected to ethical evaluation. The God of biblical faith, even though it constitutes itself in terms of the being-of-consciousness and as such has at its disposal free choice and decision, cannot exercise this free choice and decision inasmuch as the alternative option of not expressing its ontological constitution (the option whose availability would have made the exercise of choice and decision feasible) is not really available to it and not being able to exercise its capacity to freely choose and decide it cannot be subjected to ethical evaluation/judgment.

Finally, there is one further point we need address here. Namely, if the conclusion arrived at here that the God of biblical faith cannot be subjected to ethical evaluation/judgment is valid, how are we to account for the undeniable fact, already observed above, that in the religious tradition of Judaism (indeed, from its inception with Abraham challenging God on the ground of "Is the judge of all the earth not to do justice" through Job to the present-day questioning of God's silence at Auschwitz), a tradition that clearly relates to the God of biblical faith, God is subjected to ethical evaluation/judgment? Namely, if the constitution of God in terms of the being-of-consciousness cannot account for the feasibility of subjecting this God to ethical evaluation/judgment, then how could one account for the fact that the religious tradition of Judaism can subject its God to ethical evaluation/judgment? The answer to this, we would suggest, lies in the fact that although the religious tradition of Judaism (certainly in its distinctive prophetic tradition) clearly sees the essence of the divine to lie in its personhood, i.e., in the divine constituting itself as a Thou, as a being-of-consciousness, it does at the same time incorporate the being-of-power into the ontological constitution of the divine (as can be clearly seen by its attribution of omnipotence to the divine). Thus, while the essential expression of the divine continues to lie in its expression *qua* being-of-consciousness, its ontological constitution is not exclusively in terms of the being-of-consciousness but also in terms of the being-of-power. And as such, the ontological constitution of the divine becomes qualitatively (though not quantitatively) similar to that of the human—the divine becomes but "man writ large." This clearly presents serious theological problems, which obviously we cannot pursue here. But at the same time, just as clearly, it allows the divine, just as the human, to be subjected to ethical evaluation/judgment, seeing that the divine (because of the way it is ontologically constituted) has at its disposal, just like the human, not only the capacity for free decision (because of its being-of-consciousness component) but also a choice (because of the presence of both the being-of-consciousness and the being-of-power in its ontological constitution) with respect to which the capacity for free decision can express itself. Thus, the religious tradition of Judaism can indeed subject the divine to ethical evaluation/judgment but not (as intimated above) without paying a very heavy theological price.

34. Clearly, if the acting/relating is to be in terms of the subject's/agent's ontological constituent of the being-of-power, the ethical evaluation/judgment would, of course, be carried out in light of the criterion of power, which is to say, that an act/relation (the act/relation being here, of course, an act/relation of utilization) that accrues power, i.e., that increases the power of its subject/agent, will be evaluated/judged positively while an act/relation that loses power, i.e., that diminishes the power of its subject/agent, will be evaluated/judged negatively; and the greater the increase in power the more positively will the act/relation be evaluated/judged and, reversely, the greater the diminution in power the more negatively will the act/relation be evaluated/judged. On the other hand, if the acting/relating is to be in terms of the subject's/agent's ontological constituent of the being-of-consciousness, the ethical evaluation/judgment would be carried out in light of the criterion of consciousness, which is to say, that an act/relation that addresses (i.e., affirms) the other in its otherness, (i.e., affirms the other as an end in itself) will be evaluated/judged positively while an act/relation that fails to affirm the other as an end in itself (thus an act/relation that slips back into utilizing the other as a means) will be evaluated/judged negatively; and here there is no gradation in the evaluation/judgment, it is all or none. Lastly, if the acting/relating is to be in terms of the subject's/agent's all-encompassing ontological constituency, i.e., in terms of both its ontological constituent of the being-of-power and its ontological constituent of the being-of-consciousness, the ethical evaluation/judgment would have to be carried out in light of a criterion that would somehow manage to combine and represent the attributes of both the being-of-consciousness and the being-of-power and thus the dictates of both the criterion of power and the criterion of consciousness. Such a criterion, we would submit, presents itself in the notion of justice, i.e., in the notion that signifies fairness in the sense of giving each (i.e., to any and every other) its due, what it deserves.

For as such, the notion of justice succeeds in incorporating (albeit in a somewhat mitigated or partial manner) the dictates of both the criterion of power and the criterion of consciousness. It incorporates the dictates of the criterion of power (thus reflecting the state of affairs posited by the being-of-power) in that its very formulation, in trying to balance that which one gets with that which is due to it, must clearly presuppose that the acts/relations towards others which it is to evaluate/judge must lend themselves to being quantified and that, of course, means that for it the acts/relations to an other (i.e., the acts/relations to be evaluated/judged in its light as the criterion) are acts/relations that constitute themselves in terms of power—that they are fundamentally transactions in power; and as such, this, of course, means that these acts/relations are acts/relations of utilization (seeing that any transaction in power implicates, *ipso facto,* utilization), which, in turn, per force implicates that they act/relate toward the other as a means. In accepting that for it the relations to others lend themselves to being quantified, that they are thus relations of power and thus of utilization, which is to say, relations in which the other is related to as a means—in all these, the notion of justice clearly reflects the state of affairs that a being-of-power precipitates in conjunction with its presence.

At the same time, however, the notion of justice also incorporates the dictates of the criterion of consciousness in that the transactions in power, the utilizations of the other, are not left unchecked, unrestrained (as the criterion of power, left to itself, would clearly dictate—the more power one can accrue from an other, the better) but are now clearly limited, constrained, by the consideration of fairness, which is to say, by being allowed to take from or to give to the other only that which is due to it. For this means that at the same time that the other can be utilized as a means, can be related to as an object, it can also assert itself as an end-in-itself, as a subject, seeing that inasmuch as it can claim what is due to it, it is asserting rights on its behalf and in possessing such rights it clearly establishes itself as a subject and implicates that it has to be related to as an end-in-itself (indeed, to the extent that one honors these limitations on the utilization of the other, one is affirming that other as an end-in-itself). Clearly, the notion of justice also reflects the state of affairs that a being-of-consciousness precipitates in conjunction with its presence.

35. Of course, as regards both of the instances dealt with here (i.e., the instance in which the acting/relating is to an other that constitutes itself exclusively in terms of the being-of-power and the instance in which the acting/relating is to an other that constitutes itself exclusively in terms of the being-of-consciousness), it is not quite valid to intimate that in each there is available only the one other alternative mode of acting/relating cited above. Actually, as regards both instances there is yet another alternative mode of acting/relating that suggests itself, namely, the mode of acting/relating that formulates itself in terms of both the dimension-of-power and the dimension-of-consciousness (i.e., the mode of acting/relating that expresses itself in terms of utilization, but a utilization that is constrained within the bounds of justice).

But while it is true that in principle this second alternative mode of acting/relating is available (after all, a subject/agent that constitutes itself in terms of both the being-of-power and the being-of-consciousness can act/relate not only in the mode that formulates itself in terms of the dimension-of-power and in the mode that formulates itself in terms of the dimension-of-consciousness but also in the mode that formulates itself in terms of both the dimension-of-power and the dimension-of-consciousness), in actuality, given the ontological constitution of the other in both instances dealt with above, this second alternative mode of acting/relating is not really available here inasmuch as its applicability is not feasible in the two instances presented above. And its applicability is not feasible in these instances because in order for it to be feasible the other, towards which the acting/relating is directed, must constitute itself also (equally to the way the subject/agent of the acting/relating constitutes itself) in terms of both beings, i.e., the being-of-power and the being-of-consciousness. But in the two instances dealt with here the other clearly constitutes itself exclusively in terms of only one being, the being-of-power in the first instance and the being-of-consciousness in the second instance. Thus, our analysis above has not been remiss in considering only one alternative mode of acting/relating, rather than two alternative modes, in the two instances under examination above.

In this connection, it should also be noted that paralleling the difference in the rationale that underlies the inapplicability of the alternative mode of acting in the two instances before us here, there is also a significant difference in the ethical evaluation/judgment when the inapplicable alternative mode of acting/relating is applied nonetheless. For in the first instance dealt with above (i.e., the instance where the subject/agent is an entity that constitutes itself in terms of both the being-of-power and the being-of-consciousness and the other is an entity that constitutes itself exclusively in terms of the being-of-power), the ethical evaluation/judgment of an acting/relating towards that other which would formulate itself in terms of the dimension-of-consciousness would have to be taken to be neutral—such acting/relating, as said, does not make sense (and as such clearly cannot be ethically evaluated/judged positively) but it is not in any way reprehensible (and thus cannot be ethically evaluated/judged negatively). As against this, a case can be made that in the second instance (i.e., the instance where the subject/agent is the same kind of entity as in the first instance, to wit, an entity that constitutes itself in terms of both the being-of-power and the being-of-consciousness, but where the other is now an entity that constitutes itself exclusively in terms of the being-of-consciousness) the ethical evaluation/judgment of an acting/relating towards that other which would formulate itself in terms of the dimension-of-power would have to be taken to be negative. This is so because, as seen above and as will be elaborated upon below in the next chapter, the being-of-consciousness can arise only in twosomes from which would follow that a being-of-consciousness has an ethically justifiable claim on any and every other being-of-consciousness to act/relate towards it in the mode that formulates itself in terms of the dimension-of-consciousness (i.e., act/relate towards it in terms of address, affirmation) and, therefore, if any being-of-consciousness fails to so act/relate towards it, it must be ethically evaluated/judged negatively.

36. This, however, may seem to contradict our claim above that, in what

would seem to be the same circumstances (i.e., acting/relating in a mode that formulates itself in terms of the dimension-of-consciousness towards an other that is constituted in terms of the being-of-power), the ethical evaluation/judgment of such acting/relating could only be neutral but not negative. But there is really no inconsistency between our two claims. For even though it is true that in both instances the other towards which the acing/relating here (i.e., the acting/relating in the mode that formulates itself in terms of the dimension-of-consciousness) is directed is an entity that constitutes itself in terms of the same kind of being, i.e., the being-of-power, an important difference, indeed a difference that would account for the contradictory claims made in the two instances, remains nonetheless, to wit, that while in the above instance the entity that is the other is constituted in its *totality* in terms of the being-of-power, in the instance before us here it is constituted in terms of the being-of-power only *in part,* the remaining part being constituted in terms of the being-of-consciousness. For now, this difference would clearly implicate that while in the above instance the ethical evaluation/judgment has to be concerned with the effects of the acting/relating on an entity that constitutes itself exclusively in terms of the being-of-power, in the instance before us here it has to be concerned with the effects of such an acting/relating on an entity that constitutes itself no longer only in terms of the being-of-power but now also in terms of the being-of-consciousness; and this being the case, a good argument can be made that the effects of this one and the same acting/relating would differ considerably in the two instances here—not affecting adversely the entity that is the other in the above instance (indeed, not affecting it at all) while in the instance that is before us here it may well affect the entity that is the other adversely (and, of course, commensurate with this, the ethical evaluation/judgment in the above instance would have to remain neutral while in the instance before us here it would have to be negative).

Thus, for example, addressing and thus affirming (i.e., an acting/relating in a mode that formulates itself in terms of the dimension-of-consciousness) an other that is a wall would not affect the wall one way or another; as against this, addressing and thus affirming, rather than surgically excising, an other that is an inflamed appendix does affect very much the other of which the inflamed appendix is but a part, i.e., the human entity that possesses the inflamed appendix—it affects its very existence. True, it does not affect the existence of the body-part of the human other, i.e., the existence of its being-of-power constituent (the body merely undergoes changes in its functions and appearance). But it does affect the existence of the conscious-part, the personal dimension, of the human other, i.e., the existence of its being-of-consciousness constituent (the changes in the functions of the body-part terminate the existence of the conscious-part), and with this the existence of the human other *qua* human, i.e., *qua* an entity that constitutes itself in terms of both the being-of-power and the being-of-consciousness. So when a surgeon confronting a patient with an inflamed appendix proceeds to address the appendix (e.g., beseeching it to heal itself) rather than removing it, its acting/relating towards the patient affects the patient adversely in a way that a painter's talking to a wall rather than painting or plastering it does not; the acting/relating of the surgeon is clearly reprehensible and consequently its ethical evaluation/judgment would have to be negative while the acting/relating of the painter may be peculiar but it is not reprehensible and consequently the ethical evaluation/judgment is neutral.

But how can we say that the evaluation/judgment of the surgeon's acting/relating here as being negative is an evaluation/judgment that is ethical when the evaluation/judgment of the acting/relating here is carried out from the perspective of the other rather than from the perspective of the subject/agent, i.e., in terms of how it affects the other rather than in terms of how it affects the subject/agent, seeing that in our delineation of the ethical enterprise the ethical evaluation/judgment of an act/relation is to formulate itself in terms of how the act/relation affects the subject/agent rather than in terms of how it affects the other? This challenge would have been indeed most telling if it were not for the fact that, as seen above (and as will be elaborated upon in the next chapter), a being-of-consciousness, in clear contra-distinction to a being-of-power, places an obligation on any and every other being-of-consciousness not to terminate its existence (and by extension, not to adversely interfere with it) and it is in the very interest of any and every other being-of-consciousness to honor this obligation; for, as such, this means (seeing that here both the other and the subject/agent are entities that encompass within their respective ontological constitutions a being-of-consciousness, so that the other by virtue of its being-of-consciousness constituent is to place this obligation and the subject/agent by virtue of its being-of-consciousness constituent is to honor it) that the evaluation/judgment formulated above in terms of how the acting/relating affects the other at one and the same time lends itself to being formulated in terms of how it affects the subject/agent and as such it is a *bona fide* ethical evaluation/judgment.

And indeed, as indicated, this case could not have been made had the other been an entity that was constituted exclusively in terms of the being-of-power. For an entity that constitutes itself in terms of the being-of-power cannot place obligations on other entities, which, in turn, means that no equivalence could have been established here between the interests of the subject/agent of the acting/relating and those of the other towards which the acting/relating was directed, thus not allowing one to move from the interests of the other to those of the subject/agent; and, in such a context, an acting/relating that has been evaluated/judged from the perspective of the interests of the other rather than from the perspective of the interests of the subject/agent could indeed not lend itself to an evaluation/judgment that is ethical (indeed, it is worth noting that our own position above regarding the ethical evaluation/judgment of the acting/relating that is directed towards an other that is constituted exclusively in terms of the being-of-power does conform with the conclusion stated here for our position was that the ethical evaluation/judgment of such acting/relating had to be neutral and this is tantamount to saying that the evaluation/judgment here, as far as its content is concerned, is vacuous, which adds up to admitting that an *ethical* evaluation/judgment is really, in the last analysis, not available to us here). Thus, it is valid after all to note a difference with respect to the mode of acting/relating that formulates itself in terms of the dimension-of-consciousness between the case when it is directed towards an other that constitutes itself exclusively in terms of the being-of-power and the case when it is directed towards an other that also constitutes itself as a being-of-power, but this time only partially so, the other part being constituted as a being-of-consciousness; the difference being that while in the former case the possibility of an ethical evaluation/judgment that is neutral is implicated, in the latter case the possibility of an ethical evaluation/judgment that is negative is being implicated.

37. As such, let us note, the ethical evaluation/judgment here is the same as it was in the instance above where the other towards which the acting/relating was directed was an entity that constituted itself not in part but in its totality in terms of the being-of-consciousness. Thus, the case here is different from the case that obtained in the preceding instance, i.e., in the instance where an acting/relating that formulates itself in terms of the dimension-of-consciousness is directed towards an other that constitutes itself in terms of the being-of-power. Still, here too we encounter a significant difference between the two almost-parallel instances; but it is a difference that arises not with respect to the content of the evaluation (the content in both instances is the same—in both instances the evaluation is in the negative) but rather with respect to the consideration that precipitates the negative evaluation here, or, in other words, with respect to the rationale, justification that underlies the application of a negative evaluation to the act/relation that is at stake here.

Thus, in the instance above, the negative evaluation comes about not because an acting/relating that constitutes itself in terms of the dimension-of-power (i.e., an acting/relating of utilization), taken in itself as such, is evaluated to be detrimental to the other towards which it is directed (as seen, an acting/relating that constitutes itself in terms of the dimension-of-power cannot affect an other that is an entity that constitutes itself exclusively in terms of the being-of-consciousness inasmuch as an acting/relating towards an other in terms of the dimension-of-power, i.e., an acting/relating that consists in the utilization of the other, requires that the other be, to some minimal extent, an entity possessing substance, which is to say, it requires that the other constitute itself, to some minimal extent, in terms of the being-of-power, and this clearly is not the case here); rather, it comes about because the acting/relating here in terms of the dimension-of-power, being the only mode of acting/relating that is available, preempts the very possibility of acting/relating towards the other in terms of the dimension-of-consciousness and it is precisely this *absence* of this latter mode of acting/relating, i.e., the absence of acting/relating in terms of the dimension-of-consciousness, that is detrimental to the other here (the other being constituted exclusively in terms of the being-of-consciousness requires that the acting/relating towards it be in terms of the dimension-of-consciousness) and thus, in turn, necessarily implicating a negative evaluation/judgment of the acting/relating here that is in terms of the dimension-of-power. In contrast to this, in the instance before us an acting/relating in terms of the dimension-of-power (i.e., an acting/relating that constitutes itself in the utilization of the other) can affect the other, when directed towards it, seeing that a being-of-power constituent is present in the ontological constitution of the other. As such, unlike the above instance, the acting/relating in terms of the dimension-of-power can now be evaluated/judged in its own terms and not merely in terms of its ramifications (for example, that it preempts the acting/relating that constitutes itself in terms of the dimension-of-consciousness). And given the context that is presented in the instance before us, an acting/relating that constitutes itself in terms of the dimension-of-power would indeed be evaluated/judged negatively, seeing that the acting/relating here is directed towards the other not in terms of its being-of-power constituent but in terms of its being-of-consciousness constituent.

38. Clearly, utilitarianism is not the only ethical formulation that formulates itself in terms of the dimension-of-power. Many other figures in the history of philosophy present us with ethical formulations that are non-utilitarian yet, at the same time, clearly formulate themselves in terms of the dimension-of-power. Let us briefly mention here but two such figures.

One is Nietzsche who, notwithstanding his vicious attacks against utilitarianism, clearly took an ethical stance that places itself fully and uncompromisingly within the dimension-of-power. (By the way, the relation between Nietzsche and utilitarianism is a poignant exemplification of the perceptive and true observation that the closer the position between two parties, the less tolerant and accepting they are of the differences subsisting between them and the more venomous and extreme they are in rejecting each other—the bloodiest and most vicious wars are civil wars). Nietzsche's vicious attacks against utilitarianism should not fool us to think that this arose because Nietzsche is coming from a position that is far-removed and very unsympathetic to the dimension-of-power. Just the opposite is the case. Nietzsche's attacks on utilitarianism are so vicious precisely because his difference with utilitarianism is set in an underlying context of similarity. Both Nietzsche and utilitarianism formulate their ethical position in terms of the dimension-of-power with the difference that while Nietzsche focuses uncompromisingly on power in its maximal expression (the ideal of the *Übermensch* that he wants to see attained within humanity is but the human that constitutes itself exclusively and thus maximally as a being-of-power), utilitarianism, availing itself of the quantification aspect of power accepts and, indeed, formulates itself in terms of the gradation that subsists within power. And it is precisely the fact that utilitarianism accepts the "more" and thus, in Nietzsche's view, undermining and compromising the "most" in power, that utilitarianism is willing to settle and deal with fractions of power rather than insist on attaining power in its totality, that arouses Nietzsche's ire; and the ire is so violent because the difference manifests itself within the context of one and the same dimension, because both, Nietzsche and utilitarianism, play, so to speak, within the same ball park (if the two were playing in different ball parks, the clash precipitated by the difference would not have been so violent).

The other figure is Schopenhauer. Schopenhauer, in contra-distinction to

Nietzsche, is not after the maximal expression of power but rather after the maximal, i.e., the total, elimination of power. As such, his stance may indeed give the impression that it transcends in its formulation the dimension-of-power and formulates itself in terms of the dimension-of-consciousness. But this is really not so. Schopenhauer's stance formulates itself exclusively in terms of the dimension-of-power except that in this context it formulates itself in a negative manner, namely, emptying the dimension of all its contents. The dimension-of-consciousness does not enter the picture here because nothing positive in its terms is put forth as a substitute for the negation of power; all one gets is the negation, the rejection, of power but nothing else beyond it. One can see, however, how Schopenhauer could be misperceived as formulating his stance in terms of the dimension-of-consciousness, seeing that power is negated, rejected, both in the context of his stance and in that of the dimension-of-consciousness. Still, there is all the difference in the world between the two contexts.

39. Moore wants to claim 1) that there are properties/attributes that are, by their very constitution, indefinable (citing as an example the color red) and 2) that "ethical good," in similar fashion to the color red, is such a property. It would seem to us, however, that this position confuses these properties/attributes being "simple" rather than "complex" terms or universals with their being indefinable. But if this be so, then this is a mistake (though it is not difficult to see how this can come about). For "simple" in contra-distinction to "complex" signifies that an entity so qualified is not constituted in terms of other entities that, as such, form its sub-parts and that, therefore, as far as its definability is concerned, it cannot be defined in terms of its sub-parts. But this does not mean that it cannot be defined at all. Thus, "red" may well be a "simple" term and then this would indeed imply that it cannot be defined in terms of its sub-parts but not, as Moore claimed, that it cannot be defined at all. Indeed, we would submit that "red" can be defined, for example, as the sense-image that all normal-sighted persons (i.e., persons who are not color blind) have when light of a certain wave-length hits their retina. And, *mutatis mutandis,* the same conclusion would apply with respect to defining the "ethical good." The "ethical good" may indeed be a "simple" property/attribute but this should not mean that in consequence of this it is totally indefinable only that it is indefinable in terms of its sub-parts.

40. A criterion by its very definition is a point of reference in terms of which the delineation of other things is determined and as such its delineation, per force, must always constitute the starting-point in any chain of delineations while it itself cannot be a member down the line in any such chain of delineations. Indeed, it would seem to us that Moore, in resorting to the "open question argument," is shifting his grounds from delineating the ethical in terms of the presence of a certain, particular property/attribute to delineating it in terms of a certain, particular kind of evaluation/judgment. This can be seen in that the regression is propelled for him by the ever-present question of why a particular naturalistic property/attribute should be taken as the "ethical good."

41. True, it may be argued that the ontological structure here in which the

criterion is being grounded is not really, after all, available to empirical examination and validation inasmuch as it does not really lend itself to being sense-perceived. For in saying that the criterion here is grounded in the ontological structure we are really saying (as should be only too evident from our discourse above) that the criterion is grounded in one or the other of the two constituents (or in both) that make up the ontological structure here, i.e., the constituent of power and the constituent of consciousness, and clearly neither the constituent of power as such nor the constituent of consciousness as such lend themselves to being sense-perceived. Clearly, we do not and, indeed, cannot directly sense-perceive either power or consciousness. Indeed, since, as indicated above, neither the power constituent nor the consciousness constituent present themselves in the context of our formulation as substances (true, our formulation is dualistic but it is not dualistic in the Cartesian sense), it should not be surprising that neither is available to being directly sense-perceived. At the same time, however, being taken in the context of our formulation as dimensions that implicate certain kinds of acts/relations (the power constituent implicating the It kind, i.e., acts/relations that constitute themselves as acts/relations of utilization and thus as acts/relations in which the other is taken as a means, an object, and the consciousness constituent implicating the Thou kind, i.e., acts/relations that constitute themselves as acts/relations of affirmation and thus as acts/relations in which the other is taken as an end-in-itself, a subject), the existence, i.e., the reality, of the power constituent and of the consciousness constituent can be empirically validated. For clearly, the existence, i.e., the reality, of the power constituent and the consciousness constituent can be deduced from the existence, i.e., the reality, of the acts/relations that they implicate and inasmuch as these acts/relations lend themselves to being directly sense-perceived, the presence, i.e., the reality, of the power constituent and of the consciousness constituent can be empirically validated even though they, in their own terms, do not lend themselves to being directly sense-perceived.

42. Indeed, this can be clearly seen from the perspective of our formulation, according to which an utterance is defined as ethical primarily and fundamentally in terms of its evaluative function (i.e., for an utterance to be delineated as ethical it must first and foremost be evaluative). For as we have argued above, in any and every ethical evaluation an expression of the evaluator's feeling or attitude of approval or disapproval is inescapably implicated while at the same time any and every such ethical evaluation also entails a prescription—a positive evaluation of an act entailing a prescription to carry it out while a negative evaluation entails a proscription against carrying it out.

43. Such a state of affairs, as has been pointed out, may of course readily allow the positing as ethical of utterances whose content may well be totally obnoxious and unacceptable to most people. Indeed, as Nowell-Smith has suggested, the prescription to put all Jews in gas chambers may well qualify according to Hare's formulation as a valid ethical prescription—"nothing that we discover about the nature of moral judgments (in Hare's formulation)

entails that it is wrong to put all Jews in gas-chambers." This, of course, is a most serious weakness in Hare's formulation but it is not a weakness that impinges on what concerns us here. What impinges on our concern here is the weakness of relativism, the weakness with which we have dealt above.

44. The religious formulation in grounding its criterion for ethical evaluation/judgment in divine revelation certainly has a criterion that is more rigorously absolute (i.e., more firmly established in its permanence) than our formulation, which grounds its criterion for ethical evaluation/judgment in the ontological constitution of the human. For the ontological constitution of the human can and, in all probability, given enough time, will change in the course of the evolutionary process while the divine, by its very definition, is forever unchangeable. But having acknowledged this, we should hasten to add that, for all intents and purposes, the ontological constitution of the human is sufficiently absolutist as far as the feasibility of pursuing the ethical enterprise is concerned. For as we have seen above, for the ethical enterprise to be carried out in a meaningful way the present ontological constitution of the human is required—the applicability of the ethical enterprise in its full signification is possible only in the context of humans as they are presently ontologically constituted. Consequently, if the ontological constitution of the human is to be changed, the very applicability of the ethical enterprise is thrown into question. But if the ethical enterprise is not applicable to begin with (certainly, a good case can be made that with respect to humans who live in paradise the ethical enterprise is vacuous), the need for an absolute that is uncompromised would be beside the point. Thus, as long as the "absolute" here is brought into the picture because of the requirements of the ethical enterprise, the "absolute" emanating from the ontological constitution of the human is fully adequate even though in absolute terms it is not an absolute "absolute."

45. We should make clear, however, that we are not challenging the claim that the assertions of the natural law formulation lend themselves to being empirically examined and thus to there being the possibility of their being empirically validated. This evidently is the case. What we do challenge is the further, but essential, claim of the natural law formulation that this possibility is actually realized in fact.

46. Thus, for example, our formulation cannot but be extremely sympathetic and accepting of Cicero's characterization of the natural law formulation as "of universal application, unchanging and everlasting . . . And there will not be different laws at Rome and at Athens, or different laws now and in the future, but one eternal and unchangeable law will be valid for all nations and all times" (*De Re Publica,* III, xxii, as quoted in Singer 1991, 164). Indeed, it conforms precisely to the delineation of the ethical enterprise to which our formulation, by its very essence, is inextricably bound.

47. As such, we can perhaps say that, in the last analysis, both the restrictive natural law formulation and our formulation are fundamentally akin to the classical Greek, i.e., to the Platonic and Aristotelian, conception of the ethical enterprise, seeing that for both the Platonic and the Aristotelian formulation the criterion in the light of which the ethical evaluation/judgment is

to be carried out is grounded in one or another aspect, feature, of the ontological constitution of the human (and this in contra-distinction to the formulation of the sophists where the criterion is grounded in the passing and contingent feelings and interests of the individual human which as such, indeed, readily lends itself as a forerunner and a model to all subjectivist and relativistic formulations, not the least of which is the contemporary emotivist formulation). Indeed, we can perhaps put this point more specifically and say that while the restrictive natural law formulation is clearly akin to the Aristotelian formulation, our formulation, in contra-distinction, is more akin to the Platonic formulation. For while both the Aristotelian formulation and the restrictive natural law formulation view the ontological constitution of the human (as it implicates itself *qua* criterion with respect to the ethical evaluation/judgment of human acts) in terms of a single, unitary, ontological factor, i.e., the factor of reason, the Platonic formulation and our formulation view it in terms of a variety, a multiplicity, of factors—the Platonic formulation in terms of three factors (i.e., the appetites, the passions, the intellect) and our formulation in terms of two factors (i.e., power and consciousness). Thus, the kinship between the restrictive natural law formulation and the Aristotelian formulation lies in the fact that the ontological constitution of the human entity as it is implicated in the ethical enterprise (i.e., in the enterprise of ethically evaluating/judging the acts/relations of the human entity) is perceived by both to be constituted in terms of a single, unitary, ontological factor (which, indeed, is one and the same ontological factor for both, to wit, the ontological factor of reason) while the kinship between our formulation and the Platonic formulation lies in the fact that it is perceived by both to be constituted in terms of a multiplicity of ontological factors (though here, and in contra-distinction to the other kinship, the two formulations do differ with regard to the number and kind of the factors that they implicate).

But now, by the way, if this be the case, we would want to further claim that our formulation and the Platonic formulation (i.e., the formulations that implicate a multiplicity of ontological factors) have the advantage over the restrictive natural law formulation and the Aristotelian formulation (i.e., the formulations that implicate only a single, unitary, ontological factor). For we would submit that the ontological constitution of the human does implicate more than one ontological factor—no one ontological factor (no matter which one) can fully and exhaustively ontologically constitute the human. Thus, for example, as regards the ontological factor of reason, the human entity clearly manifests additional aspects, dimensions, which are not reducible to the aspect, dimension, of reason (Plato, in delineating the human, was quite right to include in addition to the dimension of reason the dimension of the passions and that of the appetites).

And if one were to object that what is at issue here is not the question of how comprehensive, how complete, is the representation of the ontological constitution of the human but rather the question of what particular aspect or aspects in that ontological constitution would lend it distinctiveness from all other possible ontological constitutions, our response would still be that even so the distinctiveness of the ontological constitution of the human cannot be validly placed in any single, unitary, ontological factor, not even when the ontological factor is to be that of reason. For although granted that the claim that the distinctiveness of the human entity from all other entities is established by virtue of the fact that the human entity alone possesses the ontological factor of reason, i.e., the capacity to think, is a claim that *prima facie* appears to be rather appealing, i.e., it appears to be rather persuasive (indeed, some very great minds held it), we must, in the last analysis, agree with those who challenge the tenability of this claim. For it would appear that the ontological factor of reason does after all manifest itself, at least to some extent, in other kinds of entities. Thus, it would appear that a good case can be made that in the class of primates other kinds of entity (such as, for example, the chimpanzee or the gorilla) may well possess to some extent the ontological factor of reason. At best, therefore, if the ontological factor of reason is to be taken as a criterion for the distinctiveness of the human entity, it can be so taken only on the basis that the distinctiveness which it can establish can only be a distinctiveness that is in quantitative but not in qualitative terms; namely, we can validly say that the ontological factor of reason is much more developed, much more complex, much more "high-powered" in the human entity than it is in all other entities but we cannot validly say that it is unique to the human entity.

A merely quantitative distinctiveness, however, is certainly not the kind of distinctiveness that the situation here requires. If already the issue of the representation of the ontological constitution of the human is to be approached here in terms of its distinctiveness rather than in terms of its all-inclusive totality, then the distinctiveness involved must be of a qualitative, and not merely of a quantitative, nature. And to get a distinctiveness for the ontological constitution of the human that is qualitative, and not merely quantitative, in nature, a certain combination of ontological factors (and not a single ontological factor) would seem to be required. A qualitative distinction can be derived here only from the particularity of a certain combination of ontological factors, which, in turn, means that a multiplicity of ontological factors (i.e., at least two) is necessarily implicated in establishing a qualitative distinctiveness for the ontological constitution of the human. Thus, in terms of distinctiveness too, a multiplicity of ontological factors is required in order to validly capture the ontological constitution of the human. We can, therefore, conclude that, in the last analysis, whether the ontological constitution of the human is to be implicated here in terms of its overall, all-encompassing, ontological make-up or in terms of its distinctiveness, formulations that perceive the ontological constitution of the human in terms of a multiplicity of ontological factors do indeed have the advantage over formulations which perceive it in terms of a unitary ontological factor.

Lastly, it may be in order here to briefly argue one further claim. Namely, we would want to argue that within the context of the group of formulations that perceive the ontological constitution of the human in terms of a multiplicity of ontological factors (this being instanced here by the Platonic formulation and our formulation) our formulation would have the advantage over all the alternative formulations within this group. This is so because the ontological factors that it identifies are, in our judgment, the most fundamental ontological factors in terms of which the ontological constitution of the human can be established.

Namely, we would submit that the ontological factors of power and consciousness are indeed the most fundamental ontological factors available to us, seeing that a good case can be made that they themselves are not further reducible to any other conceivable ontological factors and that, indeed, if anything, all other conceivable ontological factors would ultimately be reducible to them, i.e., to one or the other of these two ontological factors. Thus, to briefly illustrate this claim, let us turn to the other formulation cited here which perceives the ontological constitution of the human in terms of a multiplicity of ontological factors, i.e., the Platonic formulation. We would submit that every one of the three ontological factors introduced by the Platonic formulation is ultimately reducible to one or the other of the two ontological factors introduced by our formulation—the ontological factor of the appetites being ultimately reducible to the ontological factor of power (it being, in the last analysis, but an expression of power) while the ontological factors of the passions and the intellect being ultimately reducible to the ontological factor of consciousness (they being, in the last analysis, but an expression of consciousness). As such, notwithstanding the fact that there are any number of aspects which our formulation shares with the Platonic formulation (and because of this it is, indeed, very akin and appreciative of the Platonic formulation), an advantage over the Platonic formulation should accrue to our formulation. And, *mutatis mutandis,* a similar advantage would accrue to our formulation over any other formulation belonging to this group of formulations, i.e., the group of formulations that posit a multiplicity of ontological factors, if it can be shown (as, indeed, we have claimed it to be the case) that the ontological factors involved are, in the last analysis, reducible either to the ontological factor of power or to the ontological factor of consciousness.

48. Of course, it may be argued that in shifting the vantage point from that of the individual to that of the species we do not really escape the problematic of subjectivism inasmuch as this problematic reduces itself in our context to the problematic of temporal relativism, i.e., the problematic whereby the ethical criterion is not temporally absolute in its applicability. For while it is true that in comparison to the human individual the human species is much more enduring and unchanging, in absolute terms it too is a passing phenomenon—given enough time it too, for sure, will change and, indeed, disappear just like the human individual. Thus, in the last analysis, the difference here between grounding the ethical criterion in the human individual and grounding it in the human species is but a difference of degree, which is to say that the grounding of the criterion in the human species remains just as much within the parameters of relativism as its grounding in the human individual.

49. Clearly, if this were not the case, such formulations would be rejected out of hand. For to present a credible alternative in the context of our understanding of the ethical enterprise a formulation must appropriate this

fundamental aspect in our conception of the ethical enterprise.

50. This, indeed, is clearly the case when the ethical evaluation/judgment is established with respect to the act/relation involved, namely, when it is being established by the nature of the act/relation involved. But it would also seem that one can interpret Hume's formulation as establishing the ethical evaluation/judgment not with respect to the act/relation involved but rather with respect to the feeling that the act/relation generates within the subject/agent—a positive ethical evaluation/judgment is established when the subject/agent comes to possess a feeling of pleasure and satisfaction (though, it is true that such a feeling, in turn, is generated by an acting/relating that is in conformity with the sense of sympathy). In terms of this alternative understanding, however, it would seem that Hume's formulation loses its altruistic aspect and reverts to being an egotistical formulation. After all, it is now the state of feeling of the subject/agent which determines the ethical evaluation. Still, even so, one can argue that inasmuch as the feeling of pleasure and satisfaction is generated here by (and is thus contingent upon) a certain kind of acting/relating, to wit, an acting/relating that is in conformity with the sense of sympathy, the role of the acting/relating remains the essential and primary factor in determining the ethical evaluation/judgment and, as such, the formulation here remains altruistic. At any rate, it is towards the formulation here as it establishes the ethical evaluation/judgment with respect to the act/relation and not with respect to the feeling that the act/relation generates in the subject/agent that the observations made below are directed.

51. Two apparent exceptions to the above observation come to mind but, as we will try to show here, they do not really undermine our contention. Thus, first, it is true that many humans (though, by no means all humans) would sacrifice themselves in favor of their progeny, i.e., would act against their own interests if such acting is to the advantage of their progeny (and this is so even up to the point of giving up one's life if such an act is to save the life of the progeny). It would seem, therefore, that acting altruistically (indeed, acting altruistically in the full sense of the notion) is feasible after all. But this is not totally so. For after all, a good case can be made that progeny is, in a very real sense, a continuation of the individual self—one goes on living in one's progeny. But this being the case, the parameters of the self (and commensurately, the boundaries of the egotistical calculation) do not stop with the individual but are, so to speak, stretched to encompass the individual's progeny. And in such a context sacrificing one's interests in favor of the interests of one's progeny is not an altruistic but an egotistic act (as, indeed, one can argue analogously that the sacrifice of an organ, when this is to the advantage of the body as a whole, is an act in conformity with egotistical calculations, and not only of the body as a whole but equally so of the organ itself).

Secondly, it must be conceded, however, that there are also cases where individual humans sacrifice their interests at great cost to themselves (indeed, even to the point of giving up their lives) in favor of the interests of others who are total strangers. But such instances of acting are, relatively speaking, very few and infrequent. Indeed, such instances of acting are to be viewed as abnormal and this notwithstanding the fact that they may well be viewed positively, i.e., deemed as noble and admirable, rather than negatively, i.e., criticized or pitied—they are abnormal in the sense that they do not represent the common, universal pattern of acting characteristic of humans. By the way, we would suggest that such instances of acting come about when the individual comes to perceive/desire him/herself exclusively in terms of its Thou-being ontological constituent and in total rejection of its It-being ontological constituent and in the process, we would further submit, goes astray in understanding the aspect of being other-orientated implicated in a Thou-being. It goes astray in overlooking the all-important fact that being other-orientated which is implicated in the ontological constitution of a Thou-being is ultimately for the sake of the Thou-being ontological constituent of the self and not for the sake of the Thou-being ontological constituent of the other, thus leaving the aspect of being other-oriented which is implicated here in an egoistic and not in an altruistic frame of reference (in an authentic context the aspect of being other-orientated implicated in the Thou-being ontological constituent of the self arises in terms of a relation of mutuality with the Thou-being ontological constituent implicated in the other and not in a one-way relation from the self to the other where the self cancels itself out in favor of the other).

In any event, it is very instructive and to the point that such acting, i.e., the acting in which an individual would sacrifice itself in favor of an other, would be referred to as saintly and not as ethical, given the distinct difference in signification which the two terms carry (the significations of "saintly" and of "ethical" are by no means identical and consequently they are not to be confused with each other). Thus, while saintliness signifies a transcending of the present ontological constitution of the human as an It/Thou entity to its becoming a pure Thou entity (which is to say, a kind of a divine entity which is deemed to be a "higher" or "nobler" ontological state) ethics, certainly as formulated by us, accepts and deals with the human in terms of its present ontological constitution. But actually, even more to the point here is the contrast in signification between the derivative applicability of the "saintly" and that of the ethical. In such a derivative applicability the notion of saintly or saintliness would no longer signify a transformation in the ontological constitution of the human from being an It/Thou entity to becoming a pure Thou entity. The It constituent in the ontological constitution of the human is not abrogated here, only its expression is suppressed. The notion of saintly or saintliness now signifies a human who, while continuing to be constituted as an It/Thou entity, acts and conducts him/herself in terms of its Thou but not It constituent. In contrast to this, the notion of ethics would accept and deal with the human not only as being ontologically constituted as an It/Thou entity but as an It/Thou entity that expresses itself in terms of both its It-being and its Thou-being. Ethics does not expect or require the human to act as a saint but only as a human, albeit authentically so.

52. True, we raised the same point also with respect to Hume's formulation. But there it could be raised only when the formulation was to be

interpreted as constituting the ethical criterion not so much in terms of the conformation of the act/relation to the sense of sympathy but rather in terms of the feeling of pleasure, satisfaction, that accompanies such a conformation. Here, on the other hand, no particular interpretation of the formulation is implicated in order to establish the claim of egoism—it is given inescapably in the very substance of the formulation.

53. The suffering expresses itself in the psychological domain as a direct consequence of the "imperialistic" aspect of power. For inasmuch as power by its very nature is ever-striving to accrue more power unto itself, any entity that constitutes itself in terms of power would unceasingly strive and desire to attain more power for itself which, in turn, means that its desire can never fulfill itself and its will consequently can never come to a rest. Such an entity, to the extent that it possesses self-consciousness, must be an unhappy entity.

54. Of course, Schopenhauer's formulation can be understood differently. It can be understood as perceiving the ontological constitution of the human in the same way that our formulation does, namely, no longer exclusively in terms of power but in terms of both power and consciousness. And as such, of course, we can no longer fault it as being an invalid perception.

Indeed, the difference between Schopenhauer's formulation and our formulation is no longer a case where one presents a valid perception of a reality (the reality being the ontological constitution of the human) and the other does not. Both formulations present a valid perception of the ontological constitution of the human. Rather, the difference now is to be found in the respective evaluation of this ontological constitution by the two formulations: namely, more specifically, it is to be found with respect to where within this ontological constitution of the human they locate the problematic, the predicament, to which they are to offer the solution. As such, the difference here is not with respect to the validity of the perception but rather with respect to the evaluation/judgment that is applied to the perception, a difference which, in contra-distinction to the difference with respect to the issue of the validity of the perception, is a difference that cannot be resolved one way or another for all concerned—either evaluation/judgment can be held depending on one's disposition. Thus, Schopenhauer's formulation views the problematic, the predicament, to lie in the very inclusion, in the very presence, of the dimension of power within the ontological constitution of the human (and clearly, commensurate to this, the only viable solution, the only viable "salvation," can be secured by the total abrogation of the dimension of power). In contra-distinction, in the view of our formulation the presence of the dimension of power within the ontological constitution of the human does not precipitate the problematic, the predicament (i.e., there is no problem with the human constituting itself ontologically in terms of both the dimension of power and the dimension of consciousness, as an It/Thou entity); the problematic is precipitated by the ever-present possibility that such an ontological constitution presents, to wit, the possibility that the proportion between the respective expression of the dimension of power and the expression of the dimension of consciousness would be askew (and clearly, commensurate to this, the only viable solution, the only viable "redemption," can be secured by the ever-present vigilance and effort to re-establish the proper balance between the two dimensions).

By the way, it would seem to us that this difference between our formulation and Schopenhauer's formulation reflects the difference between the basic orientation of Judaism and that of Christianity whereby our formulation reflects the orientation of Judaism while Schopenhauer's formulation reflects the orientation of Christianity. For a good case can be made that while in the basic orientation of Judaism the presence of the It-dimension, i.e., of the dimension of power, as such, is not the source of the predicament (the source of the predicament being the disproportionate expression that the It-dimension arrogates to itself to the exclusion of the Thou-dimension, i.e., of the dimension of consciousness), in the basic orientation of Christianity, the very presence of the It-dimension, irrespective of the extent of its expression, is the source of the predicament and consequently, while in Christianity the attainment of salvation necessarily implicates a transformation in the ontological constitution of the human (i.e., the creation of a "new being"), in Judaism the attainment of redemption implicates no such transformation whatsoever within the given ontological constitution of the human, its attainment being contingent on establishing the proper balance between the expression of the It-dimension and that of the Thou-dimension (one should hasten to note, however, that any religion taken in the context of its historical expression is most likely to be a mixture of any number of different structures-of-faith which by no means need be compatible with each other and that, therefore, our attributing certain characterizations respectively to Judaism and Christianity, speaking of each as if it were a homogenous, all-inclusive religious entity that requires no further limiting qualification, would appear to be, at least on the face of it, untenable; indeed, in truth, the characterizations referred to here are really attributable to a certain strain of expression within Judaism and Christianity respectively, but in as much, as we would want to claim, the strains implicated here are the strains that capture the religious phenomenon of Judaism and Christianity respectively in their utmost distinctiveness and, indeed, in their most essential expression, referring to these religious phenomena by the all-inclusive, "umbrella" terminology of "Judaism" and "Christianity" without any further limiting qualification, may be tenable after all).

Indeed, we would submit, that from this basic difference one can readily derive a persuasive rationale for any number of other differences in the characterization that obtains between Judaism and Christianity. Thus, for example, the rationale for the difference whereby the salvific event in Christianity is a one-time, non-repetitive occurrence while the commensurate redemptive event in Judaism can be seen as a recurring, repetitive event, or the rationale for the difference whereby in Christianity the human is a passive recipient of the effects ensuing from the salvific event while in Judaism the human is an active agent in bringing about the redemptive event can be readily seen as being dictated by the inner logic emanating from the basic difference delineated above whereby the salvific event in Christianity implicates a transformation in the ontological constitution of the human while the redemptive event in Judaism implicates no such transformation but rather the proper balancing between the It-dimension and the Thou-dimension (i.e., between the dimension-of-power and the dimension-of-consciousness) that are present within the given ontological constitution of the human. For clearly a transformation in the ontological constitution of an entity is a non-recurring, one-time event and, indeed, an event that can be brought about not by the entity itself but only by an agency that exists outside the entity, seeing that no entity can act in a way that is not within the confines of its ontological constitution and that no ontological constitution could possibly implicate its own transformation, i.e., no entity can, so to speak, pull itself up by its own boot straps when the pulling implicates the transformation of its ontological constitution. At the same time, and equally as clearly, attaining and maintaining a balance between two (or more) different expressions in which at least one is ever-dynamic in striving to exclude the other (or others) is an ever-recurring, never-ending task and, indeed, a task that only the entity which is the subject of the competing expressions can carry out.

Now surely, the fact that the rationale for these differences (and, indeed, also for other differences) is so persuasively derived from the foregoing difference delineated above, namely, the difference between Christianity implicating and Judaism not implicating a transformation in the ontological constitution of the human, buttresses the validity of our claim that a difference with respect to the transformation of the ontological constitution of the human does obtain between Judaism and Christianity (that, indeed, it constitutes the fundamental difference between the two religions) and that, as such, our formulation does indeed reflect the view-point of Judaism while Schopenhauer's formulation reflects the view-point of Christianity (though it is true that in the formulation of Christianity the thrust of the transformation in the ontological constitution of the human is towards its attaining the ontological state of the pure Thou-entity while in Schopenhauer's formulation the thrust is towards its abrogating the It-dimension from the ontological constitution of the human and so in all likelihood reducing the human to a nothingness which as such would make of Schopenhauer's formulation–as indeed he himself suggested—a reflection that is much closer to the view-point of Buddhism than to that of Christianity).

One last observation may perhaps still be in order here. Namely, it may well be argued that a formulation whose diagnosis of the predicament impinges on the way the ontological constitution of the subject (the subject being here the human) is made-up and whose proffered solution, i.e., salvation, therefore, is commensurately in terms that implicate a transformation in the given ontological constitution of the subject, i.e., of the human, is a formulation which no longer belongs to the domain of the ethical enterprise but rather to the domain of the religious enterprise. For a good case can be made that the ethical enterprise by its very delineation (certainly, by the delineation put forth by us) would not locate the predicament in the way the ontological constitution of the human is made up, seeing that in its delineation the given ontological structure of the human is to serve as the criterion for the ethical evaluation/judgment and as such is the very factor which makes the ethical enterprise feasible, the very factor which enables the ethical enterprise to arise in the first place. The ethical enterprise by its very delineation must accept the ontological constitution of the human as given and proceed from there to apply itself. Indeed, strictly speaking, the ethical enterprise is not in the business of diagnosing predicaments and commensurately proffering ways of overcoming them, i.e., proffering ways of salvation—it is in the business of evaluating/judging in the light of a certain criterion (the criterion being, according to our formulation, the ontological constitution of the human). It is the religious enterprise which is in the business of diagnosing the predicaments and commensurately proffering ways of salvation and as such becoming possibly involved in implicating a transformation in the ontological structure of the human (Christianity being a good example of such an expression of the religious enterprise).

55. The one exception to this assumption of responsibility by the self for the acts of the other that Levinas acknowledges is when the acts of the other are directed not to the self but to a third party, i.e., to another other. As Levinas puts it "I am responsible for the persecutions that I undergo. But only me! My 'close relations' or 'my people' are already the others and, for them, I demand justice" (Levinas 1985, 99). Thus, in Levinas' formulation the notion of justice enters the picture only with respect to the acts of one other towards another other; it does not enter the picture with respect to the acts of an other towards the self. Justice, i.e., the possibility of holding the subject/agent of an act guilty because of the act, is available only to an other who is a third party but not to the self. Presumably, the rationale for this lies in the consideration that inasmuch as the third party is also an other, just like the subject/agent of the act, the self must assume responsibility for it just as it does for the other who is the subject/agent. The self must assume responsibility both for the persecutor and the persecuted other and in such a context the conflict between the persecuted and the persecutor can be resolved (i.e., the claims raised by the persecuted against the persecutor can be met) only by resorting to the notion of justice.

56. It is in this sense that a Thou-being is a being-for-another and an It-being is a being-for-itself. For the possibility to address or to challenge would clearly constitute a being as a being-for-another. Indeed, addressing and challenging are the two alternative ways in which a being can express itself *qua* being-for-another—it can either give affirmation to the other in the mere act of presenting itself to it or it can request/demand that affirmation be given to it by the other. By the way, it would seem that the former alternative characterizes Buber's understanding of how affirmation can be effected in the encounter between a self and an other while the latter alternative characterizes Rosenzweig's understanding.

57. This being the case, one can see, from the vantage point of our formulation, why there is much in Levinas' formulation that would strike a sympathetic note in us—after all, it shares with our formulation the

involvement with the Thou-dimension, namely, it shares with our formulation the delineation of the ethical enterprise in terms of entities that implicate the Thou-being in their ontological constitution and this is bound to present significant similarities between the two formulations.

Also, the fact that Levinas' formulation delineates the ethical enterprise in terms of the Thou-dimension (i.e., in terms of entities that implicate the Thou-being in their ontological constitution) may perhaps account for the curious fact that for Levinas ethics is a metaphysical category, indeed, one of the two fundamental categories in the domain of metaphysics, the other category being that of ontology. Thus, for Levinas, while the category of ontology is to signify the metaphysical notion of sameness within the domain of being, i.e., the all pervasive ultimate identity of all beings, the category of ethics is to signify the metaphysical notion of difference within the domain of being, i.e., the introduction of alterity, the ultimate bifurcation between self and other (not-self).

Now, it would seem to us, that the rationale for this (i.e., the rationale for both the distinction between ultimate identity and ultimate alterity within the domain of being and the use of "ontology" to refer to the former and "ethics" to refer to the latter) can be readily established if the category of ontology is to be taken (as, indeed, is generally the case) to refer to the sum-total of all substances, i.e., of all entities, that are ultimately available to being grasped by sense-perception, and the category of ethics is to be taken in the way Levinas uses it, i.e., as the assumption by the self of infinite responsibility towards the other. For in order to lend itself to being sense-perceived an entity has to constitute itself ontologically as a being-of-power, i.e., an It-being (seeing that sense-perception is constituted by transactions in terms of power thus of necessity implicating both perceiver and perceived as entities that, in turn, must implicate in their ontological constitution the being-of-power, i.e., the it-being) and, as such, this means that the category of ontology here refers to the domain of the being-of-power, i.e., to the domain of the It-being. At the same time, if our explication above is valid, Levinas' delineation of the ethical enterprise clearly implicates entities which must encompass within their ontological constitution the being-of-consciousness, i.e., the Thou-being, and as such this means that the category of ethics here is made to refer to the domain of the being-of-consciousness, i.e., to the domain of the Thou-being. Thus, the contrast between the category of ontology and that of ethics can be readily translated here into the contrast between the It-being, i.e., the being-of-power, and the Thou-being, i.e., the being-of-consciousness, and as such this means that not only the category of ontology, but equally so that of ethics, can be invested here with a metaphysical signification.

Indeed, even more specifically, they can be invested with the very signification that Levinas has attributed to the categories of ontology and ethics respectively, to wit, the attribution of the signification of sameness to the category of ontology and that of alterity, i.e., of the other, of differentiation, to the category of ethics. For inasmuch as the category of ontology formulates itself within the dimension-of-power, i.e., within the It-dimension (as noted above, it deals with the domain of the being-of-power, of the It-being), it does indeed implicate sameness, seeing that, as noted above, power by its very essence constitutes itself as a continuum and, as such, it per force excludes the very possibility of any differentiation that is qualitative, lending itself only to quantitative differentiations—in the last analysis, all entities within the dimension-of-power reduce themselves to one and the same power, differentiating themselves from one another only on the basis of embodying more or less power. In contra-distinction to this, the category of ethics, inasmuch as it formulates itself within the dimension-of-consciousness, i.e., within the Thou-dimension (as noted above, it deals with the relations that subsist between humans by virtue of the fact that the human constitutes itself ontologically in part as a being-of-consciousness), would indeed implicate alterity, seeing that consciousness in the very act of constituting itself must per force implicate a "gap," an "over-againstness," between its subject and its object (it being, by its very essence, inescapably always a consciousness *of* something or someone) thus, of necessity, implicating its object as an alterity to its subject. Thus, in the context of Levinas' formulation, "ethics" may indeed lend itself also as a category in the domain of ontology where it is to signify a reality whose ontological constitution necessarily implicates alterity while "ontology" lends itself as the category that is to signify a reality whose ontological constitution implicates an ultimate sameness.

58. As such, it would seem to us, that Levinas' formulation here of the ethical enterprise—and this, notwithstanding Levinas' mooring in his Jewish heritage (and indeed his conscious return to and adoption of that heritage)—is much more akin to the Christian than to the Jewish stance. For a good case can be made that for Christianity too the ontological constitution of the human is ultimately to be that of a pure, absolute Thou. True, Christianity would not, indeed, could not claim that in his/her present state the human is so constituted; in his/her present state the human is clearly ontologically constituted as an It/Thou-entity. But this ontological constitution is precisely what constitutes in the view of Christianity the fundamental predicament of the human, what in the theological context is signified by the notion of the Fall. Namely, the Fall in signifying the introduction of the It-being into the ontological constitution of the human, thus in signifying the ontological transformation of the human from being a pure, absolute Thou-entity (in its pre-Fall, Garden of Eden existence) to its being an It/Thou-entity (in its post-Fall, this-worldly existence) signifies the fundamental predicament of the human. And as to be expected, commensurate to this view of the predicament, the salvation that Christianity comes to offer consists essentially in the eradication of the It-being from the ontological constitution of the human thus reconstituting the human back to its pre-Fall ontological constitution of being a pure, absolute Thou-entity. Like the Fall, salvation here also signifies an ontological transformation, only this time in the reverse direction—from an It/Thou-entity to a pure, absolute Thou-entity. As such, salvation here does indeed signify the creation of a "new being," such creation being, in the last analysis, tantamount to a deification of the human, seeing that an entity which constitutes itself exclusively in terms of a Thou-

being, i.e., which ontologically constitutes itself as a pure, absolute Thou-entity, is a divine entity.

Now, given this context, it is quite understandable that Christianity would formulate its guidelines for human conduct not from the vantage point of the fallen human but from that of the saved human. Namely, it is the human ontologically constituting itself not as an It/Thou-entity but as a pure, absolute Thou that is to serve as the criterion for the guidelines for human conduct. For after all, the criterion here is with respect to guidelines for a conduct that is deemed to be the optimal, the desirable, conduct; and this being so, it is clearly called for that the criterion here be formulated in terms of the ontological constitution of the human not in its fallen but in its saved condition. But this means, of course, that for both Christianity and Levinas the right conduct for the human is formulated in terms of the human constituting him/herself as a pure, absolute Thou-entity. And this being the case, it should not be at all surprising to witness a striking parallelism between Christianity's formulation and that of Levinas. Thus, for example, do not the dicta of Christianity to turn the other cheek or to love one's enemy signify, in essence, the same kind of relatedness towards the other as Levinas' claim that the self must assume responsibility for the acts of the other, even for the acts of persecution perpetrated by the other against it? Even more, is it not the figure of Jesus, as the divine/human entity (when it functions as an agent in the drama of salvation) or as the entity representing the human in its salvific state (when it functions as the model, the paradigm, in that drama), the entity that takes upon itself the sins of others and, as such, is not the role assigned to the self in Levinas' formulation a replica of the role played by the figure of Jesus in the theology of Christianity?

This congruence of the stance taken by Levinas and that taken by Christianity is, however, in clear contrast to the stance taken by Judaism. For in the stance that characterizes Judaism the ontological status of absolute Thouness is reserved exclusively to the divine—God alone is a pure, absolute Thou-entity. The human, the self, is and always remains an It/Thou-entity. This ontological constitution (more specifically, the inclusion, the presence, of the It-being within the ontological constitution of the human entity) is not viewed in the perspective of Judaism as in any way being problematic—it does not precipitate the predicament for Judaism. And commensurate with this, the salvation (or more precisely, the redemption) for which Judaism hopes does not implicate any transformation in the ontological constitution of the human entity. Rather, as already noted above, in the perspective of Judaism the predicament is perceived to lie in the improper balance between the respective expressions of the It-being and the Thou-being within the ontological constitution of the human; and commensurate with such a perception, the redemption for which Judaism strives consists in the re-establishment of the proper balance between the respective expressions of the It-being and the Thou-being within the ontological constitution of the human, in other words, it consists in the establishment of justice. Indeed, in contrast to the dictum of "turning the other cheek" expressed by Christianity, Judaism (or, more precisely, the Hebrew bible) expresses the dictum of an "'eye for an eye" (a dictum that has been, by the way, unjustly maligned as barbaric, seeing that its intent is clearly to establish an equity between the crime committed and the punishment meted out which is after all nothing else but the upholding of justice).

But if the stance taken by Levinas' formulation is clearly not congruent with the stance taken by Judaism, seeing that in Levinas' formulation of the ethical enterprise the human (i.e., the self, the subject/agent of the act/relation to be ethically evaluated/judged) is taken as being constituted as a pure, absolute Thou-entity, the stance taken by our formulation is fully congruent with the stance taken by Judaism, seeing that in our formulation too the human is taken as being constituted as an inextricable It/Thou-entity and that, indeed, in consequence of this the ethical enterprise is formulated here in terms of the establishment of justice, i.e., in terms of establishing a proper balance between the contradictory guidelines emanating from the It-being and Thou-being respectively. Thus, the difference between Levinas' formulation and our formulation in delineating the ethical enterprise (and thus also in delineating the ontological constitution of the subject/agent of the ethical act/relation, i.e., in delineating the ontological constitution of the human self) mirrors the difference between the stance characterizing Christianity and the stance characterizing Judaism (as seen, Levinas' formulation, in unreservedly subjugating the self to the other and, as such, implicating the self as an entity that ontologically constitutes itself as a pure, absolute Thou-entity, is mirroring the stance taken by Christianity while our formulation, in balancing the claims of the self and of the other on the basis of the criterion of justice and, as such, implicating the self as an entity that ontologically constitutes itself as an It/thou-entity, is mirroring the stance taken by Judaism).

Lastly, there is one further point which may be worth making (if only very briefly), even though it is just an aside and rather speculative and hypothetical. The point is that if our claim is valid (as we believe it is) that Levinas is indeed close in his formulation of the ethical enterprise to the orientation characterizing the stance taken by Christianity, then this may well explain the further fact that of all modern Jewish philosophers/theologians Levinas felt himself drawn most closely to and was most appreciative of Rosenzweig's thought. For we would submit that a good case can be made that Rosenzweig too is very close in his thought to the orientation characterizing the stance taken by Christianity. Indeed, in his philosophy/theology Rosenzweig already asserts that Judaism and Christianity are one and the same as far as the substance of their vocation is concerned (they are different merely in the tasks assigned them within the economy of redemption). But, of course, much more importantly with respect to our claim here is the further assertion that they are the same, as we would submit, not on the basis of the stance taken by Judaism but rather on the basis of the stance taken by Christianity; namely, it is Judaism that is presented as adopting the stance arrogated (by us) to Christianity rather than, vice versa, Christianity being presented as adopting the stance arrogated (again, by us) to Judaism.

Thus, the state of salvation attributed by Rosenzweig to both Judaism and Christianity clearly implicates a stepping out of the flux of history into eternity (eternity in the sense of subsisting outside the progression of time altogether rather than of existing in the progression of time indefinitely) and this, in turn, clearly implicates the human in its salvific state as an entity that has completely extricated itself from the It-being, which is to say, an entity that ontologically constitutes itself exclusively in terms of the Thou-being, i.e., an entity that ontologically constitutes itself as a pure, absolute Thou-entity. But these implications clearly belong to the stance taken by Christianity and not to the stance taken by Judaism. Rosenzweig in attributing these implications not only to the stance taken by Christianity but equally to the stance taken by Judaism (indeed, in his formulation Judaism is the religion that, in a sense, i.e., as a presentiment, has already attained this salvific state while Christianity is still on the way towards it) is, so to speak, Christianizing Judaism. Indeed, from his perspective Rosenzweig is quite justified when he writes to his cousin Ehrenberg that he decided against conversion to Christianity because he found in Judaism what Christianity had to offer (and which indeed was what he was looking for). Given his perception of Judaism, Judaism does indeed offer the same diagnosis of what constitutes the fundamental predicament and, commensurate with this visualizes the same state of salvation as does Christianity. But be this as it may, it seems clear that both Levinas and Rosenzweig adopt the same stance (the stance in which the human in its authentic state constitutes itself as a pure, absolute Thou-entity and not as an It/Thou-entity), except that Levinas comes to it by way of his delineation of the ethical enterprise while Rosenzweig comes to it by way of his concern with the flux and thus with the relativism of temporal existence. And it is this sharing of the same stance, the stance arrogated by us to Christianity, that may account for Levinas' implicit attraction to and explicit appreciation of Rosenzweig rather than, for example, Martin Buber.

59. True, in its own terms our argument here does not lead necessarily to the conclusion that the human entity has to be taken as constituting itself as an It/Thou-entity. What it leads to is that the human entity has to include within its ontological constitution the It-being, but it has nothing to say about the inclusion or exclusion of the Thou-being with respect to the ontological constitution of the human entity. In its own terms it could just as well have led to the conclusion that the human entity constitutes itself exclusively as an It-entity, the position held by the materialistic orientation (an orientation that, indeed, has many adherents in the contemporary world). Thus, it must be granted that our conclusion that the inclusion of the It-being within the ontological constitution of the human entity leads to its being constituted as an It/Thou-entity is not derived, strictly speaking, from the argument presented here. Rather, it is derived from our previously stated dualistic view that holds that the full reduction of consciousness to a mere manifestation, a mere expression, of "blind" power (no matter how complex and intricate we allow the workings of "blind" power to be) is ultimately impossible. For as such, in contrast to the materialistic view, the ontological constitution of the human

entity in a dualistic view must include the Thou-being as an inextricable component and, therefore, if the It-being is to be also included (which is, after all, all that the argument above does claim), then the ontological constitution of the human entity will, indeed, have to be that of an It/Thou-entity and not that of an exclusively It-entity.

60. It should be noted, however, that this critical attack which we are directing here against Levinas' formulation cannot be also directed against Christianity's formulation, even though the human entity in Christianity's formulation is constituted in exactly the same way as it is constituted in Levinas' formulation, to wit, in both formulations it is constituted as a pure, absolute Thou-entity. The reason for this lies in the all-important difference that while in the case of Levinas one is dealing with an ethical formulation that is autonomous, i.e., that is grounded in itself, which is to say, that is grounded in a secularist-humanist context, in the case of Christianity one is dealing with an ethical formulation, i.e., with a guideline as to how to act and relate towards others, that clearly grounds itself in a religious context. For being grounded ultimately in a religious context makes it possible to implicate the human entity as it may be constituted at some point in the future rather than as it is constituted in the present.

61. Indeed, our strategy there in trying to establish the advantage of our formulation over the other alternative formulations consisted in trying to show that the feature, aspect, they selected as criterion was either not valid or, when valid, not as fundamental as the one to which our formulation resorted.

62. In this connection it is important to emphasize that the lack of universalizability here does not apply to the category of the prescriptions themselves (here the "religious formulation" may well claim that the prescriptions apply to any and every human subject/agent irrespective of its particular location in space and time). The lack of universalizability applies rather only to the category of the human subjects/agents; namely, it is an undeniable fact that so far (which is to say, as regards the past and the present) no specific single "religious formulation" managed to win the adherence of the totality of human subjects/agents. This, of course, means that in terms of the "religious formulation" there is no common ground applying to the totality of human subjects/agents on the basis of which the possibility of attaining a consensus embracing the totality of humanity could have become feasible. And this, in turn, clearly affects in a negative way the kind of justification that one can provide on behalf of the "religious formulation," seeing that for those humans who had not embraced the religious tradition in question, the metaphysical underpinnings of that religious tradition which inevitably would have to play an essential part in any attempt to provide a justification for the ethical expression of that tradition, these metaphysical underpinnings remain unpersuasive and hence unacceptable. As such, as regards the religious formulation of the ethical enterprise, the justification it can provide can only be partially but not universally acceptable and such a justification, if it be a justification at all, leaves much to be desired. And this being the case, it should not be surprising that the religious formulation of the ethical enterprise does not

really lend itself to any metaethical undertakings; indeed, the only ethical undertaking to which it does lend itself (and here it indeed lends itself fully and unambiguously) is that of normative ethics.

63. Though, of course, in this respect the "societal formulation" has a clear advantage over the "religious formulation," seeing that the case for the presence of a particular ethos and mores in each particular society is much more likely to be persuasively established and universally accepted than the case for the occurrence of a communication from the divine to the human (i.e., for the occurrence of a divine revelation).

Still, having made this claim, it would seem to us, that this sharp differentiation between these two ethical formulations (which, it cannot be denied, is in principle certainly valid) would have to be somewhat mitigated when these formulations are grasped by us in the context of the more immediate situation that confronts us—in this context the differentiation cannot escape being somewhat blurred. This is brought about by two considerations that are inevitably implicated here. Thus, on the one had, in as much as very few, if indeed any, proponents of the "religious formulation" would want to claim direct personal divine communication, placing instead such divine communication in the past, the divine communication must, per force, in terms of this formulation, be mediated to us through a religious tradition which, in turn, can be borne only by the on-going existence through the flux of time of a human society; but as such, the "religious formulation" would inevitably always implicate the "societal formulation." At the same time, on the other hand, in as much as any human society is most likely to be the bearer of a religious tradition (indeed, there is hardly a society in the history of humanity that was not a bearer of a religious tradition), the ethos and mores of each society would in all likelihood be shaped, molded, at least to some extent, by the particular religious tradition that it bears; but as such, the "societal formulation" would in all likelihood always implicate the "religious formulation." Thus, in terms of the concrete situation that confronts us, the demarcation between the "societal formulation" and the "religious formulation" is, in the last analysis, not all that clear. And this being the case, we should not be surprised by the observation that many (indeed if not all) of the proponents of the "religious formulation" are inclined to perceive the ethical enterprise in terms of the "societal formulation"; and, conversely, that by and large the proponents of the "societal formulation" (certainly, for example, as compared to the proponents of the "ontological formulation") are inclined to be more sympathetic towards and co-operative with the "religious formulation."

64. And as we tried to show above, as long as we remain within the parameters of the natural, i.e., within the confines of a naturalistic formulation of the ethical enterprise (thus excluding *ab initio* the availability of the "religious formulation"), such absoluteness and universality can be established only in a context where the criterion underpinning the evaluation/judgment is taken to be the ontological constitution of the subject/agent (that subject/agent being the human entity) and clearly not when it is taken to be the values and ideals of the society to which the subject/agent belongs.

65. The act of divine revelation in which the ethical enterprise here grounds itself originates in the realm of the supernatural and breaks into the flux of time but it is in no way determined or shaped by any of the characteristics of the flux. As such, the nature, the character, of the ethical enterprise here, i.e., the ethical enterprise that grounds itself in an act of divine revelation, is diametrically opposed to that of the ethical enterprise that grounds itself in the ethos of a society. For while the ethos of a society is inescapably relativistic, the content of an act of divine revelation is absolute.

66. As a peripheral observation it may perhaps be interesting to note that our formulation succeeds in gaining the advantage over the two alternative formations by situating itself, so to speak, in a middle position between the two in the sense of respectively sharing with each some of their aspects while at the same time rejecting others. For as such, it has the possibility (which it, in fact, does take up and actualize) of sharing with each those aspects that would support and validate the claim for the appellation of the "ethical" while at the same time rejecting those aspects that would undermine such a claim. In this way our formulation is left only with aspects that would support and validate the claim. Thus, with respect to the "societal formulation," it shares with it the supportive and validating aspect of grounding the ethical enterprise within the parameters of the natural world but not its undermining aspect of relativizing the evaluations/judgments (and thus also the prescriptions) which constitute the ethical enterprise; and with respect to the "religious formulation" (when it formulates itself in terms of emphasizing the act of divine revelation as such rather than its mediation and refraction through a religious tradition), it shares with it the supportive and validating aspect of absolutizing and universalizing the evaluations/judgments (and thus also the prescriptions) which constitute the ethical enterprise but not its undermining aspect of grounding the ethical enterprise in a super-natural event.

67. This, indeed, has been the case with regard to any number of formulations (as, for example, the formulations of Aristotle, Hegel, Rawls) where for many it remains unclear whether what is being done belongs to the ethical enterprise or to the enterprise of political philosophy.

68. It is, by the way, in the context of this concern that one of the most fundamental issues for the enterprise of political philosophy is precipitated, to wit, the issue of which entity, the individual or the collectivity, has the ontological/logical priority, which in other words is to say, the issue of whether the collectivity comes to be constituted by virtue of the aggregation of a multiplicity of individuals (in which case the individual and not the collectivity has the ontological/logical priority) or rather that the individual comes to be constituted by virtue of being a part of an already independently pre-existing collectivity (in which case the collectivity and not the individual has the ontological/logical priority). Reverting to the usage of analogy, the issue can be presented in terms of whether the relationship between the individual and the collectivity is to be comprehended on the analogy of a piece of machinery where the machine (i.e. the collectivity) comes into its existence by virtue of the assemblage of the various cogs, wheels and levers (i.e. the multiplicity of

individuals) or whether it is to be comprehended on the analogy of an organism where the cells and the organs (i.e. the multiplicity of individuals) come into their existence by virtue of their being part of the organism (i.e. the collectivity). Indeed, on the basis of this issue, a fundamental division is precipitated with respect to the various formulations delineating the enterprise of political philosophy—the division between the contractarian and the communitarian formulations (the former being associated with the liberal, empirical orientation and coming to the fore in modern times when indeed the individual comes to occupy center stage while the latter is being associated with the conservative/traditionalist, idealist orientation and expressing itself not only in modern times but also, and very much so, in classical antiquity and in the middle ages).

Now, we would submit, that this division between the contractarian and communitarian formulation (a division that emanates from and reflects from the division between the individual and collectivity as to which possesses ontological/logical priority) is, in turn, grounded in the even more fundamental (indeed, in the most fundamental) ontological bifurcation, the ontological bifurcation between the It-being and the Thou-being. Namely, we would submit that the contractarian formulation (i.e., the formulation that gives ontological/logical priority to the individual) can secure a rationale and justification for its position only with respect to individuals that constitute themselves as It-beings (thus being applicable only in a context where the individuals implicated are individuals that constitute themselves as It-beings) and, conversely, that the communitarian formulation (i.e., the formulation that gives ontological/logical priority to the collectivity) can secure a rationale and justification for its position only with respect to individuals that constitute themselves as Thou-beings (thus being applicable only in a context where the individuals implicated are individuals that constitute themselves as Thou-beings).

For, as we have established in a preceding section, in saying that an entity (any entity, though in the case before us here it clearly is specifically the human entity) constitutes itself as an It-being, we are actually saying that the entity constitutes itself in terms of power. Now power, as we have also argued above, or even more fundamentally motion (power being generated by motion and indeed being ultimately reducible to motion), expresses or manifests itself, i.e., becomes accessible to our sense-perception, fundamentally through what we referred to as, so to speak, an act of "sedimentation," which is to say, an act of reduction in motion. Namely, motion becomes perceptible to us when it reduces itself to being just above the point of absolute rest (i.e., Kelvin's 0° or -273.15° Celsius). Within parameters that delineate a range of motion that relative to the full range of motion is extremely narrow, motion becomes perceptible to us in the form of concrete substantial entities (the entities differentiating themselves from each other purely on a quantitative basis, i.e., in terms of the amount of power that is being "sedimented" and the extent of the "sedimentation," this being reflected in a differentiation in terms of spatial and temporal location), and it is only subsequently, once these concrete substantial entities come into existence, that they may interact among themselves thus establishing a network of relations (the interactions here being in terms of power, i.e., transactions in power, the relations are correspondingly relations of utilization). Now, it should be evident that in such a context it is the individual entity that possesses the ontological/logical primacy and not the collectivity, the collectivity being able to constitute itself only through the assemblage of a multiplicity of individual entities. As against this, in saying that an entity constitutes itself as a Thou-being, we are actually saying that the entity constitutes itself in term of consciousness, and consciousness, in turn, expresses or manifests itself, i.e., comes into existence, through an act of affirmation, namely, it comes into existence by being, so to speak, "called forth" into existence by another entity constituting itself as a Thou-being. This means, however, that in order for an entity constituting itself in terms of consciousness, i.e., for an entity constituting itself as a Thou-being, to come into existence another entity constituting itself as a Thou-being has to be implicated. Thus, an entity constituting itself as a Thou-being can come into existence only in twos and not singly (it takes two to tango). But a twosome is already a collectivity, albeit minimally so, and as such with respect to an entity constituting itself as a Thou-being it is the collectivity and not the individual that possesses the ontological/logical primacy.

Thus, the individual human, when taken in terms of its being a biological organism, a body, is independent of all other humans taken likewise in biological organisms, as bodies, and as such it is, *qua* individual, ontologically/logically prior to any collectivity of humans. On the other hand, the individual human, when taken in term of its being a conscious being, a person, is very much dependent (indeed, dependent for its very coming into existence and persevering in it) on the act of affirmation emanating from the very presence of other humans *qua* persons and, as such, the collectivity of humans *qua* persons is ontologically/logically prior to that of any individual member of such a collectivity. Thus, when the human is taken primarily in terms of its It-being, the individual human does indeed have ontological/logical priority over the collectivity of human (as indeed the liberal/contractarian formulations maintains) while when the human is taken primarily in terms of its Thou-being it is the collectivity of humans that has ontological/logical priority over the individual human (as indeed the idealist/communitarian formulation maintains).

Lastly, we may briefly observe that the ontological constitution of the human in terms of both the It-being and the Thou-being (thus allowing it to express itself and conversely to be perceived in terms either of its It-being or of its Thou-being) may provide a rationale and justification not only for the preceding claims made respectively by the contractarian and communitarian formulations, i.e., the claims made respectively on behalf of the individual and the collectivity with respect to the issue of ontological/logical priority, but also for the further claim introduced by Friedrich Tönnies that there actually are two qualitatively different kinds of collectivity, one kind to which he refers as *Gesellschaft,* i.e., society, and the other to which he refers as *Gemeinschaft,* i.e., community, the former being characterized as a kind of impersonal and competitive collectivity of isolated individuals and the latter being characterized as an organic collectivity imbued with traditional values and in which the members share a feeling of kinship and of common destiny. For clearly, given their respective characterizations, a human collectivity that constitutes itself as *Gesellschaft* is a collectivity in which the network of relations between its individual members consists of relations that are relations of utilization and of *quid pro quo* while a human collectivity that constitutes itself as a *Gemeinschaft* is a collectivity in which the network of relations between its individual members consists of relations that are relations of affirmation and of sharing. And this, in turn, necessarily implicates of course that in the human collectivity constituting itself as *Gesellschaft* the human individuals are perceived to act essentially in terms of their It-being (namely, they are taken, for all intents and purposes, to constitute themselves as It-entities) while in the human collectivity constituting itself as *Gemeinschaft* the human individuals are perceived to act essentially in terms of their Thou-being (namely, they are taken, for all intents and purposes, to constitute themselves as Thou-entities), seeing that the subjects/agents that are implicated in relations of utilization must, per force, be entities that constitute themselves as It-entities while the subjects/agents that are implicated in relations of affirmation must, per force, be entities that constitute themselves as Thou-entities. Thus, the constituting of these two kinds of human collectivity, that of *Gesellschaft* and that of *Gemeinschaft*, reflect and indeed are feasible because of the twofold ontological constitution of the human as an It/Thou-entity.

69. It may be noteworthy to point out that the attempt here to establish the claim that the ethical enterprise too implicates a collectivity is not being carried out in terms of the "societal formulation" even though this formulation, as its appellation signifies, would clearly seem to implicate a collectivity (in implicating a society it obviously implicates a collectivity). This is to be accounted for by the fact that even if this line of approach could have proven itself valid (which, as we will presently see, is not the case), it would have applied only to the ethical enterprise as apprehended in the "societal formulation" but not as it may be apprehended in alternative formulations such as the "religious formulation" or the "ontological formulation." As such, it is, so to speak, too "parochial" and cannot establish the implication of the collectivity with respect to the ethical enterprise when the latter is taken in the full range of its possible signification. As against this, the line of approach taken here, which is carried out in terms of the very structure and thrust of the ethical enterprise as delineated by us above, should apply to any and all possible formulations of the ethical enterprise.

70. Indeed, the various formulations of the ethical enterprise that one can encounter in the literature, namely, the "societal formulation," the "religious formulation" or the "ontological formulation," differentiate themselves from each other with respect to the criterion underlying the evaluation/judgment and not with respect to the object/other of the evaluation/judgment. Thus, the "societal formulation" differentiates itself from the other formulations by virtue

of the fact that for it the criterion underlying the ethical evaluation/judgment is constituted by the values of the society to which the subject/agent of the act/relation to be ethically evaluated/judged belongs while the "religious formulation" differentiates itself by virtue of the fact that for it the criterion is constituted by the dictates of the God which the subject/agent appropriates and the "ontological formulation" differentiates itself by virtue of the fact that for it the criterion is constituted by the ontological constitution which the subject/agent possesses; the object/other towards which the act/relation to be evaluated/judged directs itself remains, in contra-distinction, the same for all these formulations—it remains the individual human. And it is, indeed, because of this that all these various types of formulations belong, in the last analysis, to the domain of ethics.

71. We are, of course, needless to say, referring here to that version in Aristotle's ethical formulation that focuses on that aspect of the human that characterizes him/her as a social/political animal (for clearly, it is only by virtue of this characterization that the collectivity can be implicated). This has to be mentioned for there is no denying that another version, a version which focuses on that aspect of the human which characterizes him/her as a rational being, can also be encountered in Aristotle's ethical formulation. These two versions, by the way, need not be mutually exclusive. Indeed, they can be combined in having the rationality in the human, when it expresses itself as practical reason, being guided and directed by the values and ideals which are imposed by the community to which the individual human belongs.

Still, while not necessarily mutually exclusive, the two versions when taken in term of their own manifest signification, are clearly distinct from each other—the version where reason is taken as the distinctive characteristic of the human offers us the life of pure contemplation as the ultimate *telos* for the human (the *telos* whose actualization, by the way, would express the true nature, the true *physis,* of the being in question and, at the same time and equally so, the attainment of its ultimate happiness, of its *eudemonia*) while the version where the aspect of being a social/political animal is taken as the distinctive characteristic of the human offers us the harmonization and integration of the life of the individual human with the life of the community to which he/she belongs as the ultimate *telos* for the human. And clearly, as such, while the former version implicates the isolated individual, seeing that the life of pure contemplation involves exclusively the individual *qua* individual (it is an enterprise that can be pursued only by the individual *qua* individual), the latter version implicates the collectivity, seeing that the harmonization and integration of the individual's life with the life of its community involves not only the individual but equally so its community, which is to say, a collectivity. In as much as we are concerned here with the Aristotelian ethical theory as an exemplification of the "societal formulation" of the ethical enterprise, i.e., as an ethical formulation that implicates the collectivity, we must of course turn to the latter version of the formulation.

72. And this conclusion, by the way, is not in contradiction with Aristotle's claim that the domain of ethics is ultimately to be subsumed within

the domain of political philosophy. For it would seem to us that what Aristotle claims is that ultimately the domain of ethics is to be encompassed within the domain of political philosophy but not that his formulation is already a delineation of the domain of political philosophy rather than of the domain of ethics. If this were the case then we would indeed have had a contradiction on our hands. But this, in our judgment, is not the case. Indeed, if anything, rather than present us with a contradiction, one can argue that the claim we put forth above can provide a rationale (and thus, in a way, lend support) to Aristotle's claim. For one can argue that the very feasibility of encompassing the domain of ethics within the domain of political philosophy emerges precisely from the fact that the criterion for the evaluations/judgments that constitute the enterprise of the ethical domain, thus that the very condition for the ethical domain coming into being, is provided by a factor, i.e., the collectivity, that is intimately linked with the domain of political philosophy. Still, we should acknowledge the fact that Aristotle's claim validly makes the point that notwithstanding our attempt here to establish a distancing between the domain of ethics and the domain of political philosophy, a grey area where these two domains seem to come close to coalescing (or, perhaps, to overlapping) is also present. We will presently attempt to address this point above.

73. And clearly, only a formulation belonging to the "societal formulation" class of formulations (and not any formulation that may belong to the "religious formulation" class or to the "ontological formulation" class of formulations) can enter the picture here with regard to this consideration. For only formulations belonging to the "societal formulation" class of formulations would per force, i.e., inescapably, implicate a collectivity; formulations belonging to the other classes of formulations do not.

74. That the *Moralität* formulation is seen to suffer from the same weakness that Hegel now attributes to Kant's ethical formulation should not be surprising, seeing that the *Moralität* formulation was delineated by Hegel in the context of Kant's conception of the ethical enterprise, i.e., on the model of Kant's ethical formulation.

75. Though it should be noted that in grounding themselves not in the individual's will but in the moral will both the *Moralität* formulation and Kant's ethical formulation rise above particularity and selfishness, seeing that they are in accord with a will that is universal.

76. As such, indeed, Hegel seems to view the collectivities of the family, the civil society and the state as being encompassed within a dialectical progression that parallels the dialectical progression that encompasses the formulations of *Moralität,* of objective rights and of *Sittlichkeit.* Namely, the collectivity of the family (paralleling the formulation of *Moralität*) is posited as the thesis that proceeds to the collectivity of the civil society (paralleling the formulation of objective rights) posited as the antithesis to culminate in the collectivity of the state (paralleling the formulation of *Sittlichkeit*) posited as the synthesis. And even though the dialectic progression from the family to civil society to the state is a dialectical progression in terms of the collectivity and the dialectical progression from the formulation of *Moralität* to the

formulation of objective rights to the formulation of *Sittlichkeit* is a dialectical progression in terms of the individual (which as such would have been, according to our proposed criterion, arrogated respectively to the domain of political philosophy and to the domain of ethics), in the Hegelian system the two dialectical progressions seem to be arrogated to one and the same domain. They are a single dialectical progression that, on the one hand, expresses itself in terms of the individual and, on the other hand, expresses itself in terms of the collectivity—the dialectic in terms of the individual and the dialectic in terms of the collectivity are but two sides of one and the same coin.

77. Indeed, this coalescence can also be established from a different angle. Namely, one could argue that the ethical enterprise is not the only enterprise that evaluates/judges acts/relations; the enterprise of political philosophy also evaluates/judges acts/relations. The difference between them lies in the fact that while in the ethical enterprise the evaluation/judgment is with respect to *individual* acts/relation, in the enterprise of political philosophy the evaluation/judgment is with respect to networks of acts/relations. Still, networks of acts/relations allow themselves to be reduced to single acts/relations and as such there would indeed be an overlap, a coalescence, between the enterprise of ethics and that of political philosophy.

At the same time, however (and, indeed, in a way analogous to the delineation above on the basis of the individual versus the collectivity whereby a distinction could be introduced and maintained within an overall context of coalescence), a distinction can be established also here within the context of a coalescence between the ethical enterprise and the enterprise of political philosophy, a coalescence that bases itself in the fact that both enterprises share a common delineation, namely, the delineation of both enterprises in terms of the evaluation/judgment of acts/relations. The distinction here would be introduced by the fact that the evaluations/judgments of the ethical enterprise and the enterprise of political philosophy respectively ground themselves in different kinds of criteria. Thus, within the ethical enterprise the evaluation/judgment grounds itself in such criteria as, for example, the values and ideals of the society to which the subject/agent belongs or the structure of the subject's/agent's ontological constitution or the commands emanating from the subject's/agent's God (all being criteria which address the final ends, goals, posited for the subjects/agents that are being ethically evaluated/judged). As against this, within the enterprise of political philosophy the evaluation/judgment grounds itself in such criteria as the ordering or the regulating or the facilitating of the various acts/relations of the subjects/agents making up the collectivity (all being criteria which address the means by which to safeguard and advance the life of the collectivity). Thus, a distinction, a differentiation, can be introduced into the coalescence between the ethical enterprise and the enterprise of political philosophy—the two coalesce in that for both the enterprise consists in the evaluation/judgment of acts/relations between human subjects/agents; yet within this coalescence there is a differentiation in that in the ethical enterprise the evaluation/judgment is grounded in criteria that address envisioned ends while in the enterprise of political philosophy the evaluation/judgment is grounded in criteria that address the means needed to secure a given end.

Still, even within this differentiation between the ethical enterprise and the enterprise of political philosophy a pull backward towards coalescence between the two enterprises arises. Such a pull towards coalescence emerges from the kind of inter-relationship between the two enterprises that most of us would desire and, indeed, anticipate. Thus, in principle, there are three possible ways in which the ethical enterprise and the enterprise of political philosophy can interact with each other. First, we can have an interaction in which the evaluations/judgments in the two enterprises agree with each other or, more precisely, in which the evaluations/judgments that arise within the enterprise of political philosophy conform to the evaluations/judgments that have been established within the ethical enterprise. Secondly, we can have an interaction in which the evaluations/judgments in the two enterprises do not conform to each other but they also do not collide with or contradict each other. Rather, the evaluations/judgments arising within the ethical enterprise remain neutral as regards the evaluations/judgments that arise within the enterprise of political philosophy; it is an interaction in which the evaluations/judgments arising in the two enterprises do not connect with each other, each evaluating/judging things from a different vantage point, i.e., from a different perspective. Thirdly and lastly, it is possible to have an interaction in which the evaluations/judgments arising within the enterprise of political philosophy are clearly inconsistent with and, indeed, even contradictory to the evaluations/judgments arising within the ethical enterprise. Now, to the extent that, by and large, we (or at least, a preponderant majority of us) would have great difficulty to come to terms with the third possible kind of interaction between the two enterprises delineated here (indeed, would find it unacceptable) and would clearly favor the first kind of interaction as the desired ideal state of affairs (though many of us may be resigned to the second kind of interaction as the realistically available *modus vivendi*), a pull towards a coalescence between the ethical enterprise and the enterprise of political philosophy is clearly introduced into the picture.

Thus, we arrive here, when approaching the issue of the inter-relationship between the ethical enterprise and the enterprise of political philosophy from the perspective of what constitutes respectively the nature of these enterprises, at the same state of affairs at which we arrived above when approaching the issues from the perspective of the relation that obtains between the individual and the collectivity; namely, that there is a sense in which the ethical enterprise and the enterprise of political philosophy do coalesce and yet that within that coalescence a differentiation, a distinction, can nonetheless be established.

78. And as such, of course, Hegel's move from the *Moralität* formulation to the *Sittlichkeit* formulation (a move that was to overcome the lack of concrete content in the *Moralität* formulation with a formulation that is contentful, which the *Sittlichkeit* formulation is) does implicate, after all, a move from the domain of ethics to that of political philosophy.

By the way, we should note in this connection that it is by no means accidental or arbitrary that Hegel's *Moralität* formulation (and, for that matter, Kant's ethical formulation) is contentless and that this lack of content is overcome in his *Sittlichkeit* formulation. We would suggest that there is a consistent inner logic operating here that can account for this. This inner logic emanates from the way in which the human implicated respectively in these two formulations expresses itself. Thus, we would submit that in the *Moralität* formulation (and in Kant's ethical formulation) the human implicated is a human that expresses itself as a Thou—a human who is viewed in terms of its inward intentions and purposes and who locates itself in a collectivity that is a family (as is the case in the *Moralität* formulation) is a human that expresses itself as a Thou. But if this be the case, then indeed no contentful formulation can be applicable here, seeing that in a context where the entities involved express themselves as Thou-entities content cannot arise (the relations, interactions, between entities that express themselves as Thou-entities cannot be contentful—there can be no transmission of content between such entities). To have content, the It-dimension must be introduced into the picture, namely, the entities implicated must express themselves wholly or in part as It-entities. This is, indeed, effected in the Hegelian system by the move from the *Moralität* formulation (as thesis) to the formulation of objective rights (as antithesis) or commensurately on the institutional/collectivity level by the move from the notion of the family (as thesis) to that of civil society (as antithesis). For clearly in the formulation of objective rights and in civil society the human implicated is a human that expresses itself as an It-entity. Indeed, the human implicated here expresses itself exclusively as an It-entity (i.e., it is implicated here solely in terms of its It aspect) and as such, while indeed allowing the possibility of the introduction of content to arise, it abrogates at the same time the possibility of applying ethical evaluation/judgment, seeing that the application of ethical evaluation/judgment requires the implication of a human who also expresses itself as a Thou-entity. Thus, to have both ethical evaluation and content, one would need the implication of a human who expresses itself as an It/Thou-entity (i.e., who expresses itself both as an It and as a Thou). Now, this is effected in the Hegelian system in the next and last move of the dialectical progression that takes place in the ethical domain, i.e., the move from the formulation of objective rights or commensurately from the notion of civil society (as antithesis) to the formulation of *Sittlichkeit* or commensurately to the notion of the state (as synthesis), seeing that the human implicated in the *Sittlichkeit* formulation and in the notion of the state is indeed a human that expresses itself as an It/Thou-entity.

II
Justifying the Claim to an Ethical Right to Life

Some of the most pressing issues facing our society today, issues which sharply divide it (such issues as abortion, birth control, capital punishment, euthanasia), all implicate, in the last analysis, one and the same fundamental issue—the issue commonly referred to as the issue of the "right to life" or of the "sanctity of life." It is this issue which, in the last analysis, underlies all the foregoing issues, and if we are so sharply divided with respect to these issues, it is in no small measure due to the fact that, in the last analysis, we are not really very clear as to where we stand with respect to the issue of the right to life. Namely, we would submit that if the stances that we are to take with respect to the foregoing issues are to be buttressed by an innerly consistent rationale, then the first and most fundamental step that we have to take is to determine our stance with respect to the issue of the right to life and the rationale which we can advance in its support and justification. For clearly, the stance that we take with respect to the issue of the right to life and the rationale we advance in its support and justification will essentially determine what stances we can take with respect to the foregoing issues if we are to ground these stances in a rationale that is innerly consistent. In other words, the way we resolve the issue of the right to life, more specifically, the issue of which kind of entity can rightfully place a claim to life, will essentially determine and dictate what kind of stance we can take with respect to the other issues. Thus, centering our attention in this chapter on the issue of the right to life has the far-reaching ramifications that impinge in the most significant way on a whole array of issues that are most troubling and perplexing to our society. And to the extent that we succeed in this chapter to determine a stance and delineate its rationale with respect to the issue of the right to life, we will, in essence, have already succeeded in large measure to determine the stances and delineate their rationale with respect to the other issues even though the spelling out of these stances and their rationale (and the consideration of a great many other factors that may enter the picture with respect to these issues) must be left to the following chapter.

Before proceeding, however, with the issue that is before us here, to wit, the issue of the right to life or, more specifically, the issue of determining a persuasive rationale that can support and justify an entity's claim to possess a right to life, we need to clarify briefly a few points. Firstly, we need to explicate how we delineate the notion of a right. We delineate it as a maxim (a maxim being, according to Webster's dictionary, "an expression . . . of a general truth, especially as to conduct") that, when attributed to an entity, sanctions that entity's acting in a certain way or, alternatively, either forbids a certain acting by others being directed towards that entity or sanctions the placing of a demand by that entity upon others to act towards it in a certain way (the former instance in this alternative being referred to by some as a "negative right" while the latter instance is being referred to as a "positive right").

But in this connection we need furthermore to note that actually we do not really have rights as such, but rather rights that are qualified as certain kinds of rights. The notion of the right seems to implicate, by its very essence, a qualification so that what we really have, in the last analysis, are not rights as such, pure and simple, but rather always rights that are qualified as legal or political or natural or ethical. Now, this need for qualification and thus the subdivision of rights arises inevitably from the inescapable implication by the notion of the right as to the source which empowers it, i.e., which grants it the authority to sanction or to forbid certain acts and/or demands. For, as we have seen, a right is constituted by its capacity to sanction or forbid certain acts. But such a capacity is not built into it—it must be provided from the outside. Thus, for a right to be a right it must be empowered to sanction or forbid certain acts, and such empowerment must be provided to it from an outside source. But as such, the outside source that provides the empowerment becomes an inescapable factor (indeed, an essential inescapable factor inasmuch as it endows the right with the content of its signification) in the constituting of the right and consequently an inescapable qualifier of the right—we cannot have rights as such but only rights that are qualified by the source of their empowerment. And since one can identify a number of such sources of empowerment, one can commensurately come up with a number of different kinds of rights—legal, political, natural, ethical. Thus, a legal right would be a right that receives its empowerment from the body of positive law that is in place, while a political right would be a right that receives its empowerment from the political system that is operative, and a natural right (i.e., a right derived from natural law) would be a right that receives its empowerment from the perception of the way nature constitutes itself; lastly, an ethical right would be a right that receives its empowerment from the way the ethical enterprise is perceived to constitute itself.[1] But while this way of accounting seems at first to be applicable, on closer examination this may not be the case. For a good many acts may well be connected with more than one domain, namely, they may well belong, for example, to the political and legal domains, or to the ethical and the legal domains, or to the ethical and political domains, and so on. But if this be the case, then this alternative way of accounting for the refraction of the right as such into various qualified rights would seem to miss the mark. Furthermore, and perhaps even more tellingly, in contra-distinction to the way proposed above where the accounting is carried out in terms of the sources that may provide the right with its very empowerment to sanction or forbid and thus presenting us with an account that goes to the very core of the notion of the right, this alternative way of accounting for the refraction of the right is carried out in terms of a peripheral aspect of the notion of the right, namely, in terms of which kinds of acts the right impinges upon. In view of these considerations, this alternative way of accounting for the refraction of the notion of the right (irrespective of whatever validity it may have) cannot supplant the way of accounting presented above. Now, needless to say, our concern here is with a right that is an ethical right and not with a political or a legal or any other kind of right. Thus, our statement above, that the task before us here is to determine which kind of entity possesses a right to life (which is to say, with respect to which kind of entity can we provide a persuasive rationale that would justify such a claim), is to be understood as referring specifically to a right to life that is an ethical right, i.e., to an ethical right to life (and, indeed, all references below to a right or, more specifically, to a right to life are to be taken as referring to a right that is an ethical right when not otherwise qualified).[2]

Secondly, we must explicate more clearly what specific claim is implicated in the formulation "an ethical right to life." Namely, what specific act with respect to life does the ethical right here sanction or forbid? For the formulation as it stands can lend itself to be read as signifying three distinct and different claims with respect to life. Thus, it can be read as signifying that an entity (more precisely, a potential entity) has an ethical right to be brought into life (or put conversely, that any and every actual entity has an ethical obligation to reproduce itself, i.e., to bring other entities of its kin into life), or it can be read as signifying that an entity has an ethical right to demand from others to do, without exception, everything possible to keep it alive, or lastly, it can be read as signifying that an entity has an ethical right not to have its life terminated. Now, while all three significations are theoretically feasible and certainly merit being dealt with, it should be noted that our concern here is, in the main, with the third signification and not with the first two.[3] Namely, the task that we set ourselves in this undertaking is to determine the entity for which we can provide a persuasive rationale that would justify its claim to have an ethical right to forbid others of actively terminating its life.

Thirdly and lastly, we must further explicate why the issue of the possession of an ethical right formulates itself in terms of the notion of life, i.e., why is the possession of an ethical right raised with respect to the notion of life. For formulating the issue in terms of life fails to present it in its most fundamental or most extensive signification. For clearly, the most fundamental and extensive formulation, we would submit, would have been a formulation in terms of the notion of existence—what rationale and justification can one provide for an entity to claim a right to its existence? For the notion of existence, while encompassing fully the notion of life, clearly extends beyond it and, indeed, expresses the phenomenon before us in a more fundamental and elementary sense. The notion of life refers to a certain kind of existence. It refers to an existence that possesses certain characteristics, certain peculiarities, which other forms of existence do not possess; as such, it denotes only a subclass, a subdivision, of the all-encompassing class of existing entities. Thus clearly, formulating the issue in terms of the notion of life rather than in terms of the notion of existence implicates a limitation and a restriction of the issue before us.

But this substitution of "life" for "existence," this restriction and limitation of "existence" to "life," is not an accidental oversight devoid of significance. It is not an innocent laxness in the precision of expression using the notion of life to signify existence in general. Rather, this substitution and thus limitation is significant and is to be taken at its face value. Indeed, we would suggest, the issue is formulated in terms of "life" and not in terms of "existence" precisely because the notion of existence as such cannot provide a rationale and a justification for possessing an ethical right. For what possible rationale or justification can a number of atoms held together in a certain combination, in a certain relation to each other, provide for its having an ethical right to sustain itself in its present state? Clearly, the answer is none. There is nothing in the makeup of the atom as such or in the particular order obtaining between different atoms that can provide a rationale and a justification for its placing an ethically rightful claim on us not to have its present makeup tampered with or altered. What is there in the makeup of an atom or in the relation between atoms that would provide such a rationale and justification? Why should one kind of atom or one form of relation between atoms be preferable to another so as to justify its continuation in preference to that of the other? Indeed, the impossibility of deriving a rationale and a justification from this set of circumstances is so immediately clear to most of us (we grasp it almost subconsciously) that it is quite natural for most people to skip over confronting the issue in terms of existence as such (and quite rightly so) and move directly to the first limitation of this notion, namely, to formulate the issue in terms of an existence that is already limited to life.

Thus, indeed, for many people it is life which provides the rationale, the criterion, in terms of which we are justified in prohibiting the termination of existence—an entity endowed with life should not have its existence terminated. Indeed, it is very common for us to speak of the sanctity of life which clearly implies that the termination of the existence of any entity endowed with life would be unjustified, for surely the notion of sanctity implies preservation—the protection against being violated in any shape, form or manner and, therefore, all the more so the protection against being terminated.

But is this really so? Do we really have a convincing rationale to back up the claim that life is not to be terminated (more precisely, that the existence of an entity endowed with life is not to be terminated)? We would want to argue that the answer is no if we take "life" in terms of its primary signification, which is to say, as signifying what we may refer to as biological life, the occurrence of certain metabolic and replicatory processes. In terms of this signification, metabolism and replication delineate biological life—whenever and wherever they occur, biological life is present and if one or the other fails to occur, biological life is absent.[4] But as such, of course, the notion of biological life would encompass not only the whole range of animal life (and this means not only all multi-cellular organisms but also single-cell organisms like ameba, bacteria and viruses) but also the whole domain of plants; in other words, it would encompass not only the whole field of zoology but also the whole field of botany.[5]

But prohibiting the termination of life, when the notion of life is taken in terms of this signification, namely, as merely a collection of metabolic and replicatory processes (which is to say, as biological life), clearly implicates a number of consequences that are of questionable validity. Thus, if we take this notion of life in its maximal parameters, i.e., as including both animal and plant life, this would imply an irresolvable conflict between doing what is ethically right or, more precisely, not doing what is ethically wrong, and the very needs which human existence (and, indeed, equally so, animal existence) requires for its sustenance. Namely, if not only animals but also plants can place a moral demand on us not to terminate their existence by virtue of the fact that they are both endowed with life, then clearly human existence (not to mention the existence of all animals) is simply not possible. For human and animal existence could simply not go on without, at the very minimum, nourishing itself on plants and this clearly implicates terminating the existence of plants which, in turn, given the definition of life operating here, would necessarily implicate the termination of life. We are confronted here with the inescapable paradoxical situation whereby the concern for the preservation of life would inevitably implicate the termination of life. Thus, if human and, for that matter, animal entities are to do that which is established as the ethically right, then they must perish; they can survive only by doing the ethically wrong.[6] Clearly, the situation at which we arrive here is untenable.

Of course, this untenable situation can be somewhat attenuated by drawing the boundary of biological life not at the point of division between the domain of plants on the one hand and the domain of inanimate nature on the other but rather at the point of division between the domain of animal life on the one hand and the domain of plants on the other, thus excluding the latter domain, i.e., the domain of plants, from the category of biological life. But on the basis of what consideration is one justified in limiting the category of biological life so as to exclude the domain of plants? Is not such a limitation rather arbitrary? Certainly, on the basis of defining biological life either in terms of metabolic and replicatory processes or on the basis of the presence of DNA or RNA, such limitation of the category and the exclusion from it of the domain of plants is not justified. A different definition, a different signification, must be found for the category of biological life. But what could it possibly be? Still, there could be no question that limiting the category of biological life to the animal domain and thus excluding the domain of plants would greatly reduce and mitigate the problematic encountered in connection with this situation.

But even so, the new delineation of the category of biological life would still require us to be strict vegetarians and, indeed, if we are to have the law reflect our convictions, make the killing of an animal (any animal) an act of murder and thus punishable accordingly. Now, true, most of us would be very unhappy with these strictures. For most of us are not vegetarians and most probably would strenuously resist becoming ones. But a good case can be made that this point should not be determined by our likes and dislikes or by our present practices and inclinations, for these are clearly determined by the conditioning imposed upon us by our culture and past practices. Our present likes and dislikes, our present practices and convictions, are thus psychologically determined and this question should not be determined by psychological considerations but rather exclusively by considerations of reason and logic. Anyway, our psychological likes and dislikes, our convictions, can and do change as a result of changing our practices. Thus, if people start practicing vegetarianism it would not be very long before their likes and convictions conform to this practice, even to the point of viewing the killing of an animal as an act of murder and therefore punishable in a commensurate way to the act of killing a human being. So, our present psychological likes and dislikes do not present a problem and they can be changed.[7] No, the point here must be decided by considerations of reason, and here the problem is that there is no good reason why the category of biological life should terminate with the animal domain and not proceed to include also the domain of plants. In terms of life in the biological sense we clearly have a continuum from the domain of plants to the animal domain to the highest domain of human life.[8]

But we need not be stymied by these problems. For they actually become quite irrelevant in view of the much more fundamental problem that there is really no good convincing rationale why life in the biological sense should possess the ethical right to place upon us the claim not to have its existence terminated. What possible fact or rational consideration in a metabolic or replicatory process can support and justify a claim not to have its existence terminated? Likewise, what possible rationale or consideration is there in the make-up of a DNA or an RNA molecule to justify its claim not to have its existence terminated? Clearly, what we have here are chemical compositions with chemical processes, pure and simple, and why should such chemical configurations or chemical reactions not be terminated? There is no conceivable reasoning involved here that may persuade us that there is some justification for such a claim. Indeed, a good case can be made that in this context there is really no true termination—what we really have is but a transformation, a change, from one configuration to another or from one interaction to another (it is but a rearrangement of the same atoms).

Of course, one may argue that one must start some place and that such a starting point, by definition, must be a given that cannot be buttressed by other factors or considerations. This is true, but if the starting point is not to be arbitrary it must contain within itself some persuasiveness in support of its claim. But what possible persuasiveness is there in support of the claim for not changing a chemical configuration or a chemical reaction? So, of course we can start with this claim as we can start with any other imaginable claim. But starting with this claim would clearly be arbitrary, and if we want to get away from starting with a foundation that is arbitrary, we must look for another criterion, for another standard by which to determine what can place upon us a rightful claim not to have its existence terminated.

The next move, then, in our quest for a satisfactory rationale must be to introduce a further limitation, this time with respect to the notion of life. Thus, rather than look to the notion of life as such, i.e., to the totality of biological life, we should look to a more specific and a more limited application of this notion, and what, of course, comes readily to mind is the notion of *human* life. Thus, the claim would no longer be that it is biological life in general, but rather that it is specifically human life (i.e., human life only) that can place an ethically rightful claim not to have its existence terminated. But this means, of course, that we must look for the satisfactory rationale no longer in what the notion of life as such, i.e., biological life, may signify, but rather in what the notion of human may signify. What rationale and justification can one formulate in terms of the notion "human"? What is there in the notion "human" that would provide us with a satisfactory rationale and justification for the claim not to have its existence terminated? Thus, the task before us here is to come up with a persuasive rationale that would provide justification, no longer for any and all entities but specifically and exclusively for the human entity, to claim an ethical right not to have its existence terminated.

Now, before proceeding to present our formulation of such a rationale, it would behoove us to briefly review some alternative formulations that have been suggested and indicate why, in our judgment, they are, in the last analysis, falling short of succeeding to provide us with a fully satisfactory rationale, and this even though many of them do contain some very insightful and valid points, indeed, points that our formulation would incorporate. Thus, to begin with, we have what certainly must be characterized as the most minimalist formulation, namely, the formulation that claims that the possession by a human entity of an ethical right not to have its existence terminated must be taken as axiomatic. Namely, according to this formulation, we take it as a self-evident axiom that human life can place an ethically rightful claim not to have its existence terminated. Now, given our foregoing conclusion, this would qualify to be taken as a rationale. The significant question, however, remains: Does such a formulation really provide us with a rationale that is satisfactory and thus with a justification that is acceptable? And to this our answer must be no. For the rationale provided here clearly resorts to what Jonathan Glover, Peter Singer, and others have aptly called "speciesism," and it seems to us that they are quite right when they equate speciesism with racism. For in both cases an entity is endowed with merits or defects (given privileges, rights and advantages or deprived of rights and saddled with disabilities) merely because it is a member of a certain group. Indeed, most of us would most probably find this rationale and justification unsatisfactory, seeing that for a rationale to be acceptable most of us would want to identify a special aspect, a distinctive characteristic, in the group on the basis of which the rationale can be formulated, i.e., in which it can be grounded. But this is precisely what this formulation fails to do.[9] Finally, we may observe that in the context where the bestowal of the right to life is placed at the point where biological life (albeit the biological life specifically of the human specimen) actually begins, the turning to the onset of brain-waves rather than to the onset of motility or heart-beats as the criterion that will determine the beginning of biological life is by far the more persuasive and appealing stance to adopt. And this is so for a number of reasons, not the least of which is the reason that the onset of brain-waves is the physical-biological activity that most closely corresponds to the notion which, as we shall see below, can finally provide us with a persuasive rationale and justification for bestowing a right to life, to wit, the notion of consciousness or, to be more precise, the notion of self-consciousness.

An alternative variation on the foregoing formulation is the formulation that grounds the human right to its existence in a divine command; namely, the claim is now no longer based on the authority of what is taken to be a self-evident, axiomatic truth but rather it is based on the authority of what is taken to be a divine command. But as such, it is really, so to speak, but the other side of one and the same coin. For this formulation is informed by the same basic approach as the foregoing formulation (in this sense it belongs to one and the same coin), except that now it is expressed in a theological context rather than in a secular-human context, seeing that it opts to derive the authority for its claim not from the dictates of human reason but from the disclosure of a divine will. Now, there is no denying that grounding the claim in a divine command (similarly, indeed, to the grounding of the claim in the self-evidency of an axiomatic truth) does constitute a rationale and a justification. However, as with respect to the foregoing formulation, granting this is by no means to be taken as tantamount to further implying that we also claim that this rationale and justification are satisfactory or acceptable. Far from it. Indeed, the same basic line of criticism that was raised with respect to the foregoing formulation can also be raised here, albeit with certain adjustments and modifications due to the shift to the theological orientation. Thus, clearly, the rationale and justification offered here can be acceptable only to those who believe that God exists, and this would exclude millions upon millions of people who today do not possess such a belief. Actually, the exclusion implied here is even more radical, seeing that for this rationale to be acceptable, one must believe not only that God exists, but that this existing God has actually addressed Himself and communicated His will to the human regarding this issue, and that the number of people who today can accept such a belief is, in all likelihood, greatly circumscribed. And while this rationale may indeed be acceptable to these people, it will clearly not be persuasive and thus acceptable to the many others who do not share these beliefs. As such, this rationale cannot really be taken as satisfactory.

Clearly, we must press on in the search for a rationale and a justification that would be more widely acceptable. In this connection, an approach that readily suggests itself is the approach that would undertake to determine what other significations and connotations the notion "human" may contain in addition to its signification as a name for a certain class of entities. Can the adjective "human," in our limitation of the notion of life to that of human life, convey to us, aside from a naming of a certain class of entities, certain characteristics or aspects of life that can provide us with a rationale and a justification that may prove satisfactory and acceptable for not terminating that life?

In trying to answer this question, what comes immediately to mind is, of course, the dimension of consciousness. For surely, to be human necessarily implies not only to be biologically alive but equally to possess consciousness. To be human necessarily, and indeed essentially, implies being a being-of-consciousness. But can the notion of consciousness provide us with a rationale and a justification that would be satisfactory and acceptable? What is there in the notion of consciousness that could yield such a rationale and justification? Well, essentially, consciousness means awareness—awareness of an other. But what is there in the act of awareness that would yield the rationale and justification which we are seeking? Why should an entity which possesses the capacity to be aware of other entities be endowed with the right not to have its existence terminated while an entity which lacks this capacity be devoid of such a right? What is there in the capacity of awareness, in the capacity to be aware of an other, that would imply the right not to have the existence of that other terminated? It would seem to us that there is no persuasive answer to this question and that, consequently, the notion of consciousness as such, namely, the notion of consciousness merely as it signifies an awareness of an other, cannot provide us with the desired rationale and justification.[10]

But if this aspect of consciousness, i.e., its mere awareness of an other, fails to provide us with the desired rationale and justification, could some other aspects which clearly go beyond the mere awareness of an other, but which are feasible only on the basis of there being this aspect of consciousness, provide us with the desired rationale and justification? Thus, for example, could such aspects as sentience, i.e., emotions, or rationality provide the desired rationale and justification? Clearly, these aspects can arise only in the context of consciousness, namely, they necessarily presuppose the presence of consciousness, i.e., awareness; only an entity that is endowed with consciousness, in the sense of it being aware of an other, can also be endowed with the aspect of sentience and/or of rationality. But at the same time, it is also equally clear that sentience and rationality go beyond consciousness as mere awareness.[11] As such, the fact that consciousness as mere awareness of an other fails to provide the desired rationale does not necessarily also imply that sentience and rationality would also fail in providing a satisfactory rationale. Still, it seems to us, that the same fundamental objection that applied to the taking of the aspect of consciousness as the criterion would apply with equal force to the taking of the aspect of sentience or of rationality. For by virtue of what can we say that the aspects of sentience or of rationality are endowed with the right not to have their existence terminated? Why should an entity that is sentient or rational possess a right to claim that its existence not be terminated while an entity which in every other respect is the same, except that it is devoid of these characterizations, should not possess this right? Granted that sentience and rationality are more integrated, more advanced, indeed, that they are more precious manifestations of existence, do such considerations have within them the capacity to persuade us that by virtue of what they are they have a right to claim that their existence not be terminated in a way that entities which lack such considerations do not? An entity that is endowed with sentience or rationality has clearly a great many advantages over an entity that lacks them, but the advantage of having the right to claim not to have its existence terminated is not included among them. The right to claim not to have one's existence terminated is too elemental and fundamental to be swayed by such considerations.

This impasse pushes us to look for the criterion that can provide us with a satisfactory rationale and an acceptable justification in considerations other than those derived from features or aspects connected with the ontological constitution of the entity concerned as, indeed, was the case in our preceding attempts which focused themselves on the reality of consciousness as such—or, as Jonathan Glover puts it, on the reality of "mere consciousness"—or on its various aspects and manifestations such as rationality and sentience. (As regards references in the ensuing discussion of Glover's position regarding the issue that is before us here, see Glover 1977, chapters 3-8.) It pushes us to look for the criterion in considerations which transcend, go beyond, the ontological constitution of the human, yet whose existence is made possible only by virtue of certain considerations emanating from this ontological constitution. Namely, it pushes us to look for the criterion, not in aspects or manifestations which make up the ontological constitution of the human (and which as such are but part and parcel of it—mere expressions or manifestations of this ontological constitution), but in certain values which, although it is true, could not arise in the absence of this ontological constitution are nonetheless themselves not part and parcel of it but transcend it. In this way, "mere consciousness," while not valuable in its own terms, i.e., while not carrying the criterion in itself, is nonetheless valuable to the extent that it is needed for that which would constitute the criterion to arise. As Glover rightly notices, there is a succession of notions or considerations which, although not intrinsically valuable (i.e., which do not carry the criterion in themselves), are nonetheless valuable to the extent that they are a necessary means in a causal succession that ultimately culminates in a notion or a consideration which does carry the criterion in itself and is thus intrinsically valuable. Thus, the notion of life as such, i.e., the notion of life in the biological sense, enters the picture only because it is necessarily needed for the more specific notion of human life to arise, and the notion of human life is valuable only to the extent that it is necessarily needed in order to give rise to the notion of consciousness as such, i.e., mere consciousness. Life as such, i.e., biological life, or human life or mere consciousness matter only because they are necessary for other things. But, of course, for these notions or considerations to matter, i.e., for them to have value as precursors, one must locate the notion or consideration that is intrinsically valuable, i.e., the notion or consideration that carries the criterion itself. And so the difficult question before us here is this: Seeing that sentience or rationality fail to provide the criterion, to what else can mere consciousness lead, and would this notion or consideration be an end which in itself carries the criterion or but another means leading to yet another notion or consideration?

In answer to the above question, Glover would seem to suggest that it is a consciousness that enriches life (Glover 1977, 47). Namely, while mere consciousness, i.e., consciousness as such, as the mere capacity to perceive and experience things, cannot provide us with the satisfactory rationale (i.e., with the criterion), a consciousness that presupposes but goes beyond mere consciousness to enrich life can. In other words, a consciousness that goes beyond the mere actual perceiving and experiencing of outer reality to enrich the life of the experiencing and perceiving subject is a notion, a reality, that can provide in its own terms the satisfactory rationale (i.e., the criterion). And parallel to this, Glover also formulates his answer in a somewhat different way, this time no longer in terms of the notion and reality of consciousness but rather in terms of the notion and reality of life (thus shifting the formulation from being in terms of the causal agent, i.e., consciousness, to being in terms of the affected, receptive object, i.e., life). Now, in terms of this alternative formulation, Glover maintains that while human life as such (this being parallel to mere consciousness) cannot provide the satisfactory rationale (i.e., the criterion), a worthy life, a human life worth living (this being parallel to a consciousness that enriches life) can (pp. 51–52). So, a consciousness that goes beyond mere consciousness and enriches life, thus converting this life from being merely a life as such to becoming a worthy life, i.e., a life worth living, can establish the right for this life not to have its existence terminated. A worthy life, in contradistinction to life as such, is endowed with a right not to have its existence terminated; indeed, the very appellation "worthy" already signifies a positive valuation, namely, that the life in question is valued, approved and desired, and this, in turn, implies that, in the absence of more weighty counter-considerations, one would oppose terminating its existence.

But what makes a life a worthy life? By virtue of what is it constituted as worthy? What is the factor, the aspect, that would convert it from life as such to a worthy life? Or, to revert the question from the notion of life to that of consciousness, how can consciousness enrich life? What does it have to contain or to give in order to constitute itself as a consciousness that enriches life? To this, Glover's answer is very clear: happiness; the responsible factor is happiness. A life that is happy becomes a worthy life (it is happiness that makes life worth living), and a consciousness that is or gives happiness is a consciousness that enriches life (Glover 1977, 62–66).[12]

Now, what is one to say to this formulation that Glover proposes? Well, firstly, one would clearly have a problem with this formulation as it presently stands (and it is to Glover's credit that he is fully cognizant of it) and this is that by introducing the criterion of the "worthy life" (Glover 1977, 52) one necessarily and inescapably divides humankind into two camps, one consisting of those who possess or manifest the "worthy life" and the other consisting of those who do not. But, in such a context, the opening is clearly afforded for some human agency to play God (pp. 102–3), seeing that some human source will have to decide which humans do and which humans do not possess or manifest the "worthy life" which, in turn, means that this human source will be deciding which humans do and which humans do not have the right to claim that their existence be not terminated, i.e., which human life is protected and which is dispensable. This, however, smacks too much of the Nazi ideology of the master-race and is clearly unacceptable (pp. 52–54).

To circumvent and avoid this unpleasant and unacceptable implication, Glover suggests shifting the power of decision from the "we" (i.e., from any group within the society or, indeed, from society as a whole) to the individual concerned; namely, let each individual person decide whether or not his/her life is worthwhile, i.e., a worthy or happy life. This suggestion certainly has the great advantage of avoiding the situation in which one human being can play god over the existence of another human being. It also has the further advantage of getting us away from attempting to decide the issue of what constitutes the happy, worthy life on an objective, universal level, an attempt that is not likely to succeed. For trying to decide this issue on an objective universal level is a very difficult, if not indeed an impossible, undertaking, seeing that different people have clearly different notions of what constitutes the happy and worthy life. Under these circumstances, finding a formulation that would apply universally is almost impossible. By arrogating, however, the decision to each individual, one conveniently circumvents and avoids this problem. Rather than attempt the impossible, which is to say, attempt to find a delineation of happiness that would be acceptable universally, one lets each individual delineate his/her own notion of happiness.

But letting each individual decide whether his/her life is happy or worthy presents us immediately with the problem that not only would different individuals have a different delineation of what would constitute a happy or a worthy life but also that different individuals, because they possess different temperaments and personality traits, will evaluate and judge their lives differently in the light of what they take to be the happy or worthy life. Thus, individuals who are not by their temperament very critical or demanding of themselves would in all likelihood be more disposed to view their lives as happy or worthy than individuals who by their temperament are very critical and demanding of themselves. And while this subjectivist discrepancy may be acceptable with regard to the evaluation of a happy life, seeing that the notion of happiness, by its very essence, defines itself in a subjective context (it being an expression, a manifestation, of subjective feelings) and consequently it can indeed be determined by the individual, thus allowing different individuals (because of their different temperaments) to have different determinations of their respective lives even though the objective circumstances characterizing these lives are the same, it cannot be acceptable with regard to the evaluation of a worthy life. For the notion of worthiness does not define itself in a subjective context (if its meaning is to have any "cash value" it must be defined by consensus) and consequently its determination cannot be left to the individual—a life may indeed be worthy by the determination of the consensus while its subject (because of its overly critical and demanding disposition) evaluates it as unworthy and, vice versa, a life may be unworthy by the determination of the consensus while its subject (because of its uncritical and undemanding disposition) evaluates it as worthy. If the criterion for the claim to a right of existence is to be the possession of a worthy life, the determination of such a life cannot be left at the discretion of the individual.

But aside from this, we should not overlook the fact that Glover's proposal here to let the evaluation of a happy and worthy life be determined by the individual concerned rather than by the consensus of the "we," is really tantamount to being a proposal to let the individual concerned determine whether or not it has a rightful claim not to have its existence terminated. But if this be so, then it is highly unlikely that many people (if, indeed, any) would delineate their lives as unworthy. For what they are really determining is not so much whether or not their life is truly worthy and happy (i.e., whether or not it is commensurate with their idea of what a worthy or happy life is like) but rather whether or not they have a right to claim not to have their life terminated, and the fact is that the overwhelmingly vast majority of people would want to maintain that they have a right to such a claim. Namely, the fact is that the overwhelmingly vast majority of people (indeed, almost all people except some of those who are mentally imbalanced) would not want to have their existence terminated, and this indeed is not linked to whether or not their life is (either as an objective reality or as a subjective perception) worthy and happy. Indeed, for most people, life would have to be extremely and unbearably unhappy and unworthy (and even then only when the further proviso is added that there is no possibility whatsoever of its improvement, i.e., of its escaping this state of affairs, at any future time) before they would opt for the termination of their existence. This being the case, the notion of a worthy and happy life cannot really function as a *bona fide* criterion by which to decide whether or not a subject has a rightful claim not to have its existence terminated. For it does not allow, for all intents and purposes, a negative answer with regard to this claim, namely, its application, for all intents and purposes, would almost never lead to the conclusion that a life may be terminated (a criterion for which in 99.9% of the cases the answer can be known in advance, irrespective of its actual application, is not really functioning as a *bona fide* criterion).[13]

But it seems to us to be very questionable whether Freud's death wish really obtains in all or even most humans rather than in some isolated individuals who, therefore, can be disposed off as "abnormal" instances of human existence. And as regards the few instances of animal suicide-behavior, it seems to us that eventually it would be possible for us to account for it in terms other than an inherent death wish. Certainly, the burden of our experience overwhelmingly points to the opposite conclusion, to wit, that all biological life possesses an inherent urge to sustain itself in existence.

Indeed, what seems to be working here is not at all the notion of a worthy or happy life but rather the very elemental urge to life itself. It is the force of the urge to go on living which overcomes practically all other factors, except perhaps extreme suffering or the loss of mental sanity and balance. But if this is so, then, for all practical intents and purposes, we are no longer dealing with an attempt to decide the issue by referring it to a criterion that transcends the mere factual existence of the phenomenon of biological life; we are back to deciding the issue in terms of the very constitution of biological life—every biologically living entity is endowed with the urge to want to go on living or, to put it the other way, not to have its existence terminated. Indeed, in this context the claim not to have one's existence terminated cannot be arrogated exclusively to the class of human beings but must be extended to all classes of biological life. But this is tantamount to saying that any entity that wants to go on living is by virtue of this desire endowed with or entitled to the claim not to have its existence terminated (a version of this formulation has indeed been proposed my Michael Tooley and we shall deal with it presently). We must conclude, therefore, that Glover's proposal to shift from the "we" to the concerned individual as the agent which is to decide whether or not the criterion of happiness or of the worthy life applies does not, in the last analysis, really work. It does not work for two reasons. Firstly, in trying to make it work, one ends up inevitably in abrogating the notion of happiness or of the worthy life by reducing it to the notion of mere biological life as such. Secondly, it inevitably leads to the criterion encompassing practically the totality of normal human beings, indeed, the totality of all biological life, and a criterion that encompasses all and thus fails to introduce distinction and separation is not really functioning as a *bona fide* criterion.

Indeed, in the last analysis, Glover too realizes that shifting the decision from the "we" to the concerned individual would not really work. He advances, however, a different reason, a reason of a much more practical nature (i.e., dealing with the applicability of the criterion rather than with its signification) than the reasons we put forth. For Glover the shift is unacceptable because it makes the criterion unavailable precisely in those situations where its application would be most sorely needed. For precisely in the most crucial cases, i.e., in those cases where the decision of whether or not to preserve or prolong life would be most pressing and consequently where a determination of whether or not that life is to be deemed worthy or happy would be most sorely needed, the individual concerned would in all probability be either in no position to give us his/her assessment and determination, or his/her assessment and determination would be manifestly unreliable (i.e., clearly warped by extraneous and contingent circumstances and thus not necessarily representing the true view of the person concerned). Thus, for example, the person may be unconscious or going through a severe depression or simply uninformed (as, for example, believing and consequently being fearful that by terminating his/her life, he/she may consign him/herself to hell). Clearly, in such circumstances the person concerned cannot be invested with the power of deciding whether or not to terminate his/her life. These difficulties finally lead Glover to dismiss the possibility of letting the concerned individual be the agent who will decide this all-important question and instead lead him back to suggest that the agent here should be after all the "we," except that he now saddles this "we" with the added obligation that in making the decision they must take very seriously into consideration the concerned entity's feelings and disposition. Thus, Glover's final position is that if an entity's life is deemed worthy and happy, this being determined by the "we" who will, however, take into serious consideration the feelings and views of the entity concerned, then such an entity has a right to claim not to have its existence terminated.

Clearly, Glover is trying very valiantly to escape the pitfalls that exist in both formulations that have suggested themselves here, namely, the formulation that would let the concerned individual as such determine whether or not his/her life is worthy and happy and the formulation that would let the society in which the individual is placed make this determination. In our estimation, however, Glover's attempt is not really successful. For, in the last analysis, the fact remains that, notwithstanding all the various provisos and qualifications, we are still left with the "we" as the party that decides and determines whether or not a life is worthy and happy. And this being the case, we are faced not only with the danger of playing god but with the much more serious danger of us being the devil. For in the context of this formulation it is not at all difficult for the "we" to misuse the power given to it and to disregard or falsify the wishes and feelings of the concerned individual, making the determination exclusively in terms of their own feelings and wishes; and human nature being what it is, this is not only a mere theoretical possibility but an imminent practical danger.

Thus, Glover's formulation fails to safeguard us from the "we" misusing its powers and neither does it really succeed in extricating us from having to play god. Indeed, if anything, it places us in a position in which it is almost impossible for us not to play god. For in many of the situations where the determination has to be made (and, indeed, in most of the most pressing situations), it would be very difficult to ascertain the wishes and views of the concerned individual, and consequently, for all practical intents and purposes, the "we" willy-nilly would have to make the determination on its own and thus inescapably would have to play god. And this difficulty, i.e., the difficulty of determining who should decide whether or not a life is worthy and happy, becomes all the more problematic in view of the fact that, as argued above, there is really no consensus regarding what kind of a life would constitute a worthy and happy life, that different people clearly have different notions as to what would constitute a worthy and happy life. For in the absence of having an objective delineation of what would constitute a worthy and happy life, i.e., in the absence of having some generally accepted criteria which would determine and distinguish between a worthy and happy life and one that is not, the whole burden of determination must, perforce, fall upon the deciding agent, and consequently the difficulties connected with this issue become considerably weightier than they would have otherwise been.

But aside from all these difficulties raised thus far, by far the most fundamental difficulty, we would want to argue, is connected with the very notion that attributing to a life such aspects as worthiness and happiness can provide us with a satisfactory rationale and an acceptable justification for maintaining that such a life carries a right to claim that its existence should not be terminated. For why should a life that is worthy and happy, in contradistinction to a life that is not, have the right to claim not to have its existence terminated while the other life is deprived of such a right? What considerations or arguments can one deduce from the notions of worthiness and happiness that would lead to the conclusion that a life characterized by these notions, and by virtue of them, carries with it a rightful claim not to have its existence terminated? What the premise of the argument here (i.e., the premise that a life is endowed with worthiness and happiness) may yield is the conclusion that the subject here, i.e., the possessor of a life that is worthy and happy, would wish and desire that his/her existence would not be terminated. For one can readily appreciate the claim that a person who is endowed with a life that is worthy and happy (and that person is not, psychologically speaking, an abnormal person) would in all likelihood also be a person who would wish and desire not to have his/her existence terminated. But this, i.e., the subjective wishes and desires of the person concerned, is not the issue here. Rather, the issue is the possibility of translating such subjective wishes and desires into an objective and rightful claim upon others. But it is precisely at this point that the argument breaks down. For there is really no possibility of translating subjective wishes and desires into an objective rightful claim binding upon others. Why should someone else's wishes and desires be binding upon me? A's desire not to have its existence terminated should only imply that A itself should not terminate its own existence; it does not imply that B or C or D should accept A's wishes as binding upon themselves and consequently that they likewise should not terminate A's existence. Why should not B or C terminate A's existence, particularly if this may advantage their own existence? It certainly happens all the time in nature—the whole realm of biological life is premised on terminating the existence of others in order to sustain one's own existence.

It would seem to us, therefore, that the considerations of happiness, worthiness or the enrichment of life can no more provide a satisfactory rationale for a rightful claim not to have one's existence terminated than can the considerations of rationality or sentience considered above. This is not to say that these characterizations and attributes are not very valuable and desirable (at least for those who possess them); it is, however, to say that they fail to provide a satisfactory rationale for the justification of placing a claim on others not to terminate one's existence.

An alternative formulation within this same basic utilitarian approach, a formulation that is actually very ingenious (at least to the extent that it succeeds in getting away from the problematics of delineating what is happiness or worthiness and in avoiding the difficulties of determining who is to decide which life is happy or worthy) is the formulation put forward by Michael Tooley (see Tooley 1972). That Tooley's position is basically formulated in the context of the utilitarian approach should be quite clear. It can be seen in the fact, for example, that ultimately, in the context of his position, the moral obligation is reduced to and is grasped in terms of desires and wishes; that it is determined via the mediation of a calculus, i.e., by weighing opposing wishes and considerations, calculating their relative strengths and giving the race to the strongest; or indeed, it can be seen in the explicit statement that, morally speaking, there can be no difference between actually killing a person, on the one hand, and not taking any action to save a person in danger of being killed, on the other, between not sending food to starving people and actually killing people, in short, in the explicit rejection of the claim "that the obligation to refrain from killing someone is a more serious obligation than one's obligation to save lives (p. 59).[14]

Now, in view of our criticism above of these points which characterize the utilitarian approach in ethical evaluation (in particular the last point, i.e., the point which maintains that there is no difference in ethical evaluation between actively perpetrating an ethically reprehensible act and passively neglecting an ethically laudable act), it should be clear that, in the last analysis, we cannot find Tooley's position acceptable. Thus, for example, we would want to argue that there is a difference between the killing of an other and not saving the life of an other in that the former implicates that the other possesses an ethical right not to have its life terminated while the latter implicates that the other possesses an ethical right to have its life sustained, and clearly these are two different rights implying two different obligations on the ethical agent—the obligation not to terminate the life of an other (in the former case) and the obligation to sustain the life of an other (in the latter case). Now, it may well be that the obligation not to terminate the life of an other can be justified and thus validated while the obligation to sustain the life of an other could not, and if this be the case, then the ethical evaluation of the two acts clearly cannot be identical as Tooley wants to claim (though, admittedly, if the obligation to sustain the life of an other could be justified and thus validated, a good case could be made that the justification and thus the validation of the obligation not to terminate the life of an other would necessarily ensue, and in this case the ethical evaluation of the two acts would be identical).

Further, we would want to maintain, contra Tooley, that ethical evaluation is not determined exclusively (or, indeed, even essentially) by the objective outcomes of acts but rather by the intention/motivation that generates or accompanies the acts. And if this be so, then clearly the mere fact that the objective outcomes of two acts are identical by no means insures that their respective ethical evaluation would likewise be identical (as Tooley wants to maintain). The outcomes may be identical but if the intention/motivation is different, the ethical evaluation would be different. Indeed, depending on what intention/motivation is being implicated, four different comparative ethical evaluations may be called for. We may have a negative evaluation for both when, in both the case of the killing of an other and in the case of not saving the life of an other, the intention/motivation is indeed to see that other dead; or, secondly, we may have a positive evaluation for both when in both cases the death of the other occurs unintentionally or, indeed, in spite of an intention to help the other (thus, for example, with regard to the case of killing an other, not knowing, and having no way of knowing, that the other is deathly allergic to a drink which one has served to that other, or the surgeon who, in trying to heal a patient, loses, through no fault of his/her own, the patient's life in the course of the operation; alternatively, with regard to the case of not saving the life of an other, e.g., not providing food to a starving person, it may be that one has no knowledge that the other is on the brink of death because of starvation, or that one believes that withholding food is medically beneficial to that other, not realizing, and having no way to realize, that because of a certain concealed peculiarity in the physiology of that other, the deprivation of food would result in sudden death); or, thirdly, we may have a negative ethical evaluation for the case of the killing of an other and a positive ethical evaluation for the case of not saving the life of an other when the intention/motivation in the former case is to have that other dead and the intention/motivation in the latter case is not to have that other dead or even indeed to help that other (see the examples provided in conjunction with the second possibility); or, fourthly, we may have reversely a positive ethical evaluation for the case of the killing of an other and a negative ethical evaluation for the case of not saving the life of an other when the intention/motivation in the latter case is to have that other dead and the intention/motivation in the former case is not to have the other dead or even indeed to help that other (see same examples provided in conjunction with the second possibility).

Finally, we would submit, that there is a significant distinction between the two cases whereby the killing of an other implicates the agent as active while the not saving of the life of an other implicates the agent as passive which, in turn, implicates that in the former case responsibility for the death devolves exclusively on the agent while in the latter case an additional factor must inescapably be involved and indeed the direct responsibility for the death clearly devolves on it and not on the agent (responsibility devolves on the agent only inasmuch as it fails to block the activity of the other factor). And this being the case, the agents in both cases cannot possibly be held equally responsible irrespective of the fact that the objective outcomes in these cases are identical.

But while we must find Tooley's position in its final conclusion unacceptable, this is not to say that we may not identify any number of interesting penultimate points that he makes with respect to the utilitarian context, the very context in which he formulates his position. Thus, for example, Tooley has some very pertinent and valid observations to make regarding some aspects of the methodology that is implicated in the utilitarian enterprise, and on the basis of these observations he can subsequently proceed to invalidate some of the alternative utilitarian formulations that have been put forth. In the main, he makes the valid methodological point that for a formulation to be acceptable, it will have to make its case on the grounds of what can be "readily viewed as a basic moral principle" (Tooley 1972, 50). And this leads him to argue that for a formulation to be acceptable and valid, its case will have to be made in terms of a certain property or properties that the entity concerned possesses and where by virtue of such a property or properties a moral right can be established—"one should be prepared to point to some property that is morally significant" (pp. 50–51)—which, in turn, implicates that the proper approach for a valid, acceptable formulation to take is the approach in which "the basic issue to be discussed is what properties a thing must possess in order to have a serious right to life" (p. 37). For a formulation, therefore, to be valid, the crucial question that must be decided is whether or not there is a property or a set of properties possessed by the entity concerned that can be taken as morally significant (i.e., being able to provide an acceptable rationale and justification for granting the entity concerned a moral right). In the absence of such a property or a set of properties, a formulation cannot make its case, and if it tries, it can only prove itself to be invalid.

To illustrate this, Tooley refers to the formulation which tries to make its case on the grounds that the entity concerned belongs to one species rather than another. Such a formulation, he rightly argues, cannot be valid or acceptable for a "difference in species is not *per se* a morally relative difference" (Tooley 1972, 51). "The fact that human beings belong to the human species is in itself totally invalid and unacceptable as a ground for claiming that human beings possess the right to life or, in other words, equating human beings with persons, where person is in my definition that being which has a (serious) moral right to life" (p. 49). It seems to us that the point Tooley makes here can be clearly applied against the position taken by such people as Wertheimer and Brody and even also against the position taken by Judith Jarvis Thomson (see Thomson 1971). For the position taken by these people (Wertheimer and Brody putting it forth on the claim of its self-evident validity while Thomson conceding it for the sake of making a case against a different point) is that being a human being is *a priori* equivalent to being a person on the exclusive ground, apparently, that belonging to the human species is tantamount to being a person—a human being, exclusively by virtue of its membership in the human species, is a person, i.e., an entity which possesses a right to life. Tooley rightly rejects this position as untenable. One must point to a property or a set of properties that would be "morally relevant" (we take this to mean properties that would yield a satisfactory rationale for such a claim), and the mere belongingness to one species rather than another is not such a "morally relevant" property (Tooley 1972, 41). The equation between human being and person cannot be established in an *a priori* way (i.e., by mere definition as these alternative formulations propose). The equation between human being and person cannot be assumed or taken for granted as self-evident—it is precisely the task that has to be performed, it is precisely what has to be shown.

Finally, Tooley makes the obviously valid point that we must distinguish between determining the valid moral principle, i.e., determining what properties are morally significant, and determining which entities may or may not possess these morally significant properties. And clearly, it is the former and not the latter which constitutes the task for the moral enterprise, i.e., for moral reflection and argumentation; the latter merely raises a question of fact—it presents us with the task of determining facts as, for example, which entity does or does not possess this or that property.

Now, on the basis of this methodological approach, Tooley proceeds to make his case. Clearly, the fundamental and crucial move that needs to be made here is to define the notion of right, namely, to delineate what we mean when we say that someone has a right to something. And once having done this, we can readily move to clarify what we mean when we say that someone has a right specifically to life, to wit, when the something for which someone has a right is life. Finally, on the basis of the foregoing two moves, we should be able to proceed to the third and final move, the move which consists in carrying out the very task called for by the enterprise here, namely, the task of determining what kind of properties can implicate a claim to a right to life so that the attribution of such properties to an entity would endow that entity with a right to life. For in carrying out this move we would have attained everything that we need in order to decide whether or not we have in the subject of the claim a property that is "morally significant."

So, firstly, how is the notion of right to be understood? For Tooley to say that "A has a right to X" is tantamount to saying that "if A desires X then others are under *prima facie* obligation to refrain from actions that would deprive him of it" (Tooley 1972, 45). Right is clearly defined here in terms of desire—it is a desire, but a special kind of desire, to wit, it is a desire that, at least *prima facie* (i.e., in the absence of other overriding considerations), should not be deterred or frustrated by the actions of others. And this being the understanding of the notion of right, it of course follows that in claiming a right to life we are actually stating that if someone desires life, this desire, in the absence of other overriding considerations, should not be blocked or frustrated by the actions of others. All that one has to do is to substitute for the X in the definition of right a definable and contentful object that in this case is the notion of life. But now, secondly, how is the notion of life to be understood? For obviously the notion of life bears more than one signification, and what signification is actually involved would therefore have a significant bearing on the implications that can be drawn from the claim. For Tooley and, one suspects, for most other people dealing with the claim of a right to life as it impinges specifically on the human subject, the notion of life signifies not merely the existence of a biological organism but rather the existence of a subject of experiences and other mental states. As such, the claim of a right to life includes not only the right (i.e., a desire which is not to be countermanded) to "continue the existence of a biological organism but the right of a subject of experiences and other mental states to continue to exist" (p. 46).

Thirdly and finally, with the notions of right and life being clarified, Tooley can proceed to the kind of properties that can be attributed to the subject that is involved in this kind of situation, namely, he can undertake to determine what kind of a subject (i.e., a subject possessing what kind of properties) could place a claim to a right to life. Tooley comes up with three properties. Firstly, the subject must be such that it can possess a concept of an entity that is a subject of experiences and states of mind. Secondly, the subject must be such that it can and does believe that it itself is such an entity, i.e., that it believes itself to be a subject of experiences and states of mind. And thirdly, that it must be an entity that possesses the desire to go on being such an entity (Tooley 1972, 51).

There is no gainsaying the validity of the logic behind this deduction—it is clear and indeed convincing. For, as we have seen, according to this argument the notion of one's right is established in terms of one's desires (seeing that it signifies one's capacity to lay claim not to have one's desires frustrated). Thus, clearly, for one to be able to place such a claim and so institute one's right, one must possess some desires. But if one does indeed possess some desires, then one must, at the very least, also possess a concept of an entity endowed with desires. For how else can it be an entity that actually possesses such desires if it does not at the same time have a conception of such an entity, i.e., a conception of an entity that possesses desires?[15] But having a conception of an entity that possesses desires necessarily has to presuppose having a conception of an entity that is a subject of experiences and states of mind. Thus, in order to establish a right on behalf of any entity, that entity has to possess desires and as such be a subject of experiences and states of mind. Still, having a conception, a consciousness, of such an entity in general, i.e., having a conception that there is such an entity possessing desires (and thus being a subject of experiences and states of mind) somewhere out there in the world, is obviously not enough; what is needed is that one should possess a conception, a consciousness, of itself being such an entity, i.e., an entity possessing desires and thus a subject of experiences and states of mind. For the claim to a right to life is being placed not by some other entity out there in the world but by this particular entity, and consequently all talk and considerations must be in terms of this particular entity and not in terms of some other entity. Finally, not only must this particular entity possess a conception of such an entity, it must actually be that entity. For the desires must actually be expressed (and not be a mere capacity, a mere possibility) in order for the claim to have force and validity. Thus, Tooley's three-fold deduction with respect to the kind of properties the entity in question must possess is quite valid. Of course, in the last analysis, what the possession of these properties signifies is that the entity involved here, i.e., the entity that can place a claim to a right to life, must be not only a conscious entity but a *self*-conscious entity. The bottom line, then, is that only an entity which possesses self-consciousness can place a claim to a right to life, i.e., can place a claim not to have its existence terminated.

Now, it must be granted that Tooley's formulation is consistent, namely, that every step taken in its development is consistent with and flows from the preceding established step. Thus, given his formulation of the notion of right in terms of the notion of desire, and his delineation of the notion of desire in terms of intentions, i.e., as acts of consciousness rather than behavioristically, it consistently follows that an entity which possesses a right to life must be an entity possessing the property of self-consciousness (and this, one might add, is tantamount to saying that only a human being possesses this right, seeing that only the human being, as far as we know, is being endowed with self-consciousness). But, of course, we must realize that Tooley can consistently arrive at this conclusion only on the basis of his delineating desire (i.e., the desire for life) in terms of an act of intention and not behavioristically. For only when desire is delineated as intention and not behavioristically, can it provide the implication that the entity possessing it must also possess self-consciousness (and thus, that only the human being is such an entity). For indeed, desire when delineated as intention is by its very essence constituted as an expression of self-consciousness and as such can arise only in an entity possessing self-consciousness; as against this, when it is delineated behavioristically it is constituted as a certain pattern of action and behavior, and this in no way need implicate self-consciousness—the pattern of action and behavior may well be "blind," mechanistic, instinctive. Thus, when desire is delineated behavioristically, it does not lead to the conclusion that self-consciousness is necessarily implicated, and that consequently the human being is the exclusive entity to possess desire, i.e., a desire for life, and therefore, according to this formulation, also a right to life.[16]

But this state of affairs, where the desire for life and thus the right to life is not limited to the human but extended to all living entities (due to its being delineated behavioristically rather than in terms of intention) is apparently not amenable to Tooley (seeing that he is not disposed to extend the right to life to any entity other than the human), and so he avoids it by delineating the desire for life in terms of intention and not of behavior, thus allowing him, as we have seen, to posit self-consciousness as a necessary property and consequently arrogate the desire for and the associated right to life exclusively to the human. It would seem to us, however, that this move by Tooley is inconsistent with the utilitarian stance that he adopts. For in the context of the utilitarian stance, a delineation in terms of intention is not really applicable, seeing that the calculus on which the utilitarian stance bases itself is a calculus that is carried out exclusively in terms of overt acts—in the last analysis, what counts in the utilitarian calculus is outward behavior and not inward intentions. Consequently, for any factor to count in the utilitarian calculus (specifically for us here, this being the desire for life), it has to be delineated in terms of overt behavior and not in terms of inward intention. Thus, for Tooley's formulation to adopt the utilitarian stance (this being a fundamental and not a mere peripheral move on the part of Tooley's formulation as, indeed, it would be on the part of any other formulation) and at the same time proceed to delineate the desire for life in terms of intention seems to us to introduce a fundamental inconsistency into the formulation and consequently throw its validity into question.

To make things worse, this is not the only problem we have with Tooley's formulation. Thus, we have the further and more serious problem that, in our judgment, the right to life that Tooley's formulation delivers to us is only a relative but not an absolute right. For as will be recalled, the notion of right in the context of "A has a right to X" is explicated in this formulation as stating that "if A desires X, then others are under a *prima facie* obligation to refrain from depriving X from A," the "*prima facie*" being tantamount to stating "in the absence of other overriding desires, i.e., other overriding considerations." Now, we would submit that the introduction of this qualification relativizes the right to life. For in introducing this qualification, the determination of the right to life here is no longer dependent merely on the determination of whether a certain characteristic (i.e., the desire for life) is or is not present. It is now also dependent on the further determination of whether other desires or considerations present may or may not have the power to override the characteristic in question (and it is only when the latter is determined in the negative that the right is established). Indeed, seeing that the characteristic in question here (i.e., the desire for life) is most likely almost always to be present, the real crux for the determination of the right to life lies here in the latter determination, i.e., in the determination of whether other considerations present may or may not have the power to override the characteristic in question here. And this, in turn, necessarily implicates a further factor in the determination of the right to life, to wit, the criterion for selectivity. For clearly, one would need a criterion by which to determine which desire, which consideration, is to be the overriding one (for Tooley, as for any good utilitarian, it is the consideration that produces the greater benefit). Indeed, the relation between a desire and a right is no longer to be grasped as a straightforward, simple one-to-one relation—a right arising as the direct, uncomplicated consequence of a desire. Rather, a right arises as the consequence of a desire that has emerged victorious from a clash of desires. A right is, strictly speaking, not the expression of a desire, pure and simple, but the expression of an *overriding* desire. And an overriding desire is constituted not only by its content but also by the criterion of selectivity that establishes it as overriding. Thus, desire is not the only basic factor determining the right; the criterion of selectivity is also a basic, and in a sense perhaps even a more basic, factor determining the right.

But this means that we cannot have a determination of the right to life that is carried out in its own terms and is as such determined to be absolute and permanent; rather, the determination that we can have is a determination that is dependent on external considerations and as such is only relative and transitory. For the determination now depends on ascertaining whether or not there is another consideration present which can claim to be the overriding consideration, and this obviously may change from situation to situation. It is certainly possible that while in situation A a desire could constitute a right because there are no other overriding considerations, in situation B the very same desire would not constitute a right because another consideration that does prove itself to be overriding enters the picture. Thus, the notion of the right here is such that it does not affix itself permanently. It is not the case that once possessed by an entity, it is possessed permanently; rather, it is something that may come and go as the situation changes. But is such a notion of the right really acceptable? Is this really what the notion should signify—merely the relative advantage, the relative superiority, of a certain desire in comparison to the other competing desires present in the situation (the situation itself being contingent and transitory)? The failure to provide a right to life that would be inherent and absolute betrays, in our judgment, a serious weakness in Tooley's formulation.[17]

Furthermore, it would seem that the introduction here into the delineation of the right of the qualification that there be no other overriding consideration present would inevitably implicate the introduction of the utilitarian calculus into the delineation. For, as we have just seen, what would determine in the context of this delineation whether or not an entity has a right to life is no longer pure and simple, whether or not it has the desire to go on living (after all, every normal living entity would have this desire) but rather whether or not another desire (i.e., another consideration, another factor) that can be judged to be overriding the desire to go on living is present. And such a judgment, we would submit, can be established, in the last analysis, only on the basis of the utilitarian calculus, namely, on the basis of which factor, which desire, can produce the greater good. But the utilitarian calculus can lead, it would seem to us, to some very problematic and, indeed, untenable situations. Thus, consider, for example, the following possible scenario. Suppose A has a desire to kill B and that the only consideration to the contrary is B's desire to go on living. In the context of Tooley's formulation, what one would have to do to determine the morality of the proposed act would be to determine which consideration, which desire, is the overriding one. Now, suppose that B's life is of very little value (assuming, of course, that we have agreement as to how to determine what constitutes a more or less valuable life) and, furthermore, that A's desire to kill B would be of very great benefit not only to A but also to a great many others and that, therefore, on the basis of the utilitarian calculus it is not B's desire to go on living but A's desire to kill B that is really the overriding consideration. In the context of Tooley's formulation, therefore, A's desire, i.e., intention, to kill B in these circumstances will have to be morally approved. But can we really accept this conclusion as valid? Is there not something dreadfully wrong in giving moral approval to such an intended act?[18]

Lastly, a problem arises for us in connection with Tooley's formulation delineating the notion of the right in terms of the notion of desire, namely, with its explication of "A has a right to X" to mean "A desires X and is not to be frustrated, blocked, in having X if no other desires, factors, that are overriding and counter-indicative are present."

For we would want to question whether it is really valid to say that the notion of the right is delineated by the notion of desire, namely, that one's right to something is established by one's desiring that something, provided only that there are no other overriding considerations. After all, we clearly can cite examples where we would want to say that one's right to a certain something is clearly established even though the one may not desire that something. Thus, for example, the right of King George VI to the throne of England was clearly established even though he may very well have not desired it. True, had he not desired it sufficiently, he could have abdicated the right. But this precisely makes our point. The lack of desire in itself, as such, does not abrogate the right. Abrogation of the right is effected only by the additional, separate and distinct act of abdication. The lack of desire may lead to the act of abdication but precisely as such it cannot be identified with it. But if the lack of desire in itself does not as such cancel out the right, the presence of desire in itself (in the absence of other overriding considerations) cannot as such constitute the right either. Indeed, it is difficult to see or appreciate how, for example, a right to any title, to possession or to inheritance can be constituted in terms of desire. Rather, it seems clear that in these instances the right is established on the basis of some other consideration or principle that has nothing to do with desire, and that desire enters the picture here only inasmuch as it may lead the subject to abdicate that right.

So, we clearly have any number of important instances where the way we use the notion of the right does not lend itself to our delineating it in terms of desire; rather, it points to its delineation in terms of something that is objectively and permanently inherent in the very structure of the relation or the entity in whose context the notion of the right arises. But if this criticism is valid, then one would have to conclude that Tooley's formulation cannot be taken as descriptive of the way we use the notion of the right but, at best, only as a prescriptive, and even then its persuasiveness would in all likelihood be very questionable, seeing that what it prescribes is not what generally one would want to claim.

But one may respond to this by noting that Tooley's formulation is intended to apply to the notion of a right that is moral (rather than, for example, to the notion of a right that is legal or political), i.e., the notion of a right that is to be delineated in terms of desire is to be specifically and exclusively the notion of a moral right. And this being the case, then clearly resorting to rights of title, possession or inheritance should not be taken as a valid argument against Tooley's formulation, seeing that they cannot be counted as moral right and, therefore, as valid counter-examples against the right to life which is clearly to be taken as a moral right. Namely, one may well retort in defense of Tooley's delineation of the right to life in terms of desire (i.e., in terms of the subject's desire for the continuation of its life) that while legal and political rights may indeed not be delineated in terms of desire, moral rights (thus the right to life) may be so delineated. Thus, one would have to concede that, in the last analysis, this line of criticism is not really effective.

There is, however, another line of criticism (indeed, a line of criticism that goes more deeply to the very heart of the issue here) which, in our judgment, does throw the validity of Tooley's delineation of the right to life in terms of desire into serious question. Namely, one must question whether a right to life delineated in terms of desire can really be taken to constitute itself as a *moral* right. Can one really take this delineation of the notion of the right in terms of desire as a delineation that, to quote Tooley, can "plausibly be viewed as a basic moral principle" (Tooley 1972, 50)? For is it really plausible to maintain that what the notion of a moral right signifies is nothing else but the granting of permission, in the absence of any other overriding considerations to the contrary, for someone to realize his/her desire, whatever that desire may be? Can this possibly constitute a basic moral principle? We may perhaps be able to accept that in such circumstances, i.e., when there is no other overriding consideration to the contrary, a legal or political right may be implicated to the effect that one is not to be blocked from realizing his/her desire (though, as we have seen, this is really a statement which is devoid of any "cash value," seeing that it is self-evident), but that this right is a *moral* right would be very difficult to accept. What is moral about the realization of desires regardless of what those desires are?[19]

Thus, in light of the problems raised here, we must conclude that, in the last analysis, Tooley's formulation is really not acceptable to us, and we say this even though there is no denying that in many ways it is a very ingenious and intriguing formulation. It is certainly very valuable to us in making the two all-important points which we would fully embrace (although, again, we cannot accept the definition or the rationale which Tooley provides for them), namely, firstly, the distinction and clear separation that it establishes between the term "human being" and the term "person," and secondly (and this is by far the more substantial and significant point made), the identification of self-consciousness as the property by virtue of which the claim for a right to life can be established (for rejecting the equation of "person" with "human being" see Tooley 1972, 41; for identifying self-consciousness as the morally significant property see pp. 47 and 62).[20] The second difference is much more substantial and significant. It refers to the role that the notion of self-consciousness plays in establishing the rationale for the claim to a right to life. For Tooley, self-consciousness plays a role because he sees it as being necessarily implicated by the positing of such properties as desiring and conceiving; namely, he rightly perceives that an entity that manifests desires and conceptions is necessarily an entity that is self-conscious. But self-consciousness as such does not impinge directly upon the claim to a right to life—the rationale and justification for such a claim are not made in its terms; rather, they are made in terms of the positing of certain desires, and self-consciousness enters the picture only because such positing necessarily presupposes the presence of self-consciousness. For us, on the other hand, the rationale and justification for the claim to a right to life are to be made, as we shall see below, by the very terms of the notion of self-consciousness. It is the very notion of self-consciousness that is to provide the rationale and justification. Thus, it is by virtue of the very possession of self-consciousness as such (and not by virtue of the presence of some other properties whose presence, in turn, implicates the presence of self-consciousness) that the rationale and justification for a claim to a right to life are to be established. Needless to say, the rationale and justification obtained in the context of our approach would differ greatly from that which is obtained in the context of Tooley's approach.

Lastly, before proceeding to put forth our formulation, we still have to briefly examine the excellent essay by Mary Warren (1982) entitled "On the Moral and Legal Status of Abortion" (the references to this essay here are to this reprint). Although the main manifest thrust of this paper is directed to the issue of abortion as such (i.e., to the issue of whether or not a fetus can be aborted), it is inevitable that this issue would implicate the further and more fundamental issue of the right to life (i.e., by virtue of what does an entity have a right to life). This is indeed the case in this essay and consequently the essay does indeed imply a stance that one may take with respect to the issue of the right to life. In essence, the stance implied in Warren's position seems to be very close and similar to the stance implied in Tooley's position. But Warren spells out her case and its rationale in much greater detail than Tooley, in this way buttressing her case but also leaving herself open to a more extensive line of criticism. Thus, Warren's essay makes by far the strongest case for the stance that comes closest to the stance which we would want to adopt (and which we would put forth presently) while at the same time it also places its weaknesses in much greater relief.

Warren follows Tooley in subscribing to the important distinction between the characterization (i.e., the category) of being a human being and the characterization of being a person. For Warren the former characterization is delineated by genetic consideration while the latter characterization is delineated by moral considerations (Warren 1982, 255); to the extent, however, that the former characterization is interchangeable with the latter characterization, the term "human" comes to carry two significations, genetic and moral. But clearly, it is only in terms of the moral signification, i.e., in terms of the signification of "human" as person when "the concept of a person is in part a moral concept . . . a member of the moral community," that the case for a right to life can be made (p. 256). For it is only to the extent that "human" signifies a moral agent, i.e., a being carrying moral obligations and consequently also endowed with moral rights, that the case for the specific right to life can be made. But Warren proceeds beyond Tooley to spell out the property or properties by virtue of which a being can be designated as a person, i.e., as a moral entity, an entity endowed with rights, specifically the right to life. She cites five traits which she considers to be the most central traits by virtue of which an entity can be transformed into a person (and thus specifically by virtue of which a human being in the genetic sense can be transformed into a human being in the moral sense). These five traits are as follows: 1) the possession of a consciousness of external and/or internal objects and events, in particular the possession of a capacity to feel pain; 2) the possession of a reasoning capacity to solve problems; 3) the capacity to instigate self-motivated activity; 4) the capacity to communicate; and 5) the possession of self-concepts and of self-awareness in its individual or racial signification (p. 256). But while these five traits are indeed the most central traits that characterize an entity as a person, they are not all necessarily needed to be present, according to Warren's further argument, in order for an entity to be designated as a person. Indeed, according to Warren, traits 1 and 2 in themselves "may well be sufficient" in order to transform an entity into a person, and the presence of traits 1 and 3 in themselves would "quite probably" be also sufficient for this purpose (p. 256). Thus, according to Warren, while traits 1 and 2 are definitely sufficient in themselves and traits 1 and 3 are probably sufficient in themselves, traits 4 and 5 are clearly not sufficient in themselves to constitute personhood. Traits 4 and 5 are central characterizations of personhood but in themselves are not sufficient to constitute it.

Now, what is one to say to this? As granted above, we certainly consider it a most significant and valid advance in overcoming the misunderstandings connected with the issue before us here when a distinction between the notion of a human being as such and the notion of a human being *qua* person is clearly established and when the dimension of consciousness is introduced into the picture as the factor by which the distinction is established. And this being the case, we would certainly award Warren (as indeed also Tooley) high credit for their respective formulations. Still, even so, we cannot, in the last analysis, accept Warren's formulation as the final word, i.e., as the formulation that succeeds in providing us with a fully satisfactory rationale and justification for the claim to a right to life, and this for the following two considerations. Firstly, as we have seen, Warren formulates her rationale in terms of consciousness and reason, i.e., traits 1 and 2, or in terms of consciousness and self-motivated activity, i.e., traits 1 and 3 (we are identifying traits 1, 2 and 3 and not traits 4 and 5 as the traits in terms of which Warren formulates her rationale because what is necessary for establishing a rationale are traits that are needed and sufficient to constitute a person and not merely traits that are valued as central traits). But what is there in the manifestation of consciousness as such or of rational activity or of self-motivated activity that would provide an explanation, let alone a justification, for the claim to a right to life? By virtue of what can they provide a rationale for such a claim? None is offered by Warren and, as far as we can see, none is available. And secondly, a clear consequence of taking traits 1, 2 and 3 as the determining criteria in formulating the rationale for the claim to a right to life is that some animals may well qualify as persons, i.e., as entities possessing a right to life, while some human beings may not. Indeed, Warren is aware of this as she states very clearly that some entities which are, genetically speaking, clearly human are nonetheless not persons while there may be entities that are persons but are not, genetically speaking, human beings. Thus, according to Warren, defective, unreasoning, i.e., imbecile, humans are not to be regarded as persons while advanced robots which are self-aware are to be regarded as persons (p. 257). And if the case can be made for robots it can also be made, it would seem to us, for certain animals.[21]

But is this really acceptable and convincing? Do we really want to say that a dolphin or a chimpanzee or, even more so, an advanced robot has a right not to have its existence terminated but a human being who is a moron does not? Clearly, something must be wrong if we end up with this kind of a conclusion and inasmuch as the process of reasoning here seems to be consistent and valid, the wrongness must lie in the premises, i.e., in the properties or the traits selected as the criteria by which to justify the claim to a right to life. But if this is so, then, for all intents and purposes, we are faced with three possible options by which to proceed. We can, firstly, search for another trait, not mentioned thus far, which will be able to provide us with a rationale and a justification that would be convincing and thus acceptable. Or, secondly, we can turn to a trait that has been already mentioned in one of the foregoing formulations but where its potential to provide a convincing and thus an acceptable rationale and justification for the claim to a right to life was not adequately explicated (so that what is called for in order to secure a convincing and thus an acceptable rationale and justification is a more adequate explication of the trait). Or, thirdly, if both preceding alternatives prove unavailing, we may have to resign ourselves to the fact that we cannot establish a convincing and thus an acceptable rationale and justification for the claim to a right to life and that consequently the claim can have no validity and our whole effort to establish it and resort to it is patently untenable.

Now, it would seem to us that we do not have to succumb to the third option. There is a valid claim to a right to life and therefore a convincing rationale and justification for it must ultimately also be attainable. True, we must concede that the first option fails us rather badly in this matter—we certainly cannot come up with any additional traits that could provide us with a satisfactory rationale and thus an acceptable justification for the claim to a right to life. But we still have the second option, and here in the context of this option, we would want to claim, a possibility for establishing such a rationale and justification does present itself. Thus, we would submit that while a convincing rationale and thus an acceptable justification cannot indeed be established in terms of most of the traits referred to in the foregoing formulations (thus, that it cannot be established in terms of such traits as self-motivated action or sentience or rationality or even consciousness as such), there is one trait in terms of which a convincing rationale and thus an acceptable justification can be established. This is the trait of *self*-consciousness, a trait that, as will be recalled, does appear in Tooley's formulation. True, in spite of the presence of the trait of self-consciousness in Tooley's formulation, the formulation, in our judgment, fails to provide the rationale and justification that are called for. But this is so because, as already pointed out above, the formulation fails to properly utilize the trait of self-consciousness.[22] If, however, the trait of self-consciousness is to be properly utilized, as we hope proves to be the case in our presentation below, then the trait of self-consciousness will provide us with a convincing rationale and thus an acceptable justification for the claim to a right to life. So, let us proceed to lay out how our formulation utilizes the trait of self-consciousness in formulating its rationale and justification for the claim that an entity can possess an ethical right to life, i.e., an ethical right not to have its existence terminated, by virtue of the fact that it possesses the trait of self-consciousness.[23]

Thus, to begin with, we would submit that for self-consciousness to come into existence and, indeed, maintain itself in existence, it requires that it be affirmed from the outside by an other—it can come into existence only by being called forth by an other and it can maintain itself in this existence, i.e., it can fend off its disintegration, only by the affirmation being periodically renewed. As oxygen is required for biological existence, so is affirmation required for the existence of self-consciousness. Indeed, this observation constitutes the very foundation from which a rationale, a justification, for our claim that an entity possessing self-consciousness is endowed with an ethical right to life, i.e., with an ethical right not to have its existence terminated, can be derived. For clearly, an entity which constitutes itself in terms of self-consciousness would adopt the characteristics possessed by self-consciousness, which is to say that any entity constituting itself in terms of self-consciousness would require by its very ontological constitution that, in order for it to come into existence and maintain itself in it, it be affirmed from the outside by an other, and this is tantamount to saying that such an entity would be endowed with a right, indeed, with an ethical right (seeing that the right grounds itself here in the very ontological constitution of the entity that bears it) to request/demand that it be affirmed. But now, affirmation, by its very signification, clearly implicates, in turn, the preclusion of terminating the existence of an entity to which affirmation has been extended. For after all, does not the notion of affirmation signify, in the last analysis, the acknowledgment of the existence of the other, i.e., of the entity to which affirmation is extended, as an end-in-itself, which is to say the acknowledgment of the other in its otherness (after all, can anything else be affirmed of an entity if the affirmation of its existence is not already implicated)? But if this is so, then it would be logically contradictory to affirm the existence of an entity and at the same time terminate its existence. It is not possible, at one and the same time, to affirm and to terminate the existence of one and the same entity. Thus, if an entity constituting itself in terms of self-consciousness is endowed with an ethical right to request/demand that it be affirmed, then it also follows, of necessity, that it is endowed with an ethical right to life, i.e., with an ethical right to request/demand that its existence not be terminated—an ethical right to request/demand affirmation necessarily implicates an ethical right to request/demand not to be terminated. Thus, being constituted in terms of self-consciousness does endow an entity with an ethical right to life.

Indeed, as far as we can see, one cannot make the foregoing case on behalf of any other ontological constituent beside self-consciousness. Namely, we would submit that no other ontological constituent can bestow upon an entity an ethical right to request/demand to be affirmed and thus an ethical right to request/demand not to have its existence terminated. Thus, the case cannot be made on behalf of power as an ontological constituent, for clearly, power, being "blind" (i.e., being totally devoid of awareness and therefore of needs or desires), does not require to be affirmed in order for it to come into or maintain itself within existence. And likewise, though perhaps less readily apparent than in the instance of power, the case cannot be made on behalf of consciousness as such (i.e., of consciousness devoid of self-consciousness) as an ontological constituent. Consciousness as mere awareness of an other (and such an other can be any external object to the act of awareness, and this would encompass the physical body of the bearer of consciousness), in contra-distinction to a consciousness of itself, to a consciousness of being conscious, i.e., to self-consciousness, does not require to be affirmed from the outside in order to establish itself in existence. The rationale behind this claim may lie in the fact that when the other for an act of consciousness is anything else but the act of consciousness itself, such an other would be, in principle, always accessible to being validated within our experience. The only instance where the other is not so accessible is when the other is the act of consciousness itself, and consequently its validation must be provided by an act of affirmation from the outside.

But whether or not the rationale advanced here in connection with the three-fold claim (i.e., the claim that power and consciousness as such do not require affirmation from the outside in order to come into and maintain themselves within existence while self-consciousness does) is, in the last analysis, valid, common experience does seem to substantiate it. Thus, experience clearly shows that such entities as rocks or metals or vegetation, namely, entities that constitute themselves exclusively in terms of power, do not require any affirmation from the outside in order to come into existence or maintain themselves within existence, and consequently such entities cannot be (and, indeed, are not) endowed with an ethical right not to have their existence terminated.[24] Lastly, we should note that even in a context where the notion of termination is not taken in its radical signification (i.e., when it is not taken as signifying a total abrogation of existence) but only in its less radical signification (i.e., when it is taken as signifying merely a change in the level of manifestation of the "stuff" constituting the entity), and where therefore the notion of termination in this latter signification will be applicable only to entities which constitute themselves in terms of power, a claim to an ethical right to life, even when the ethical right to life is to implicate here the notion of termination not in its radical but only in its less radical signification, will not be available to such entities, i.e., to entities constituting themselves in terms of power. For inasmuch as the right signifies now a request/demand not to have the level of the manifestation of the "stuff" constituting the entity changed, i.e., diminished, such a right is still in conflict with the very nature of the "stuff" constituting the entity to which it is applied, seeing that that "stuff" is power and that power by its very essence implicates motion and that motion, in turn, by its very essence implicates change. Entities that constitute themselves in terms of power cannot therefore possibly escape being in the grip of continuous motion and consequently being subjected to continuous change. And this being the case, a request/demand not to be subjected to change is clearly inapplicable to such entities. Likewise, experience also shows that such entities as animals, namely, entities that constitute themselves in terms of consciousness as such (or, more precisely, entities whose ontological constitution encompasses, in addition to power, also consciousness as such), also do not require affirmation from the outside in order to come to possess or maintain their consciousness as such—animals can come to possess or maintain their consciousness as such while being completely isolated from their fellow animals (thus, for example, a tiger or a deer or any other animal could develop and retain in complete isolation from all other members of its class the capacity to be aware of things outside itself). And this being the case, animals too cannot be (and indeed are not) endowed with an ethical right not to have their existence terminated.

In contra-distinction to this, however, experience also shows that in the case of humans, namely, in the case of entities whose ontological constitution encompasses not only power and consciousness as such but also self-consciousness, self-consciousness cannot arise nor, once having arisen, maintain itself, if the human entity is completely isolated from its fellow human entities.[25] Thus, there seems to be sufficiently persuasive data that point to the conclusion that when human infants are totally isolated from any and all contact with other humans, they fail to develop as persons, i.e., as bearers of self-consciousness (indeed, even more fundamentally, there seems to be evidence pointing to the fact that such infants, even though they do receive all the needed nourishment and medical care, do not survive physically for very long). And even more definitively, there is very convincing evidence to buttress the claim that when adult humans are placed in solitary confinement for a long enough time, they sooner or later (depending on how strong is their capacity to retain the memory of past affirmations) disintegrate as persons, which is to say that the capacity of self-consciousness is withdrawn from them. Thus indeed, humans are the only entities encountered in our experience who, because of their ontological constitution, require affirmation from the outside in order for them to come into existence and maintain themselves within it, and who consequently (given our delineation of what the notion of ethical right signifies) are endowed with an ethical right to life, i.e., with an ethical right to request/demand that their existence not be terminated.

There is, however, another entity which, by virtue of its ontological constitution, would require affirmation from the outside in order for it to come into existence and maintain itself within it and which as such would be endowed with an ethical right to request/demand that its existence not be terminated. The entity to which we are referring here is an entity that constitutes itself exclusively in the context of the dimension-of-consciousness as it expresses itself in terms of self-consciousness (i.e., being conscious of one's own conscious activity as the object of the act) but which as such is also to say, at one and the same time, as it also expresses itself in terms of consciousness as such (i.e., being conscious of entities outside of oneself as the object of the act), seeing that while the arising of consciousness as such does not necessarily implicate the arising of self-consciousness, the arising of self-consciousness inescapably implicates the arising of consciousness as such as the necessary precondition for its own arising. Thus, the entity to which we are referring here is like the human entity in going beyond the expression of the dimension-of-consciousness exclusively in terms of consciousness as such (as is the case in the animal entity) to its expression also in terms of self-consciousness, but unlike the human entity, in which (like in the animal entity) the dimension-of-power continues to express itself, the entity here transcends any and every expression of the dimension-of-power.

Namely, in contra-distinction to the animal entity whose ontological constitution encompasses the expression of power and of consciousness as such, and in contrast to the human entity whose ontological constitution encompasses the expression of power, of consciousness as such and of self-consciousness, the ontological constitution of the entity here encompasses only the expression of consciousness as such and of self-consciousness but not of power. Clearly, the entity to which we are referring here is the entity delineated by Buber as a pure Thou entity (i.e., an entity that constitutes itself exclusively in terms of the dimension-of-consciousness) and identified by him as the divine entity that is encountered in biblical faith (i.e., the divine entity encountered in the various historical expressions of biblical faith, to wit, the Hebrew Bible and the various historical religions that ground themselves in the Hebrew Bible such as Judaism, Christianity and Islam).[26] Thus, while with respect to the It-god, i.e., the god encountered in paganism, dependency would indeed undermine its divinity, with respect to the Thou-god, the god encountered in biblical faith, not only would dependency not undermine its divinity but it is an inextricable, necessary requirement for its very ontological constitution. And now, seeing that in our analysis above we were dealing with the god of biblical faith, indeed, with the god *par excellence* of biblical faith, i.e., the Buberian pure Thou-god, implicating dependency to it should in no way be viewed as problematic.

We have thus far established that only entities which possess self-consciousness (which is to say, only humans and a Thou-god) can claim an ethical right to request/demand that they be affirmed as ends-in-themselves, which is tantamount to saying that they have an ethical right not to have their existence terminated (and, indeed, not to be related to in terms of utilization). But, of course, nothing in our analysis thus far has in any way established that there are others who would be under an ethical *obligation* to acknowledge and honor such requests/demands for affirmation. And in the absence of establishing the availability of such others, the ethical right to request/demand affirmation which can be ascribed to humans and to a Thou-god must per force remain unfulfilled, vacuous. To give the claim to an ethical right to life, so to speak, "cash value," i.e., to be able to make it operable, to invest it with actuality, we must be able to establish that there are others who would be under an ethical obligation to satisfy such a claim, i.e., to extend such an affirmation. For an ethical right to life to have "cash value" we must establish not only that there is such an ethical right but equally that there is an ethical obligation to honor such a right. It is to this undertaking that we must now turn.

Indeed, it would seem to us that there are two ways by which an ethical obligation to honor the ethical right to life can be established. One way would base itself on the implicatory relation that obtains between the notion of right and that of obligation. Namely, it would seem self-evident that if an entity claims the right to request/demand that it be affirmed by an other, it should at the same time assume, in return, the obligation to extend the same affirmation to that other upon its request/demand for such an affirmation. And conversely, if an entity is placed under an obligation to extend affirmation to an other, it should at the same time have the right (assuming, of course, that its ontological structure would allow this) to request/demand that affirmation be extended to it from that other. This mutual implicatory relation between the notion of right and that of obligation is not only grounded in an elemental sense of fairness (i.e., repaying in kind for what one has received or receiving in kind for what one has paid out) but equally in egotistical calculations based on self-interest. For clearly, if my existence is contingent on my request/demand for affirmation being met by an other, it is to my interest to meet, in return, the request/demand for affirmation of that other if its existence is contingent on its request/demand being met. As such, the notions of right and obligation are but two sides of one and the same coin. The two are inextricably linked together—one cannot possess a right without at the same time assuming the commensurate obligation, nor can one be subjected to an obligation without at the same time being invested with the commensurate right.[27]

But clearly this implicatory relation between right and obligation can be obtained only in a context where both the subject and the other involved in this implicatory relation are entities possessing the same ontological constitution or, more specifically and accurately, where both the subject and the other possess the factor of self-consciousness in their respective ontological constitutions—it is only by virtue of possessing self-consciousness that an entity can be endowed with a right to request/demand that affirmation be extended to it, and likewise it is only by virtue of possessing self-consciousness that an entity can be saddled with the obligation to extend affirmation to an other.[28]

Indeed, as such, the act of validation here is radically different from the other act of validation that is most relevant to our discussion here, namely, the validation of an act of consciousness as such. For the validation in this latter instance is mediated in terms of its consequences (thus, for example, whether the sighting of a blue patch in the distant horizon of the desert is actually water or a mirage would be validated by the consequence of whether or not one's thirst can be quenched by it). But with respect to self-consciousness, there are no consequences. The actuality of self-consciousness can be validated only by direct affirmation from the outside and such affirmation can be extended only by an entity which itself possesses self-consciousness, for only such an entity can empathize with another entity possessing self-consciousness and thus intuit and affirm its actuality. If animals, therefore, do not possess self-consciousness, as we would want to argue, then they really cannot extend affirmation for the actuality of self-consciousness in an other. That domestic animals are sometimes taken as substitutes for other humans as sources of affirmation is made feasible by the recipient human entity extending, by wishful interpretation, its affirmation as a means to some further end to signify its affirmation as an end-in-itself. Thus, we can conclude that we can establish a right to be affirmed and an obligation to affirm (thus safeguarding the right to be affirmed from being vacuous) but only in a context where both the subject and the other are personal entities, namely, entities that encompass the Thou-dimension, the dimension-of-consciousness, in their ontological constitution, in other words, only in a context where the implicated entities can only be human entities or the Thou-god. But this limitation is quite acceptable and, indeed, fully agrees with our contention made in the previous chapter that the parameters of the ethical enterprise are confined to the domain of relations between personal entities.

The second way would establish the obligation to acknowledge and respond to the right to life, i.e., to the right to request/demand to be affirmed, in terms of the very mechanism by which affirmation is extended from one entity to another entity (the entities here are, of course, as established above, personal entities). For, we would submit, the mechanism is such that the putting forth of the request/demand to be affirmed and the extending of affirmation are placed in one and the same act.[29] How is this done? The key lies in the fact that an entity possessing self-consciousness is also, at one and the same time, inescapably an entity that possesses consciousness as such. Now, as an entity that possesses consciousness as such, it inevitably extends affirmation to the other of which it becomes conscious, seeing that the act of becoming conscious of an other necessarily implicates an act of cognition of that other and the act of cognition, in turn, necessarily implicates an act of affirmation of that other. At the same time, as an entity that possesses self-consciousness, it continuously puts forth a request/demand to be affirmed. But putting forth a request/demand to be affirmed by an other and extending affirmation to that other are not two separate acts here. Rather they are contained in one act—one and the same act simultaneously extends affirmation to an other and puts forth a request/demand to be affirmed by that other. It is one and the same act/relation that accomplishes both, and as such the request for and the extension of affirmation are clearly linked in a synchronic and not in a diachronic manner.

But the considerations brought forth thus far do not as yet safeguard the right to request/demand from being vacuous even though they place the extension of affirmation in one and the same act/relation in which the request/demand for affirmation has been placed. For the extension of affirmation has to come not from the subject, i.e., from the entity putting forth the request/demand for affirmation, but from the other, and what has been established here thus far is that, with respect to the subject, there is a linkage between the request/demand for and the extension of affirmation (i.e., that one and the same entity, the subject, in one and the same act/relation both requests/demands and extends affirmation) but not that there is a linkage between a request/demand for affirmation emanating from the subject and an extension of affirmation emanating from the other. It is this latter linkage that must be established, and it is to this task that we must now turn.

The first move in the pursuit of this task is to recognize that the other here is also constituted as an entity possessing self-consciousness (indeed, as the subject is constituted here). For as such, the other, just as was the case with the subject, would in one and the same act put forth a request/demand to be affirmed and extend an affirmation to other entities. And in such a context, of course, the request/demand put forth by the subject can be met by the extension of affirmation from the other.

Still, this situation leaves us with a problem, indeed, with a fairly serious problem. For does not this situation in which the subject puts forth a request/demand for affirmation and the other meets the request/demand by extending its affirmation present us with a diachronic rather than a synchronic state of affairs between the request/demand put forth by the subject and the affirmation extended by the other? And if this is so, then we do not really have here the assurance that the linkage between the request/demand for affirmation and the extension of such an affirmation is inextricable, an assurance that we certainly require if a right to request/demand affirmation (i.e., a right to life in the sense of not having one's existence terminated) is not to remain vacuous and which we thought to have established above.

For the inextricable linkage between a request/demand for affirmation and an extension of such an affirmation which was indeed established above was established within the parameters of one and the same act emanating from one and the same entity (that entity being either the subject or the other) and not within the parameters of two different acts emanating from two different entities—the request/demand for affirmation being signified by one act emanating from one entity, i.e., the subject, and the extension of affirmation being signified by a second act emanating from a second entity, i.e., the other. But it is precisely an inextricable linkage in terms of the latter parameters (i.e., where the request/demand for affirmation is signified by one act emanating from one entity and the extension of affirmation is signified by another act emanating from another entity) that one needs in order to safeguard the right to request/demand affirmation from remaining vacuous.

Thus, the crucial question before us here is whether we can overcome this problem. Can the discrepancy between the fact that the request/demand for affirmation and the extension of affirmation are arrogated to two separate acts/relations emanating from two separate entities and the need to have the linkage between the request/demand for affirmation and the extension of affirmation be a linkage that is inextricable and which as such would implicate that both the request/demand for affirmation and the extension of affirmation have to be encompassed in one and the same act/relation be bridged? We think it can, so let us proceed to try and make our case.

We must begin by reiterating what has already been established, namely, that we as humans are ontologically constituted in terms of both the dimension-of-power, the It-dimension, and the dimension-of-consciousness, the Thou-dimension, and consequently can view things from the perspective of either dimension. Now, as such, the diachronic state of affairs which we encounter in our common experience whereby the request/demand for affirmation and the extension of affirmation are arrogated to two separate acts/relations emanating from two separate entities, the latter succeeding the former, and where as such no inextricable linkage between the two can be established (and thus failing to safeguard that the request/demand for affirmation would not be left vacuous), is clearly due to our perceiving things from the vantage point of the dimension-of-power. For from the perspective of this dimension, the primary, most fundamental expression of reality, i.e., of reality constituted in terms of power, manifests itself in terms of the entity which then secondarily may or may not proceed to act/relate to another entity. Now, in such a context a request/demand for affirmation (which clearly constitutes itself as an act/relation) would necessarily have to implicate a foregoing entity in place which would initiate, i.e., bring forth, this request/demand, and likewise the extension of affirmation would necessarily have to implicate a foregoing entity in place which would initiate, i.e., extend, such an affirmation. This, in turn, means, however, that the request/demand for affirmation and the extension of affirmation would indeed have to be arrogated here to two separate acts/relations emanating from two separate entities which, as such, would, of course, implicate that the relation between the request/demand for affirmation and the extension of affirmation would have to be diachronic and not synchronic, thus undermining the possibility of providing us with a safeguard that the right to request/demand affirmation (i.e., the right to life in the sense of being a right not to have one's existence terminated) would not remain vacuous. The perspective of the dimension-of-power cannot present us with a mechanism which would provide any such safeguard and thus to the extent that we are bound to see things in terms of the dimension-of-power (seeing that the world given in our common sense-experience is a world that constitutes itself in terms of power), we must be left with the problematic that we cannot have at our disposal a mechanism that would safeguard that the right to life would not remain vacuous.

But this problematic is not, in the last analysis, as serious as it may appear at first sight (i.e., on a more superficial level). Indeed, in a way it is not serious at all. For a more careful reflection should persuade us that the phenomenon with which we are dealing here, i.e., the phenomenon of affirmation (whether it be in requesting/demanding it or in extending it), cannot arise within the context of the dimension-of-power; in terms of power it simply makes no sense to speak of requesting/demanding or of extending affirmation. The phenomenon of affirmation can arise only within the context of the dimension-of-consciousness. It makes sense to request/demand affirmation or to extend affirmation only when these acts are directed towards entities that possess self-consciousness. And this being the case, the question of whether or not an inextricable linkage between the request/demand for affirmation and the extension of affirmation can be established has to be resolved not within the context of the dimension-of-power but within the context of the dimension-of-consciousness. The relevant question here is not whether the dimension-of-power but whether the dimension-of-consciousness can provide us with a mechanism that would safeguard the right to life from being left vacuous. Thus, to deal in a relevant manner with the question that is before us here, we must turn to examine the ontological structure that characterizes the dimension-of-consciousness.

Now, as has been argued above in greater detail, in the context of the dimension-of-consciousness, and in contrast to that of the dimension-of-power, the primary, most fundamental expression of reality (reality constituting itself here in terms of consciousness rather than of power) manifests itself (as Buber rightly maintained) not in terms of the entity but in terms of the relation.[30] The primary ontological expression here is the relation, the entity arising secondarily as one of the two poles delineating the relation by establishing its border, its limit, on either side.[31] As such, seeing that the relation here in the context of the dimension-of-consciousness is the most fundamental, ultimate, expression (the expression being here, of course, the expression of consciousness) and that, therefore, it does not emanate from any preceding entity nor "moves" towards an already existing other entity, the "movement" of the relation here must be self-enclosed within itself and consequently any and every relation that arises within the context of the dimension-of-consciousness must constitute itself as a two-way relation, as a relation of mutuality.

It should be clear, however, that mutuality here is not attained by having two one-way relations "moving" simultaneously in opposite directions imposed on each other. True, this is the only way by which a relation of mutuality can and does arise when the context is that of the dimension-of-power. For in this context the relation can constitute itself only as a one-way relation (seeing that it arises here as a secondary expression emanating from the entity and therefore is capable of "moving" only in one direction, to wit, in the direction of another entity) and consequently a relation of mutuality can constitute itself here only by the imposition of two one-way relations "moving" in opposite direction upon each other. Of course, as such, we cannot really have here a single relation of mutuality. In the last analysis, what we do have are two separate relations. The relation of mutuality here is a composite relation made up of two separate relations. As against this, within the context of the dimension-of-consciousness, the relation being the most fundamental, ultimate expression within that dimension, there is no entity from which it can emanate (for this would ground the relation within the entity thus making the entity a more fundamental expression). In the context of the dimension-of-consciousness, the relation is the ground of everything else and as such it itself is not grounded in anything else—it can be grounded only in itself. And this being the case, both opposite "movements" must be contained simultaneously in the single "movement" of a single relation. Such a state of affairs may perhaps be grasped by visualizing the relation as vibrating or oscillating between its two poles. In this way it directs its signification simultaneously to both entities, each constituting itself at either pole; and the signification here is nothing else but the extension of affirmation to either entity.

By the way, it should be noted that our claim is that the signification here consists exclusively of the extension of affirmation thus excluding that it consists also of the request/demand for affirmation. This is justified by the fact that in the perspective that formulates itself from the vantage point of the relation itself, i.e., from the vantage point of the in-between (and this after all is the perspective that arises within the context of the dimension-of-consciousness), the request/demand for affirmation does not arise. For with respect to the relation itself, to the in-between, there can be no need for affirmation that, in turn, may dictate a request/demand for affirmation. A need for affirmation can and does arise only with respect to the entity that constitutes itself at the pole of the relation, more specifically, at the pole of the relation that is an I-Thou relation, a relation of address (and not an I-It relation, a relation of utilization). For the entity constituting itself at the pole of an I-Thou relation (and clearly the relation here is an I-Thou relation, seeing that it arises within the context of the dimension-of-consciousness) is an entity that possesses self-consciousness and such an entity, as we have argued above, does indeed require affirmation for it to come into, and maintain itself within, existence. But if this be so (namely, that in the perspective that formulates itself from the vantage point of the in-between of the relation, and not from the vantage point of the pole of the relation, one encounters only the aspect of the extension of affirmation but not also the aspect of the request/demand for affirmation), then the whole question of whether a linkage between the extension of affirmation and the request/demand for affirmation is synchronic or diachronic and thus whether or not such a linkage can indeed be inextricable, is really beside the point—having only the extension of affirmation, the question of linkage does not arise (though the implication would seem to be that if the request/demand for affirmation were somehow to be introduced into the picture here, its linkage with the extension of affirmation would be synchronic and not diachronic, thus making the linkage inextricable, seeing that we have here only one relation and not a multiplicity of relations inasmuch as the relation precedes ontologically the entity, thus precluding the possibility of having a multiplicity of entities, each emanating a single relation, which as such would have indeed introduced a multiplicity of relations).

Further, it may be relevant to our discussion here to also point out that since the "stuff" which makes up the reality within the dimension-of-consciousness constitutes itself in terms of consciousness and consciousness, unlike power, does not implicate motion and, indeed, commensurate with this, seeing that the primary, most fundamental expression of consciousness is in terms of the self-enclosed relation of authentic mutuality (i.e., the relation as delineated above and not a relation made up of two one-way relations moving in opposite directions imposed on each other), a good case can be made that here with respect to such a relation of authentic mutuality (and in contra-distinction to the primary, most fundamental expression within the dimension-of-power, i.e., to the entity with its one-way relation protrusions) a transcending of temporality, of the flux, takes place. As Buber rightly observed, the relation of authentic mutuality, the I-Thou relation, subsists in an eternal present—there is no earlier and later, past and future, seeing that there is no motion and consequently no passage of time (time cannot arise in the absence of motion) either beyond or within the relation. There can be no motion beyond the relation inasmuch as it is the ultimate expression here and therefore it itself cannot be grounded in anything beyond it—the relation itself cannot be placed within a flux. Likewise, there can be no real motion within the relation inasmuch as the relation here is in no way a one-way relation (which as such would have indeed implicated a movement from one point to another)—the vibration, the oscillation, characterizing the relation here is at best, so to speak, a movement in place. And this being the case, it means that within the context of the dimension-of-consciousness no mechanism can arise that would yield a linkage that is diachronic; the only mechanism that can arise within the context of the dimension-of-consciousness is a mechanism that would yield a linkage that is synchronic. And this, in turn, means that the only linkage that can be established within the context of the dimension-of-consciousness is a linkage that is inextricable. Thus, the bottom line is that within the context of the dimension-of-consciousness (and this after all is what really counts, in the last analysis, with respect to the issue of affirmation) we do not, and indeed cannot, have a diachronic linkage between the request/demand for and the extension of affirmation (either because both are grounded in one and the same relation or, more accurately, because only the extension of, but not the request/demand for, affirmation find expression here), which means that if a linkage between the request/demand for and the extension of affirmation can be established here at all, such a linkage would have to be inextricable and this, in turn, means that the right to request/demand affirmation is safeguarded in this context against being left vacuous.

But it must be admitted that the dimension-of-consciousness, when taken exclusively in its own terms (when it is, so to speak, in a pure state, i.e., a pure dimension-of-consciousness), is not really available to us in our common experience. Indeed, in our common experience we can have no direct encounter with it. For in order for anything to be encountered in our common experience, that thing has to be mediated to us by or, put slightly differently, "refracted" for us through, the dimension-of-power (without the mediation of our body and its senses, and these are clearly expressions of the dimension-of-power, nothing can present itself in our common experience, and such mediation necessarily implicates the "refraction" of the mediated by the conditions characterizing the mediator). Indeed, what is given to us in our common experience is not the pure dimension-of-consciousness but the dimension-of-consciousness that is already "refracted" through the dimension-of-power; and it is only from this "refracted" dimension-of-consciousness that we can, through inference, catch glimpses of what the state of affairs is really like in the pure dimension-of-consciousness, i.e., in the dimension-of-consciousness when it is not "refracted" through the dimension-of-power.

Now, the "refraction" here is effected by a shift in perspective, a shift from a perspective that emanates from the vantage point which grounds itself in the in-between of the relation (i.e., in the very essence of what constitutes the authentic relation of mutuality) to a perspective that emanates from the vantage point which grounds itself in the pole of the relation (i.e., in the entity constituting itself at either pole of the relation). This shift brings about a number of significant changes. Thus, to begin with, it introduces the aspect of the request/demand for affirmation into the picture here so that now, in addition to the aspect of extending affirmation (this aspect emanating from the very signification of the relation which arises within the context of the dimension-of-consciousness, the relation, by its very essence, being here a relation of affirmation), we also have the aspect of the request/demand for affirmation; and indeed, not only does the shift introduce the aspect of the request/demand for affirmation, but it gives it precedence over the aspect of extending affirmation, seeing that from the vantage point of the entity at the pole (such an entity with respect to the relation here being of necessity an entity which possesses self-consciousness) the request/demand for affirmation is its primary expression inasmuch as its very coming into existence and its ability to sustain itself within it is contingent on its receiving affirmation. From the vantage point of the entity at the pole, it is the request/demand for affirmation which in its turn implicates the need for the extension of affirmation and not the other way around, and this clearly gives the priority to the aspect of the request/demand for affirmation over the aspect of the extension of affirmation.

Furthermore, the shift here from the in-between of the relation to the pole of the relation "fractures" the single two-way relation into two one-way relations—we get now one one-way relation proceeding from pole A to pole B requesting/demanding affirmation and a second one-way relation proceeding from pole B to pole A extending affirmation. But clearly, such a "fracture" introduces a diachronic linkage between the two one-way relations and thus between the request/demand for affirmation and the extension of affirmation, which, in turn, means that, the linkage between the two is not inextricable and that consequently there is no guaranty that the right to request/demand affirmation would not be left vacuous.

Now, in a way, this is certainly a heavy price that the dimension-of-power exacts for "refracting" the non-"refracted" dimension-of-consciousness. At the same time there is also a great benefit to be derived here, seeing that the "refraction" here enables us to gain a glimpse into the state of affairs that obtains within the non-"refracted" dimension-of-consciousness and, indeed, as such enabling us to ascertain that in the non-"refracted" dimension-of-consciousness there obtains a mechanism which excludes the possibility of a diachronic linkage and thus safeguards the right to request/demand affirmation from being left vacuous (the point here is being presented in the negative, namely, stating the exclusion of the possibility of a diachronic linkage rather than the establishment of a synchronic linkage, because, as we have seen, in the non-"refracted" dimension-of-consciousness the aspect of the request/demand for affirmation may not arise to begin with and consequently the very issue of linkage is beside the point). For after all, seeing that the very notion of affirmation can arise only within the context of the dimension-of-consciousness, establishing that the set-up within such a context, when it is not "refracted," would exclude the possibility of a diachronic linkage, thus also excluding the possibility of the right to request/demand affirmation being left vacuous, is a significant datum.

Clearly, the issue of the right to request/demand affirmation being left vacuous can really arise and be relevant only in the context of a "refracted" dimension-of-consciousness. Still, even so, notwithstanding the fact that the "refraction" seems to introduce a set-up which would preclude the safeguarding of the right to request/demand affirmation from being left vacuous (as for example, in its splitting of the one two-way relation into two one-way relations that are in a diachronic relationship), a case can be made that the "refracted" dimension-of-consciousness does manage nonetheless to retain a synchronic linkage between the request/demand for affirmation and the extension of affirmation, thus safeguarding after all the right to request/demand affirmation from being left vacuous. The "refracted" dimension-of-consciousness brings this about, even though it splits the single two-way relation into two one-way relations, by not dividing the request/demand for affirmation and the extension of affirmation between the two relations, arrogating the request/demand for affirmation to one relation and the extension of affirmation to the other relation (and, of course, as such clearly establishing a diachronic linkage between the two). Rather, it arrogates both the request/demand for affirmation and the extension of affirmation to both relations. Each of the two one-way relations that were split from the original single two-way relation is invested with both the request/demand for affirmation and the extension of affirmation. The split of the single relation into two relations does not entail here a parallel split between the request/demand for affirmation and the extension of affirmation—the two remain linked but now expressing themselves in two relations rather than in one (in splitting the single two-way relation into two one-way relations the "refracted" dimension-of-consciousness does, so to speak, do the bidding of the dimension-of-power, while in arrogating both the request/demand for affirmation and the extension of affirmation to each of the two one-way relations, the "refracted" dimension-of-consciousness preserves its non-refractory character). In this way the "refracted" dimension-of-consciousness retains a synchronic linkage, and thus a linkage that remains inextricable, between the request/demand for affirmation and the extension of affirmation despite the fact that it splits the single two-way relation into two separate one-way relations.

Now, the mechanism within the "refracted" dimension-of-consciousness that can bring about such a state of affairs, i.e., that can arrogate both the request/demand for affirmation and the extension of affirmation to one and the same one-way relation, may perhaps be grasped in the following way. As we have already seen above, an entity which possesses self-consciousness (and the entity constituting itself at the pole of a relation signifying affirmation is, per force, an entity which possesses self-consciousness) is forced by its very ontological constitution to request/demand affirmation, seeing that its very coming into existence and its maintaining itself within existence is contingent on its receiving affirmation. But now, and here lies the twist that makes such double arrogation to one and the same relation feasible, the way in which such an entity goes about expressing, i.e., communicating, its request/demand for affirmation is by extending affirmation to any and all other entities (we can perhaps see this process taking place in little children who, before maturing enough to anticipate which kind of entity is likely to respond, relate to any and all other entities as personal entities). Entities devoid of self-consciousness would of course remain unaffected by such extension of affirmation, and this clearly would put an end to the process here. On the other hand, entities possessing self-consciousness would, so to speak, pick up, i.e., acknowledge, the affirmation extended to them and in so doing extend, in return, their affirmation to the sending entity, this extended affirmation implicating, in turn, its own request/demand for affirmation (notwithstanding the fact that such affirmation has already been extended).[32] In this connection we may also submit that our delineation here of the mechanism implicated in the attainment of affirmation may perhaps suggest an analogue (albeit not in every respect) in the mechanism implicated in the workings of radar. Thus, for example, like the mechanism implicated in the workings of radar where the radar waves are projected to any and all objects in space, so too in the mechanism implicated in the attainment of affirmation, the affirmation is extended to any and all other entities. Or again, like the mechanism implicated in the workings of radar where the object makes its presence known to the sender by, so to speak, picking up and returning the radar waves that have impinged upon it, so too the other in the mechanism implicated in the attainment of affirmation makes its presence as an entity possessing self-consciousness known to the sender by picking up, i.e., acknowledging, and thus extending to the sender, in return, the affirmation extended to it; and conversely, when an object does not pick up the radar waves and deflect them back to the sender (as is the case, for example, with the stealth bomber), it remains undetected, so too an other possessing self-consciousness who chooses not to acknowledge the affirmation extended to it remains unknown to the sender as a bearer of self-consciousness. True, a fundamental difference between the two mechanisms does remain nonetheless inasmuch as in the case of radar the relation between sender and receiver is clearly a one-way relation while in the case of attaining affirmation the relation is a two-way relation where the receiver is at one and the same time, also the sender. Still, the parallelism between the two mechanisms suggested here may hopefully be of some help to us in grasping more clearly the mechanism implicated in the workings of attaining affirmation. In this way, in each of the two one-way relations that the "refraction" presents us with, i.e., the relation from sender to receiver and the relation from receiver to sender, the request/demand for affirmation and the extension of affirmation are synchronically linked, thus establishing a linkage between the two that is inextricable and so safeguarding the right to request/demand affirmation from being left vacuous.

We may conclude, therefore, that a right to request/demand affirmation, which is tantamount to being a right to life (in the sense of being a right not to have one's existence terminated), can be established, and that furthermore such a right is not left vacuous, which is to say, that an obligation to extend affirmation to the other can equally be established (and as we have seen, it can be established not only on the basis of fairness but also on the basis of the mechanism operating within the dimension-of-consciousness, the dimension to which the phenomenon affirmation properly belongs). The one proviso that must be introduced here is that such establishing of both the right to request/demand affirmation and the obligation to extend affirmation, which is to say, the right to request/demand that one's existence not be terminated and the obligation to honor such a request/demand, can take place only in the context where both the entities claiming such a right and the entities placed under obligation to honor it must be entities possessing self-consciousness, i.e., entities that ontologically constitute themselves, at least in part, as Thou entities, which is to say, that they can only be human entities or the biblical God. But such a limitation should present no problem for us, seeing that we had already to conclude in the preceding chapter that the enterprise of ethics can, in the last analysis, take place only with respect to acts/relations that subsist between humans and, for our purposes here, we can add between humans and the biblical God. The biblical God was excluded from the delineation in the preceding chapter inasmuch as the ethical enterprise was delineated there in terms of evaluation/judgment (which, in turn, implicated prescription) and for this to have, so to speak, "cash value," the option and the capacity to act/relate in more than one way must be available, an option and a capacity that are not available to the biblical God, seeing that it constitutes itself exclusively as a pure Thou entity.[33] Thus, the positing of the biblical God as an It/Thou god, wile allowing the biblical God to be encompassed within the ethical enterprise, carries with it two serious weaknesses, the first being that it precipitates the problematic of theodicy, and the second being that the solution for overcoming the problematic that can be offered within its context is unacceptable. But with regard to our concerns here, namely, the concern with the establishing of a right to request/demand affirmation and the concern with the imposition of an obligation to extend affirmation, the biblical God is clearly to be included. After all, the biblical God is the Thou entity *par excellence* and as such it, more than any other entity, is endowed with the right to request/demand affirmation and, at the same time and equally so, is constrained with the obligation to extend affirmation.

We may conclude, therefore, that with respect to entities who possess self-consciousness, i.e., entities who at least in part of their ontological structure are constituted as Thou-beings, and only with respect to such entities, a right which is an *ethical* right to request/demand affirmation (thus an ethical right to life in the sense of not having one's existence terminated) and, commensurate to this, an obligation which, again, is an *ethical* obligation to extend affirmation, thus safeguarding the ethical right here from being left vacuous, can be established.

Notes

1. A possible alternative way to account for the refraction of the notion of the right as such into the various qualified rights such as the legal, political, natural or ethical rights is to suggest that the qualifications indicate and, indeed, come about because of the various kinds of acts upon which the right can impinge (rather than because of the various sources of empowerment that suggest themselves). Thus, for example, a legal right would be a right that impinges on acts that fall within the purview of the law (e.g., the right to a *habeas corpus* or the right to a trial by one's peers) while a political right would be a right that impinges on acts that pertain to the political domain (e.g., the right to vote, to hold office or to assemble) and so on.

2. Of course, as we have seen, there are a number of different perceptions of how the ethical enterprise constitutes itself and this, in turn, would clearly present us with different sources for the empowerment of the ethical right. Thus, for example, in a positivist perception (i.e., that which is tantamount to what we referred above as the "societal ethics" formulation) the source of empowerment would be placed in custom and convention while in a religionist perception (i.e., that which is tantamount to what we referred above as the "religious ethics" formulation) the source of empowerment would be placed in divine revelation. However, neither of these sources can enter the picture here, seeing that neither of these two perceptions underlying the two sources here has been embraced by us. Clearly, the source that would enter the picture here is the source that is implicated by the perception underlying our delineation of the

ethical enterprise, a delineation which clearly intimates that the source of empowerment for the ethical right is to be located in the ontological structure of the entity claiming for itself an ethical right.

3. Actually, it is with the first signification particularly (i.e., the signification whereby a potential living entity is to possess an ethical right to demand that it be brought into life) that we have no occasion at all to deal with. As regards the second signification (i.e., the signification whereby a living entity is to possess an ethical right to demand of others that every effort be made to sustain it in life), we do actually have occasion below to deal with it in connection with the issue of withholding and/or terminating life-support. But this signification comes here into the picture, so to speak, by the side door, and our dealing with it is rather peripheral.

4. For a very lucid and incisive presentation of this thesis readily accessible to the layman, see Dyson 1988, 54–73.

5. The differences by which life in the animal domain is differentiated from life in the domain of plants, such differences as, for example, mobility versus fixation or metabolism in terms of carbon compounds versus metabolism in terms of photosynthesis, are clearly secondary to the common characteristics of metabolic and replicatory processes which define biological life and which are clearly present in both the animal domain and the domain of plants. As such, the distinction between the animal domain and the domain of plants merely signifies subdivisions within the category of biological life.

6. Animals of course are not bothered by this consideration of ethical right and wrong and therefore will presumably go on surviving by doing the ethically wrong, i.e., consuming other animals or plants. Man, however, is the entity that is faced with this irresolvable dilemma. He is damned if he does and he is damned if he does not. In either case he must kill and the killing will be viewed as murder. In order to exist he must bring the existence of some entities endowed with life to termination and this is tantamount to murder; and if he is to refrain from committing such murder, then he of necessity brings his existence to termination, i.e., he indubitably commits suicide, and this is tantamount to an act of murder. Even more paradoxically, if the rationale is to be derived from the notion of life as a biological category, it is very likely that one would be called upon to commit a killing in order to prevent a killing that is deemed as murder. Namely, inasmuch as animals, in all probability would not be much bothered by this ethical consideration of right and wrong (i.e., concerned about doing the right act and avoiding doing the wrong one) and consequently would consume plants or other animals in order to sustain themselves in existence, they would have from the vantage point of this rationale to be viewed as aggressors and murderers and therefore, from the ethical vantage point, it would be incumbent upon one to proceed and kill those animals in order to save the existence of their potential victims from being terminated. For in terms of this rationale, plants possess life in the same sense as animals or humans do and consequently have the same right to have their existence protected from murder in the same way that animals or humans do. But surely this conclusion, though logically consistent, is quite absurd. It means

that if this world is to conduct itself by the dictates of ethics, neither humans nor animals could exist in it; only plants, ethically speaking, could rightfully exist in this world, seeing that plants to not need to consume another source of biological life in order to sustain themselves in existence.

Of course, in the competition for water and light, plants often can cause the termination of the existence of other plants. But the termination of existence here is not the result of a direct act of consummation by the offending plant (let us refer to it as plant A). Rather it comes about as a byproduct of the activity of it towards a third party, e.g., water or light (and let us refer to this as C) which both it and the other plant (let us refer to it as plant B) need for their respective existence. Namely, the termination of B's existence is not the result of A's consummation of B (as is the case with carnivorous animals). Rather it is the result of both A and B requiring C for their existence to continue and A pre-empting C so that B is left devoid of C (as, for example, if there is not enough water to go to B or A, by virtue of its location and size, blocks the sunlight from reaching B). Clearly, we have here, ethically speaking, a different case in the termination of B's existence by A than we have in the case of carnivorous animals. The ethical right to life, as we delineated it, would not quite apply to B here. For given our delineation of the ethical right to life, B's possession of such a right would entitle it to claim that its existence should not be terminated by a direct act of A. It does not entitle it to claim that A should not procure the things it needs for its existence or move its location or change its size so that it can go on existing. Thus, the situation is, in the last analysis, different in the plant domain than it is in the animal domain. Indeed, the difference expresses itself most fundamentally in the fact that while in the animal domain for an entity to go on existing it must consume, i.e., terminate the existence of, another biological entity (another animal or plant), this is not the case in the plant domain. Here, in the plant domain, what an entity requires in order to go on existing, to with, water and light, is clearly something which is not biological life. In this sense, plants are the only form of biological life that does not need to terminate the existence of other biological life in order to survive and in this way it is the only form of biological life that can exist and survive without having to commit the ethically wrong act.

7. What we do have a right to expect is that whatever criterion is being used (regardless of how the criterion is being determined, whether it be determined by illegitimate psychological considerations or by legitimate logical considerations), the application of the criterion must be consistent. Thus, if one is to use life in the biological sense as the criterion and it is determined that this criterion encompasses the animal domain, then one must indeed practice strict vegetarianism. Specifically, this means that to be logically consistent, those who oppose abortion on the basis of defending life in the biological sense must also be strict vegetarians. Namely, if one is to oppose the termination of the existence of the fetus on the grounds that it manifests life in the biological sense, then one must at the same time also oppose the termination of the existence of the cow or chicken on the same ground that they manifest life in the biological sense, and if the former act is an act of murder, so is the latter

act.

8. Indeed, one may even attempt to argue that there may not be a legitimate boundary between the realm of biological life and that of inanimate nature, and that the continuum is thus to be also extended downward to include the realm of inanimate nature. Thus, by the same token that we have a problem to determine whether an ameba or a bacteria is a plant or an animal life we would also have a problem to determine whether it is merely a protean molecule (thus belonging to inanimate nature) or a primitive form of plant or animal life.

9. By the way, however, it is interesting to note that a great many of the proponents of a more extreme and rigid anti-abortion stance (i.e., proponents of the prohibition of abortion from a moment very early in pregnancy if not, indeed, from the very moment of conception) do seem to accept the rationale provided by this formulation as satisfactory. Namely, they indeed seem to take it for granted that it is self-evident that being a member of the human species endows one with the right to life, with the rightful claim not to have his/her existence terminated. Thus, for example, see the position implied in Wertheimer 1971, or that implied in Noonan 1968, or that implied in Brody 1978a, 1978b. Indeed, given the very conservative position regarding the issue of abortion taken by these authors (the first two reflecting the Catholic stance while the last reflecting the conservative trend in Jewish Orthodoxy), it is understandable, we would submit, that they should want to take it for granted that the sanctity of human life, the right of each and every human not to have its existence terminated, is a self-evident given. For by doing this, they clearly avoid the thorny and difficult task of having to come up with a rationale and a justification for why humans, but not other living entities, have the right not to have their existence terminated (thus conveniently avoiding having to deal with a question that may well doom their conservative position regarding the issue of abortion); instead, they provide themselves with a task that is much more tractable and amenable to their conservative position, to wit, the task of determining the point at which human life begins, i.e., the point at which an entity becomes human. For clearly, since they take it for granted that a human being *ipso facto* carries with it the right not to have its existence terminated, the instance a human life comes into existence, its sanctity, i.e., its right not to have its existence terminated, is also automatically established. Consequently, what is crucial and all-important in this context is to determine the point at which human life begins.

Indeed, this shift by which the question "at what point does human life begin?" becomes the central and all-determining question (rather than the question "by virtue of what does human life have a rightful claim not to have its existence terminated?") is a shift that actually plays right into the hands of the conservative anti-abortion position by clearly opening up the possibility for a very early determination of the beginning of human life. For inasmuch as the adjective "human" is taken here to signify nothing else but a membership in a certain class of entities (it being claimed that this membership as such and by itself bestows the right to life!) and inasmuch as the members of this class, as indeed the members of all other classes of entities which likewise manifest the characterization of life, are inescapably embedded in an unceasing continuous process of change, of development (precisely because of the characterization of life that they manifest—life means change), it is really not feasible to have *within* this continuum any point that can signify such a qualitative change, i.e., the beginning of membership in the class of humans. *Within* a continuum, every antecedent point differs only quantitatively and as such, of course, the ongoing difference is reducible to an infinitesimally minute quantitative change so that at any point the immediately preceding point is almost indistinguishable. Thus, in looking for the beginning point, where membership in the class of humans is to be instigated, by retracing the steps backward from the state of the adult human, there would be no point within the continuum that would qualify until we come to the point of conception. It is only here, it may be argued, that we can, for the first time, step out of the continuum. For it is only from this point, the point of conception, that we have an entity that can be arrogated to the class of humans, seeing that if the human is to be taken as such, i.e., if it is to be defined exclusively in terms of its biological constitution (and after all the proposal here is to ground the justification for a right to life in the mere fact that the entity in question belongs to the class of humans as it is defined biologically), then it is defined exclusively by virtue of its possession of a certain complement of genes (an ever so slightly different complement would define a different class of entities) and that such a complement first presents itself at the point of conception. Thus, indeed, the phenomenon of humanness (perceived in biological terms) and the continuum that characterizes it do begin at the point of conception and consequently the only points from which a stepping out from this continuum would be feasible would be those which precede the point of conception.

But is this really so? Is the point of conception really the first instance where the complement of genes defining the class of humans first presents itself? Is not the complement of genes defining the class of humans already present at a point prior to conception as, for instance, in the male's sperm or in the females's ova? And, if this be the case, then why stop at conception and not proceed further down the continuum and claim a right to life for the sperm or the unfertilized ovum? Indeed, if we are not mistaken, such a claim on behalf of spilt human sperm was put forth by some Christian theologians in medieval times and certainly the biblical text of Leviticus, which condemns masturbation, may be seen as making the same claim. Of course, one can counter this claim by arguing that, while it is true that sperm and ova do indeed already present the complement of genes that define the class of humans, they in themselves cannot be viewed as separate, distinct members of that class but only as parts, organs, of their bearers (similarly to other organs such as the liver or the kidneys), the bearer being the member of the class of humans. And this is so, not so much because they cannot have an independent existence outside their bearers' bodies (anyway, this would not really apply to the sperm which can be ejaculated), but because the sum-total of the genes contained in their complement of chromosomes is exactly identical to that which constitutes the complement of chromosomes of their bearers. For the status of being a distinct, separate member of the class is defined by the possession of a distinct, unique, combination of genes that no other member possesses. And such a distinct, unique, combination of genes first arises only at conception. At conception, an entity (i.e., a zygote) comes into existence that possesses a set of genes that is uniquely its own (a new and unique selection from two antecedent sets) and as such it constitutes itself as a distinct, separate, member of the human class and not just as an additional organ or a growth in the mother's body. It is only from this point, from the point of conception, and not prior to it, that a new member of the class of humans comes into existence, and since the claim is that the right to life is bestowed on members of the class of humans but not on any of their organs or parts, it is only from the point of conception and not from any point prior to it that a right to life can be established in this context, i.e., in the context of the position that claims that the mere membership in the class of humans endows an entity with the right to life. (By the way, on this logic, if a human individual were to be cloned, something which in principle, if not in practice, is already feasible, the cloned entity is not to be viewed as a distinct, independent member in the class of humans but rather as an extension, an organ, of the human individual from whom it was cloned and consequently as an entity devoid of the right to life; but is the cloned entity still to be viewed as an organ rather than as a distinct, independent entity and thus as an entity devoid of the right to life after the "parent" entity ceases to exist?)

We should be clear, however, about the role that the factor of uniqueness plays here in providing the rationale for the claim to a right to life. Directly, it plays no role—the rationale is made here exclusively in terms of the factor of membership in the class of humans. The factor of uniqueness (i.e., uniqueness in terms of the set of genes defining the individual and not just in terms of the spatio-temporal location of the individual, a uniqueness which characterizes each and every individual) does not play any role here in providing a rationale for the claim to a right to life. It is an accompaniment, an inescapable accompaniment, to being a member in the class of humans (i.e., it is an inescapable characterization of any and every member of the class of humans), but the rationale for a right to life made on behalf of humans is not formulated here in its terms—it is formulated in terms of the belongingness as such to the class of humans.

But, of course, this is not to say that one could not, so to speak, move beyond the mere notion of membership and attempt to formulate the rationale for a right to life in terms of the notion of uniqueness that characterizes any and every member of the class of humans. Indeed, such a move has been undertaken by the eminent Christian ethicist Paul Ramsey, who has claimed that a right to life on behalf of the human individual can be established and justified on the basis that each human individual is qualitatively unique and therefore irreplaceable.

But this formulation does not, in our judgment, fare any better than the preceding formulation, i.e., the formulation in terms of membership in the class of humans. For what is there in the notion of uniqueness that can provide a persuasive rationale and justification for not terminating the existence of entities which possess it? Why allow terminating the existence of entities that are not unique but not of entities that are unique? One possible retort that comes readily to mind is that with respect to entities that are unique, no replacement is possible. This is true. But then, so what? Why is it important to have these entities represented in existence? And anyway, eventually they will have to die a natural death and will not be replaceable. There is no escape from lacunae occurring with respect to unique entities.

And if the retort is to be that we derive the rationale and justification for the claim to the right to life not so much from the fact that we desire this particular unique entity to be *always* present in existence but rather from the fact that we place the highest value on enriching creation in the sense of wanting to have the greatest degree of variety of entities to have existed at one time or another, then aside from having to question whether we really have or ought to have such a desire and, even if we did, whether such a desire really deserves to be invested with the highest value, the further basic question remains of whether the claim to a right to life on behalf of entities that are unique really safeguards and promotes the richness of the variety of entities, seeing that these unique entities, even if they were devoid of the right to life would have already existed prior to the termination of their existence and thus would have had occasion to add their unique, so to speak, "ontological flavor" to the richness of the ontological variety of creation (though in fairness to Ramsey, he is speaking of terminating the life of the fetus which is viewed as a being not yet fully developed, completed, but only a potential of its full-fledged being, so that the termination of its existence, i.e., the interruption of its development, would indeed deprive creation of its "ontological flavor," seeing that it is unique and therefore irreplaceable). In addition, it would not be amiss to point out that on the basis of this rationale and justification which ground themselves in the notion of uniqueness, one would, in all probability, have to extend such a right to life to the individual members of a number of other classes in the animal kingdom (seeing that in the more advanced classes, e.g., among chimpanzees, one can discern uniqueness in individuals just like among humans) while, at the same time, having to deny such a right to life to a human individual who is a paternal twin, seeing that he/she is not qualitatively, i.e., genetically, unique. Clearly, a rationale in terms of uniqueness cannot be persuasive if it entails such ramifications.

But to return to the main point we are trying to make here, we have seen that by making the mere membership of an individual in the class of humans tantamount to bestowing upon it the right to life, we are also, for all intents and purposes, fixing the point of such a bestowal very early in the process of pregnancy. Indeed, to the extent that in determining the beginning of human life the emphasis in the notion of "human life" is placed on the "human" (i.e., on the instigation of membership in the class of humans), the point of bestowing the right to life must be as early as conception (this being, by the way, the position of the Catholic Church); on the other hand, however, if the emphasis in the notion of "human life" is shifted from the "human" to "life," the bestowing of the right to life would clearly shift to a point where some indication of biological life, such as motility, a heart-beat or a brain-wave, would manifest itself and this, in turn, clearly means that the bestowal of the right to life would now come at a point somewhat later than conception, though still, relatively speaking, quite early in the process of pregnancy. Indeed, it is precisely in terms of this differentiation (i.e., the differentiation between emphasizing "human" as against emphasizing "life" in the notion of "human life") that we can see why Brody recommends using the onset of brain-waves as the point marking the beginning of human life while Wertheimer and Noonan recommend using conception—clearly for Brody the emphasis in the notion of "human life" is on "life" while for Wertheimer and Noonan it is on "human."

10. In addition, by the way, it should be noted that this capacity of consciousness, i.e., the capacity to be aware of an other, is by no means unique to the human. Certainly, the more advanced animals, such as primates and certain mammals, do possess this capacity. As such, if the aspect of consciousness could indeed be taken as the source which can provide us with the desired rationale and justification, then the right to life, i.e., the right not to have one's existence terminated, would have to be extended and attributed not only to the class of humans but also to the classes of the more advanced animals. Indeed, inasmuch as these animals manifest more clearly the attribute of consciousness than human fetuses, and even than human infants (certainly in the first months of their lives), and seeing that the right to life is to be determined by the manifestation of this attribute, these animals should have a weightier claim to this right than human fetuses or infants in their first months of life. In this respect, the case that Peter Singer makes on behalf of animals' rights is quite persuasive (see, for example, Singer 1980).

11. By the way, the case can also be made that the aspects of sentience and rationality are much more specifically and exclusively human than the aspect of consciousness as mere awareness of an other, though this is not completely so. Namely, while consciousness as mere awareness of an other is quite prevalent in the animal kingdom, sentience and rationality are noticeably less so. Still, even so, a case can be made that in the more advanced animal species these aspects of sentience and rationality are in some sense present and thus that they too are not the exclusive possession of the human species. These aspects, like the aspect of consciousness, fall within a continuum that operates within evolution, and from this perspective the human can be seen as included within the animal kingdom—the most advanced animal thus far. So, while it is true that sentience and rationality are more characteristically human than consciousness as mere awareness is, the difference is not qualitative but only quantitative.

12. Not surprisingly, Glover's position betrays the eudemonistic-utilitarian approach that characterizes so much of the ethical thinking done in the context of Anglo-Saxon analytic philosophy. Much of the interesting contemporary work in ethics is done in the context of this philosophy and, therefore, one must take it very seriously; we should, however, admit up front that, in the last

analysis, we do not find the approach taken by this philosophy acceptable. Of course, here is not the place to undertake a thorough and careful analysis of this approach so as to substantiate our conclusion. But since we shall be dealing in the text below with criticism directed at Glover's proposed answer, and since this answer is clearly formulated in the context of this approach, i.e., in the context of the eudemonistic-utilitarian approach, we should briefly present here our criticism of two basic features which characterize this approach (in the text below, in connection with our specific criticism of Glover's position, some additional criticism of this approach would be presented).

The first feature is the exclusive emphasis that this approach places on the bottom line, on the end result, irrespective of any differences that may obtain with respect to the means by which it is attained; specifically, it is the neglect, nay, the actual rejection, of the claim that, ethically speaking, there is a significant difference between a means implicating an active involvement and a means implicating a passive involvement in the bringing about of the end result. Thus, for example, Glover and other utilitarians fail to see any difference of an ethical significance between the person who actively murders another person and a person who could have saved another person from death but fails to do so (Glover 1977, 92–94, 98–99, 116). There is no difference between actually drowning another person and not jumping into the lake to save a drowning person (assuming, of course, that one can swim and could have saved the drowning person). Since the end result is the same, it is immaterial, ethically speaking, whether it is brought about because of one's active agency or because of one's passive failure to prevent it from occurring.

The second feature consists in the quantification of the criterion of the good or of happiness, thus introducing a calculus into the picture here on the basis of which one can compare alternative states of happiness with regard to the degree of happiness they implicate and on the basis of this, in turn, choose between the competing alternatives and decide what trade-offs may or may not be acceptable. Thus, for example, if one has to choose between saving the life of an old, ordinary, run-of-the-mill, simple person and the life of a young, extremely talented person, one would opt, according to this calculus, for the latter alternative, seeing that it clearly yields the greater quantity of a life worth living. Or alternatively, if one is confronted with a trade-off between providing the cost for the prolongation of the life of an old ordinary person and using these same resources to provide food and shelter to needy young children, one may well opt for the latter alternative on the basis that it provides the greater quantity of happiness (Glover 1977, 57–58; for the former example see Singer, while for the latter example see Glover 1977).

But surely, neither the first nor the second feature that this approach necessarily implicates would be acceptable to our ethical sensitivity. For as regards the first feature, in making the ethical evaluation dependent exclusively on the objective end result that is obtained, this feature overlooks the significant bearing which the inward intention accompanying the act has on the question of ethical valuation. But the inward intention should have a significant bearing on the question of ethical evaluation. Thus, for example, an act whose intention was to help others but because of an unforeseen turn of events—or even if the turn was in principle foreseeable but the agent was not endowed with the capacity to actually foresee it, or even if he/she were so endowed but somehow did not foresee it—results in the killing of that other (e.g., the giving of a medication that normally heals but because of the presence of some factor that is not foreseen turns lethal) should not be viewed as an act that is ethically reprehensible.

Indeed, while neglect of the intention accompanying the objective act may be understandable with respect to decisions made in the context of the law (though even here it is so only partially and up to a point), it is certainly unacceptable with respect to judgments and evaluations made in the context of ethics; for while the law, by and large, deals with judgments regarding happenings in the external objective reality, ethics essentially deals with judgments regarding occurrences in the realm of intention. And this being the case, it is clearly possible that judgments in the law need not be commensurate with ethical judgments. For it is certainly possible that in two instances the end results occurring in the external objective reality would be the same and yet at the same time the respective accompanying intentions be marked by significant differences. Thus, for example, take the following scenario: In two separate instances a person dies (thus the end result in objective reality is the same in both instances), though in the one instance the person dies in consequence of being drowned by an other while in the other instance the person dies in consequence of not being saved from drowning by an other. Now, ethics should judge these two instances differently (even though the end result in objective reality is the same). And this is so not only or, indeed, primarily because we have a difference between activity and passivity—the difference between actively doing something wrong and passively not doing something right. For with respect to this difference one could argue that, in the last analysis, the difference really cancels itself out with regard to the end result, seeing that the opposition of doing and not doing, of activity and passivity, is with respect to diametrically contradictory acts—action with respect to a wrongful act (the act of drowning an other) and passive with respect to a rightful act (the act of extending a helping, saving hand)—and clearly the doing of a wrongful act equals the not doing of a rightful act (the plus, i.e., the adding, of a minus quantity equals the minus, i.e., the subtracting, of a plus quantity). What is really the significant cause here, what really constitutes a difference that cannot be canceled out, is that we have operating here two different intentions that are irreducible to each other and the ethical evaluation is carried out essentially with respect to the intentions that accompany the objective act.

One can, perhaps, see this more clearly if we shift the ground from being a difference between intentions to being a difference between the corresponding rights that the negative evaluations of these intentions implicates. Thus, the negative evaluation of the intention to kill an other implicates that other's right not to have its existence terminated, while the negative evaluation of the intention not to extend a helping, saving hand to an other implicates that other's right to have its existence sustained and prolonged. But these two rights are clearly not the same and, therefore, there can be, at least *prima fascia*, no canceling out between the respective ethical evaluations regarding the violation of these rights. We may, indeed, condemn equally the violation of either right (thus letting them, indeed, cancel each other out), but this is not inherently necessitated (and this is the crux of the matter) by the very formulation of the rights involved. We may just as well condemn the violation of the former but not the violation of the latter, or condemn the violation of both but not in equal measure. As such, although the external, objective end result is the same in both instances, it by no means follows that the ethical evaluation must equally be the same.

And as regards the second feature, namely, the introduction of a calculus with respect to the notions of happiness and the good whereby we can proceed to establish priorities of preference which, in turn, would allow us to introduce comparisons and trade-offs between various claims, many of us would find this approach completely unsuitable as regards the claim that is before us, namely, the claim of an entity to its right of existence (either in the signification of not having its existence terminated or in the alternative signification of having its existence sustained and prolonged). For this claim (regardless of what position we may take with respect to other claims) does not lend itself, we would submit, to degrees of validity or of value and thus to comparisons and trade-offs with other claims. Rather, it presents us with an all-or-none alternative, which is to say that if it is established and accepted at all, then it simply cannot be placed in the same league and consequently in any competition with any other possible claim (it being such a fundamental and, indeed, a *sui generis* claim). The situation here is in a way analogous to that which obtains with respect to truly great, creative art. Great paintings or pieces of music cannot be compared so that we can say A is greater than B (e.g., Bach is greater music than Mozart or vice versa) or, even more poignantly, being able to say that A is greater than B by 20, 30 or what have you percentage points. The very idea of establishing such a calculus and thus enabling one to trade off and balance between various values and claims seems absurd and offensive—no doubt because it is guilty of instituting a complete mismatch between the kind of object confronting us and the kind of approach we propose to apply to it. Thus, the claim to a right to existence cannot countenance a quantitative and consequently a comparative approach. But this is precisely the approach Glover, in conformity with the utilitarian orientation, applies to this claim (Glover 1977, 57).

13. True, some would no doubt want to question whether the urge to sustain oneself in existence is indeed as universal as we claimed here. We certainly have Freud's counterclaim expressed in his theory of the death wish which he arrogates to all humans. We also have some instances of animals seeming to periodically commit mass suicide, as, for example, is the case with lemmings.

14. By the way, this last observation is a sure give-away for a utilitarian position, seeing that it is only in the context of utilitarianism that such a position can be maintained. Indeed, for the utilitarian position, the only thing

that counts, in the last analysis, is the bottom line, and therefore if the bottom line of the two positions comes out to be the same, then there can really be no difference of substance between the two positions—like in arithmetic, if two methods lead to the same result, both methods are valued.

15. Of course, this linkage between having desires and having a conception of an entity that possesses desires is valid only on the basis that having desires is determined in the context of intentions, i.e., in the context of inward consciousness, and not in the context of outward behaviorism. If desires are to be the expression of intentions and consciousness and not just a strange, roundabout way of talking about "blind," mechanical patterns of behavior, then clearly one cannot have desires without at the same time having also a consciousness, i.e., a conception, of an entity that possesses such consciousness and intentions. Tooley is aware of this and indeed makes it clear that he conceives of desires in terms of intentions and inward consciousness and not in terms of behavioristic patterns (Tooley 1972, 45).

16. This same conclusion can be arrived at from a different angle. Thus, when a desire to life is delineated in terms of intention, one can very clearly perceive it as a desire for the prolongation of life, a holding on to life, in distinction from being a fear, an avoidance, of or an escape from the threat of death. But when it is delineated behavioristically, this distinction is not available. For this distinction can be established only in the context of inward intention, of consciousness, and as such it can be relegated only to the human being; in the context of outward behavior, the distinction does not manifest itself—the one and the same outward act can signify either—and as such it can no longer be confined exclusively to the human but must be extended to encompass all biologically living entities, certainly all species of the animal kingdom (and in the context of Tooley's proposal, they would consequently all have to be granted the right to life). Indeed, it is we humans, operating from the vantage point of intention, who interpret the behavior of animals as signifying an escape from a perceived threat to life rather than a desire to prolong life. But since, from a behavioristic vantage point, this distinction does not obtain to begin with, we cannot use it to exclude the animal kingdom and establish the case of the human as unique.

17. Before leaving this point, we should note (and, indeed, emphasize) that Tooley's qualification of his delineation of the right to life in terms of the desire for life by the stipulation of there being present no other overriding desire does not really add anything new which is not already per force included as self-evident in the very substance of the formulation itself. For clearly, there can be no rationale or justification for anyone to frustrate or obstruct someone's having that which it desires if there is no other overriding desire present. The qualification therefore merely makes explicit what is already inescapably implicit in the substance of the formulation. And this being the case, there would be no point in offering to remove the qualification in order to escape the problematic of being saddled with a right to life that is not absolute but merely relative. Removing the qualification would not remove the problematic of having a right to life that is merely relative. For the problematic of ending up

with a right to life that is relative is not introduced by the qualification—it is inbuilt into the very substance of the formulation and the qualification merely brings it to the fore. As such, the problematic here is inescapable, seeing that it is located in the very core of the formulation.

18. And if one were tempted to bring as a counter-argument the hypothetical case where the object of the intended act to kill (i.e., entity B in our discourse above) is to be a Hitler and where as such the intended act to kill would not have seemed to implicate that something dreadfully wrong is involved in giving moral approval to the intended act to kill, our response is that the two cases, even though on the surface they may appear to be the same, are in truth not at all similar. This is so because the evaluation of the intended act to kill in the two cases bases itself respectively on two totally different criteria. In the case above it bases itself on the utilitarian calculus—the intended act to kill is morally approved because, in the last analysis, it will yield the greater good and as such it is given the overriding consideration. In the case here, however, where the object of the intended act to kill is Hitler, the evaluation of the intended act does not base itself on the utilitarian calculus. Rather, it bases itself on 1) the wish to stop the perpetration of evil and 2) the wish to mete the appropriate punishment for crimes committed. As such, indeed, there is no contradiction between our feeling in conjunction with the evaluation above, i.e., the evaluation based on the utilitarian calculus, that something is dreadfully wrong with the evaluation and our feeling in conjunction with the evaluation here that the evaluation is morally acceptable. There is no contradiction between feeling that it is morally wrong to kill an innocent person in order to receive a greater good and feeling that it is morally right to kill an evil person in order to stop his/her evildoing and to mete to him/her the appropriate punishment. By the way, the valid analogy to the case above is not the case where the object of the intended act to kill is a Hitler but rather the case where the object is an innocent person who, as in some primitive societies, is sacrificed in the belief that this would induce the gods to bestow benefits on the whole society. And indeed, our reaction to this case is the same as it is to the case above—something is dreadfully wrong in morally approving these acts.

19. Indeed, this problem with Tooley's delineation of moral right in terms of desire can be restated somewhat more poignantly. Namely, we would submit that with regard to a moral right, in contra-distinction to a legal or political right, the right implicates not only its empowerment to sanction or forbid but also the approval and embracement of its content (i.e., what it sanctions or forbids). With regard to a legal or political right, one can concede that it possesses empowerment to sanction or forbid and yet, at the same time, disapprove of its content (i.e., disapprove of what it sanctions or forbids) and, indeed, attempt to cancel it out either by persuasion or by force. This, however, cannot apply to a moral right—one cannot disapprove of its content and want to cancel it out while, at the same time, accepting it as a moral right. Thus, a moral right does of necessity implicate its approval and embrace. But, as we have seen above, Tooley's delineation of the moral right in terms of desire

cannot provide us the rationale for its needed approval and, this being the case, one would have to conclude that, in the last analysis, it fails to establish a right that is a *bona fide* moral right.

20. It may be instructive to briefly spell out our differences with Tooley's formulation on these two points. First, let us turn to the less significant and really not so important difference, namely, the difference in defining the notion of person (the definition which provides the basis for a separation and distinction between the notion of person and that of human being). Thus, in contra-distinction to "human being," which is defined in terms of membership in a certain class of entities, "person," according to Tooley, is to be defined not just as an entity that possesses rights in general but rather as an entity that possesses specifically the right to life—a person is that entity which "has a (serious) moral right to life" (Tooley 1972, 40; by the way, this specificity which is introduced into the definition is, of course, necessary and significant for, clearly, there can be entities that may possess all sorts of rights but not the specific right to life—not everything that has rights must also have a right to life or is, according to this delineation, a person). This move with respect to the definition of "person" in contra-distinction to that of "human being" is extremely valuable and helpful in that it brings clearly to the fore the fact that one cannot go automatically from merely signifying membership in a certain class of entities (that is what the term "human being" signifies—an entity that belongs to the class of humans) to signifying that that entity also possesses a right to life. This move, this linkage, cannot be established by the mere fiat of a definition; rather, it must be argued and demonstrated. In establishing this, Tooley renders very valuable service for he exposes and blocks, as already pointed out, the all too facile and rather dubious attempts by people like Wertheimer or Brody to slip by us such definitional identities.

Tooley, however, does it by letting "human being" be defined in terms of the starting point (i.e., being a member of a certain class of entities called "human") and "person" be defined in terms of the desired end result (i.e., being in possession of a right to life). We, on the other hand, would propose to define "person" not in terms of the desired end result but rather in terms of the specific property that an entity must possess in order to be able to establish the desired end result, i.e., the right to life—a person is that entity which possesses the property that can provide us with a satisfactory rationale for the claim to a right to life. Both definitions are clearly alike in establishing a separation between the signification of "human being" and that of "person," thus establishing the all-important separation between being a human entity and being an entity that has a right to life. But they accomplish this separation differently. For while for both definitions the notion of human being stays the same, i.e., a notion signifying the starting point (to what kind of entity are we referring, i.e., to what class of entities does it belong), the notion of person is arrogated by Tooley's definition to signify the entity that is in the state of the desired end result, i.e., the entity that possesses a right to life, while in our definition it is arrogated to signify the entity that possesses the property by virtue of which the desired end result can be established. The resulting difference is that while

Tooley's definition fails to give us any inkling as to how one is to get from the starting point to the desired end result (it merely establishes that the starting point does not already contain within it the desired end result), the definition we propose to adopt clearly spells out the strategy by which one is to get from the starting point to the desired end result, to wit, one would start by showing how the property identified by the definition can provide us with a satisfactory rationale for the claim involved in the desired end result and then proceed to empirically determine whether a certain entity does or does not possess this property. But as such, we would submit, our formulation possesses a significant advantage which is gained precisely in that it refers itself not to the desired end result but rather, so to speak, to the bridge that links the starting point with the desired end result—because the notion of person is delineated not as the entity that is in the state of the desired end result but rather as the entity that is in the in-between (i.e., while not being in the state of the desired end result, possessing nonetheless the capacity to get there) and thus as the entity that links the starting point with the desired end result. Still, it is true that as to the most fundamental point in the issue that is before us here, i.e., the rejection of the axiomatic identification between the starting point and the desired end result (between being a human entity and being an entity that possesses a right to life), there is really no difference between the two definitions.

21. True, as regards the trait of rational activity, the advanced robots may have the advantage. Still, there are certain animals, like chimpanzees, gorillas or dolphins, which certainly manifest what can be taken as rational activity, thus satisfying this criterion (in any case, Warren's delineation of rational activity as the capacity to solve "relatively complex" problems is too imprecise—where is one to draw the line between relatively complex and relatively uncomplex problems?). On the other hand, however, as regards the trait of consciousness, animals would seem to have the advantage over robots.

22. Still, even so, Tooley's formulation, by virtue of the fact that it includes the trait of self-consciousness, and includes it in a very basic way (seeing that the basic trait implicated by an entity desiring to go on living is the trait of self-consciousness), is much closer to our stance than alternative formulations. Specifically, it is clearly closer than Warren's formulation. For Warren seems to withdraw from the trait of self-consciousness towards the trait of consciousness as such, making the latter the central and predominant trait in her formulation of the rationale and justification for the claim to a right to life. This can be clearly seen from the fact that while trait 5, i.e., the trait of possessing a self-concept and a self-awareness, is completely neglected when she speaks of the traits that are not only manifestations of personhood but are necessary for constituting personhood, trait 1, i.e., the trait of possessing consciousness as such (consciousness of external and/or internal objects and events), is the one trait that constantly appears when Warren speaks about traits that are necessary for the constitution of personhood. It is the one trait that appears both when she speaks about traits that "may well be sufficient" and also when she speaks about traits that "quite probably . . . are sufficient."

23. Before proceeding, however, with this task, we should note one further

difference between our formulation and Tooley's. This difference arises with regard to the definition of the notion of the person in distinguishing it from the notion of the human being (the difference revealing the much more fundamental role assigned to the trait of self-consciousness in our formulation). Namely, in contra-distinction to Tooley's formulation which defines the notion of the person as signifying an entity that possesses a right to life, our formulation would define it as signifying an entity that possesses self-consciousness, i.e., an entity that is constituted by self-consciousness—any entity manifesting self-consciousness would qualify to be designated as a person. Thus, in terms of our formulation, the distinction between the notion of the human being and that of the person would lie in that the former signifies a belongingness to or a membership in a specific species, i.e., the human species (the same signification as in Tooley's formulation), while the latter signifies the possession or manifestation of self-consciousness (a signification different from that delineated in Tooley's formulation). And in terms of this distinction in signification between the notion of the human being and that of the person, we can trace the main outline of the argument by which our formulation would attempt to establish its claim that a human being possesses a right to life in the following way: A human being has a right to life because it is a person, and a person has a right to life because it is an entity endowed with self-consciousness. Thus, in the last analysis, it is in terms of the notion of self-consciousness that we must formulate the rationale and justification for the claim to a right to life. And, of course, whether or not the formulation succeeds will depend on whether or not the rationale and thus the justification that we can put forth in terms of the notion of self-consciousness proves to be persuasive. So, it should be clear that in our formulation everything comes to depend ultimately on whether or not we can establish that the trait of self-consciousness can provide the rationale and justification for a claim to a right to life, i.e., the right of a bearer of self-consciousness not to have its existence terminated.

24. In a way, the very notion of terminating the existence of an entity that constitutes itself in terms of power may well be, in the last analysis, rather misleading. For one can make the case that the existence of entities constituting themselves in terms of power can never be really terminated—they can only be transformed, seeing that such entities place themselves in a continuum of power where the only way by which they can distinguish themselves from one another is in terms of the degree of power manifested in them, the distinction that is thus available here being only of a quantitative but not of a qualitative nature. As such, the disappearance of an entity constituting itself in terms of power (i.e., the termination of its existence) does not really mean the termination, the disappearance, of that which constitutes it, i.e., the power manifested in it, but only its transformation to different levels of manifestation, either through its disintegration into entities manifesting smaller degrees of power or through its incorporation into an entity manifesting a larger degree of power. But in either case its power (i.e., the "stuff" in terms of which it constitutes itself) does not disappear—it merely rearranges itself in different configurations.

As such, indeed, terminating the existence of an entity constituting itself in terms of power is quite a different proposition from terminating the existence of an entity constituting itself in terms of self-consciousness, seeing that the notion of termination in its radical signification (i.e., when it signifies the disappearance from existence of the very "stuff" in terms of which the entity constitutes itself) is applicable only in the latter but not in the former case. Thus, if it is the notion of termination in its radical signification that is implicated when we undertake to establish what kind of an entity can be endowed with an ethical right to request/demand not to have its existence terminated, then clearly an entity constituting itself in terms of power would not qualify, seeing that a notion of termination carrying this signification, i.e., its radical signification, would not be applicable to such an entity. (By the way, it is worth noting that these considerations give rise to yet another significant distinction, namely, the distinction whereby in the context of self-consciousness, i.e., in the context where entities constitute themselves in terms of self-consciousness, each entity constitutes itself as a unique entity, while in the context of power, i.e., in the context where entities constitute themselves in terms of power, the entities do not constitute themselves as unique; and this is so inasmuch as entities which constitute themselves in terms of self-consciousness constitute themselves in terms of the content of the self-consciousness and the content of the self-consciousness in each entity is unique, while entities which constitute themselves in terms of power constitute themselves in terms of the level, of the degree, of power manifested in them and the level, the degree, of power that is manifested can be shared by any number of entities—entities constituting themselves in terms of power can be cloned.)

25. To be more precise, we should, most probably, add the further claim, not with regard to the aspect of the arising of self-consciousness but with regard to the aspect of self-consciousness maintaining itself in existence, that the human, i.e., the entity bearing self-consciousness, has to be isolated also from animals that bond with humans as, for example, dogs. For experience does show that animals such as dogs can substitute, up to a point, for the presence of other humans in supporting a bearer of self-consciousness, i.e., a human entity, in maintaining its self-consciousness. There is much validity in the common observation that such animals do serve as companions to humans. And the rationale for this, we would submit, lies in the fact that entities whose ontological constitution encompasses consciousness as such (in addition, of course, to encompassing power) do possess a capacity to extend affirmation to others, even though they themselves, in turn, do not require affirmation from the outside for their consciousness as such to arise or to maintain itself in existence. It does, of course, follow from this that, according to our claim here, all entities possessing consciousness as such, i.e., all animals, could serve as sources of affirmation. This, in principle, is indeed so. In practice, however, such affirmation could be extended only in instances where the entities possessing consciousness as such interact in a positive way with human entities, and hence the limitation introduced into our claim whereby it is only

the entities possessing consciousness as such, i.e., the animals, which bond with humans that can be taken as sources extending affirmation to human entities and thus being capable to supplant, up to a point, the presence of other human entities.

26. At this point, three brief observations with respect to Buber's identification of the pure Thou entity with the divine entity which is encountered in the various historical expressions of biblical faith may be in order. Firstly, taken at face value, it would appear that Buber's divine entity constituting itself ontologically as a pure Thou entity is not at all congruent with the ontological constitution characterizing the divine entity which is encountered in the various historical expressions of biblical faith and that consequently Buber's claim that the divine entity which is encountered in the various historical expressions of biblical faith is an entity which ontologically constitutes itself exclusively in terms of the Thou-dimension, i.e., as a pure Thou-god, is rather dubious. True, the various historical expressions of biblical faith do introduce the Thou-dimension into the ontological constitution of the divine. Indeed, we would submit, that it is precisely this introduction of the Thou-dimension into the ontological constitution of the divine which distinguishes biblical faith from paganism where the ontological constitution of the divine is exclusively in terms of the It-dimension, i.e., exclusively in terms of power, thus presenting a divine entity that is a pure It-god (and as such, indeed, this does signify a most fundamental breakthrough in the history of religions). But at the same time, it is also true that the various historical expressions of biblical faith do not go all the way in supplanting the It-dimension by the Thou-dimension so as to end up with a pure Thou-god. They, so to speak, get stuck midway so that the divine entity that can be encountered in them is not a pure Thou-god but an It/Thou-god.

Still, a case can be made that, notwithstanding the foregoing observation, there is merit and validity in the claim that the divine entity implicated by the inner logic of biblical faith is, in the last analysis (i.e., when taken in its fullest, ideal manifestation), to be an entity that is ontologically constituted as a pure Thou entity. For the inner logic operating here, as it manifests itself in the act of partially introducing the Thou-dimension into the ontological constitution of the divine (and thus partially supplanting the It-dimension in terms of which it was constituted), points towards the ultimate culmination of this act in the act of fully introducing the Thou-dimension and thus totally supplanting the It-dimension by the Thou-dimension, ending up no longer with an It/Thou divine entity but with a pure Thou divine entity. After all, inasmuch as the distinctive feature of the various historical expressions of biblical faith lies in their introducing the Thou-dimension into the ontological constitution of the divine entity, why stop midway and not proceed all the way in supplanting the It-dimension by the Thou-dimension? Indeed, this point receives added force from the fact that a good case can be made that the various historical expressions of biblical faith not only introduce the Thou-dimension into the ontological constitution of the divine entity but that they further turn to the Thou-dimension for it to define the essential orientation of their respective religious structure (a good example of this, particularly in the case of Judaism, as Gershom Scholem has pointed out, is the insistence *sine-qua-non* that the relation between the divine entity and the world be theistic and the corresponding uncompromising rejection of its being pantheistic) thus relating to the Thou-dimension as, so to speak, the senior partner in the It/Thou ontological constitution characterizing their divine entity. Thus, there is after all a sense in which one could claim that Buber's pure Thou-god validly represents, albeit in the fullest, maximal degree (and thus in an idealized fashion), the divine entity of biblical faith.

Secondly, in comparing the two ontological constitutions ascribed to the divine entity of biblical faith with which we are dealing here (i.e., that of the pure Thou ascribed by Buber and that of the It/Thou ascribed in the various concrete historical expressions of biblical faith), a good case can be made that, with one exception (though admittedly a not insignificant exception), the advantage from the perspective of the Thou-dimension and thus also from the perspective of biblical faith (for after all, as argued above, even in the various concrete historical expressions of biblical faith, where the divine entity is presented not as a pure Thou but as an It/Thou entity, when there is a clash between the dictates of the Thou-dimension and those of the It-dimension, it is the dictates of the Thou-dimension which take priority and prevail over the dictates of the It-dimension) lies with the divine entity which is represented as a pure Thou rather than as an It/Thou entity.

The one significant exception lies in the fact that in a divine entity which is perceived to constitute itself as an It/Thou entity we have the mechanism, due to the presence of the It-dimension in the ontological constitution of the divine entity, by which communication between the divine entity and the human entity (namely, both the communication from the divine to the human, to wit, revelation, and the communication from the human to the divine, to wit, worship *qua* address) is in principle comprehensible and feasible. This is so because, as established above, all communication which we as humans can come to receive from others and to convey to others has to be mediated, "refracted," through the dimension of power, the It-dimension, seeing that it must be mediated through light waves or sound waves. Indeed, the communication between an It/Thou divine entity and a human entity should be, in principle, just as feasible and comprehensible as the communication between one human entity and another human entity. But clearly the same cannot be said if the divine entity that is to be implicated in a communicative relationship with the human entity is a divine entity that ontologically constitutes itself as a pure Thou entity. For here, in the ontological constitution of a pure Thou divine entity, the dimension-of-power, the It-dimension, is not present, and consequently both the feasibility and the comprehensibility of a communicative relationship between such a divine entity and the human entity must, in principle, remain wrapped up in an unresolved mystery. The claim that such a communicative relationship is nonetheless feasible and in fact has taken place at certain points in time can be taken only on the basis of faith in the biblical sense of *emunah* (and not in the Greek sense of *pistis*), which is to say that it can be taken only on the basis of an act of trust which, in principle, could never be replaced, overcome, by an act of knowledge. Now, seeing that biblical faith grounds itself in the act of revelation and in the act of worship *qua* address, the fact that an It/Thou divine entity can provide feasibility and comprehensibility to these acts while a pure Thou divine entity cannot clearly give the advantage to the It/Thou divine entity with respect to this issue.

As against this, however, we have at least two very significant advantages that go to a divine entity that constitutes itself ontologically as a pure Thou entity over a divine entity that constitutes itself ontologically as an It/Thou entity. The first advantage lies in the consideration that the failure to encounter a divine entity in our common concrete experience can be counted as a valid argument against the existence of such an entity when this entity is an It/Thou divine entity but not when it is a pure Thou divine entity. This is so, for inasmuch as an It/Thou divine entity does include in its ontological constitution the It-dimension, i.e., the dimension-of-power, it can, in principle, be encountered in our common, concrete experience, and consequently the fact that an encounter with such an entity is not available in our common, concrete experience can be taken as an indication that such an entity does not exist. In contra-distinction to this, a pure Thou divine entity does not include in its ontological constitution an It-dimension, i.e., a dimension-of-power, and, therefore, it, in principle, cannot be encountered in our common, concrete experience, and consequently the fact that an encounter with such an entity is indeed not available in our common, concrete experience cannot be taken as an indication that such an entity does not exist. Needless to say, that this being the case bestows a considerable advantage on the pure Thou divine entity over the It/Thou divine entity in the enterprise of natural/rational theology and, even more so, in the enterprise of apologetics.

The second advantage lies in the consideration that while an It/Thou divine entity can have, in terms of its ontological constitution, only a quantitative distinction from the human entity, the pure Thou divine entity has a qualitative distinction. As such, while the It/Thou divine entity remains, in the last analysis, but "man writ large" and as such allows, in principle, the possibility of both the divination of the human (i.e., apotheosis) and the humanization of the divine (i.e., incarnation) which, in turn, implicates a pantheistic orientation, i.e., the ultimate identity of the divine entity with the world, the pure Thou divine entity constitutes itself as a "wholly other" entity, thus implicating an unbridgeable "gap" between itself and the human entity and rejecting, in principle, the possibility of both apotheosis and incarnation entailing, in turn, a rejection of the pantheistic orientation and an insistence on the theistic orientation (by the way, in this connection it should be clear that Feuerbach's reduction of religion to humanism, i.e., his presentation of the divine entity as but a projection of the human entity is, in the last analysis, really applicable only to religious formulations in which the divine entity is constituted as an It/Thou entity and not when it is constituted as a pure Thou entity).

Now, these distinctions between the It/Thou divine entity and the pure

Thou divine entity are the most relevant distinctions by which the advantage, from the vantage point of biblical faith, of the pure Thou divine entity over the It/Thou divine entity can be established for they all emanate from the most fundamental and essential distinction by which the religious orientation of biblical faith differentiates itself from the religious orientation of paganism. Namely, we would submit, that the most fundamental and essential distinction between the religious orientation of biblical faith and that of paganism lies in the fact that in the religious orientation of biblical faith the ultimate entity, i.e., the entity which one ultimately encounters, thus the divine entity, is a personal entity (an entity which incorporates consciousness, awareness), while in the religious orientation of paganism it is blind power, and that it is, indeed, from this fundamental distinction that the foregoing distinctions delineated here, to wit, the distinction of "gap" versus continuum, of theism versus pantheism, of the rejection of apotheosis and incarnation versus their acceptance, emanate and receive their rationale. As such, indeed, a pure Thou divine entity represents in the fullest and maximal way the ultimate entity that one can encounter in the context of biblical faith, while an It/Thou divine entity is already a mitigation of the fullest, maximal representation of this ultimate entity, an attempt to synthesize, to hold on to the religious orientation of both biblical faith and paganism, and clearly as such the advantage, from the vantage point of biblical faith, goes to the divine entity which is delineated as a pure Thou entity.

At the same time, however, it should be noted that since none of the three concrete historical expressions of biblical faith, to wit, neither Judaism nor Christianity nor Islam, has, so to speak, gone all the way to embrace exclusively the Thou-dimension to the exclusion of the It-dimension as is reflected in the fact that the divine entity in all of these three concrete historical expressions is constituted as an It/Thou and not as a pure Thou entity, a gradation among these three concrete historical expressions of biblical faith can be introduced on the basis of what degree of relative dominance is allotted respectively to the It and Thou components in the ontological constitution of the divine or, in other words, on the basis of how far tilted away from paganism towards biblical faith are these expressions respectively. Indeed, a convenient criterion by which to determine such gradation is the respective stances that these three concrete historical expressions of biblical faith take with regard to the issues of apotheosis and incarnation, namely, how accepting or rejecting they are of the feasibility of these phenomena—the more accepting any one of these expressions is, the closer is its link to the religious orientation of paganism and, reversely, the more radical any one of them is in its rejection, the closer is its link to the religious orientation of biblical faith.

Now, on the basis of this criterion, we would submit that it is mainstream Judaism and mainstream Islam, i.e., the prophetic, non-mystical expressions within Judaism and Islam, which come closest to the religious orientation of biblical faith, seeing that both incarnation and apotheosis are radically rejected by these two concrete historical expressions (at the same time, however, a case can be made that while regarding the issues of incarnation and apotheosis,

Judaism and Islam are equal in their tilting away from the orientation of paganism towards that of biblical faith, regarding other issues Islam may revert much more extensively than Judaism away from the orientation of biblical faith back to that of paganism, a good example of this being the respective positions of Judaism and Islam regarding the issue of divine providence where Islam takes a much more fatalistic stance than Judaism, ascribing any and all occurrences to divine intervention, thus reverting to a divine entity where the It-dimension, the dimension-of-power, is given greater dominance). Christianity, on the other hand, does not come as close to the orientation of biblical faith (which, as such, is to say that it is more retentive of aspects characterizing the orientation of paganism), seeing that in all its expressions, not only is the feasibility of the act of incarnation accepted but the actuality of its having occurred is asserted (indeed, a good case can be made that any expression which does not assert the occurrence of incarnation, and, for that matter, of resurrection, cannot be taken as an authentic expression of Christianity). Not only that, but in its oldest and most extensive expressions, i.e., in Catholicism and Eastern Orthodoxy, in addition to the acceptability of incarnation (which, by the way, receives an additional concrete form of expression in the presentation of icons), the feasibility of apotheosis is also accepted and its actual occurrence asserted as, for example, in the canonization of saints. No wonder that Christianity, at least in terms of its Catholic and Eastern Orthodox expressions, is widely and rightly seen as the great attempt at the synthesis of Judaism and Hellenism, i.e., of biblical faith and paganism; but precisely as such it is, per force, also less close to the orientation of biblical faith.

True, it must be conceded that in the remaining significant expression of Christianity, i.e., in Protestantism, apotheosis is not accepted. Also, incarnation, which is accepted (as argued here, Protestantism could not have been an authentic expression of Christianity, which it is, had it rejected incarnation) is, at the same time, nonetheless somewhat compromised and obscured in its expression, seeing that its expression in the presentation of icons (which Catholicism and Eastern Orthodoxy fully embrace) is excluded in Protestantism. Indeed as such, one might well want to argue that Protestantism is the expression of Christianity that comes closest to the orientation of biblical faith, that the Reformation is indeed to be viewed as the major counter-pull within Christianity, moving it from its Hellenistic/pagan pole to its Judaic/biblical faith pole; and that if this be so, then indeed Christianity, in its expression in Protestantism (if not in its expression in Catholicism and Eastern Orthodoxy) would have to be accorded the same degree of closeness to biblical faith that one encounters in Judaism and Islam.

But, alas, the conclusion of the argument here is not really valid in the last analysis. For first of all, Protestantism, if it is to be an authentic expression of Christianity, must, as argued above, accept incarnation, if only in the unique case of Jesus. Thus, the exclusion of iconography in Protestantism cannot be taken as its rejection of incarnation (the most it can be taken to signify is the uneasiness in Protestantism with the taking of incarnation in too concrete a fashion). But if incarnation is accepted in Protestantism, even if only in principle and thus in a very limited way, then Protestantism cannot be placed on the same level of closeness to biblical faith as Judaism or Islam. But moreover, in accepting incarnation but rejecting apotheosis, Protestantism falls into a fundamental inconsistency. For in accepting incarnation, Protestantism accepts the feasibility of moving from one kind of ontological constitution to a qualitatively different kind of ontological constitution (in the case of incarnation from a pure Thou ontological constitution to an It/Thou ontological constitution); and once the feasibility of such a movement is accepted, the feasibility of its moving in the opposite direction (as it is in the case of apotheosis, where it moves from an It/Thou ontological constitution to a pure Thou ontological constitution) should be just as acceptable. If a movement from a divine entity to a human entity, i.e., incarnation, is feasible, there is no inherent reason why a movement from a human entity to a divine entity, i.e., apotheosis, should not be equally feasible.

True, rationally, movement between entities possessing qualitatively different ontological constitutions should not be possible, seeing that there is a "gap" between them that cannot be traversed. But if a claim is nonetheless made that the "gap" can be traversed, then, unless by an arbitrary fiat that dictates otherwise, it has to be a two-way street. Thus, if incarnation is acceptable, apotheosis too must be acceptable and, vice versa, if apotheosis is acceptable, incarnation too must be acceptable. Put somewhat differently, one can argue that the making of such a movement feasible (and this regardless of what its specific direction may be) necessarily implicates abrogation of the "gap" and the substituting of a continuum in its place and that, in the context of a continuum, movement cannot, in principle, be one-directional but must be bi-directional—if the continuum allows you to move from A to B, it must also, in principle, allow you to move from B to A, which is to say that if it allows a move from the divine to the human (i.e., incarnation), it must also, in principle, allow a move from the human to the divine (i.e., apotheosis). Indeed, in the multiple expressions of paganism, the two go hand in hand together; we never encounter one without the other—humans, for example, heroes or kings, become deities and deities become humans. Likewise, with respect to Catholicism and Eastern Orthodoxy, incarnation and apotheosis also go hand in hand together, and while it is true that, by virtue of holding on to both of them, these expressions clearly tilt away from the orientation of biblical faith towards the orientation of paganism, it is also true that by the same token (i.e., by virtue of holding on to both incarnation and apotheosis) these expressions safeguard the consistency of their formulation. Protestantism, on the other hand, by holding on to incarnation only and not also to apotheosis, tilts back (though not all the way) from the orientation of paganism to the orientation of biblical faith, but at the cost of introducing inconsistency into its formulation.

Of course, alternatively, there is the possibility of arguing that, in the last analysis, Protestantism too is consistent in its formulation in that after all it too does hold on not only to the notion of incarnation but also to that of apotheosis as can be seen in the fact that Protestantism does embrace the notion of the "new being," i.e., the feasibility of transforming the present ontological constitution of the human entity to some other ontological constitution, that other ontological constitution being, one may well argue, an ontological constitution that defines an entity no longer as human but as divine. As such, Protestantism appears here, as far as substance is concerned, to tilt away from the orientation of biblical faith to that of paganism to the same extent that Catholicism and Eastern Orthodoxy do. The only difference between Protestantism, on the one hand, and Catholicism and Eastern Orthodoxy, on the other hand, would lie here in the way they respectively express their embrace of the notions of incarnation and apotheosis—Catholicism and Eastern Orthodoxy (and here, it would seem, Eastern Orthodoxy even more than Catholicism) are fully explicit and up front in expressing their embrace of these notions (and particularly in expressing their embrace of all the aspects implicated in these notions as, for example, iconography and sainthood), while Protestantism, on the other hand, is much more circumspect and less forthcoming in its expression; indeed, if anything, it seems to want to obfuscate the expression of this embrace as can be seen in its rejection of iconography and sainthood. Thus, in the context of this interpretation, the difference between Protestantism, on the one hand, and Catholicism and Eastern Orthodoxy, on the other hand, is only in terms of expression but not of substance. Still, closing an eye to the many reservations and qualifications one can introduce into the analysis here, we can generalize and say that a gradation can be introduced here whereby Eastern Orthodoxy, Catholicism, Protestantism, Islam and Judaism are tilting away from paganism towards biblical faith in an ascending order.

The third and last observation to be made here is with respect to the assertion made above to the effect that a divine entity which constitutes itself as a Thou entity is dependent, as regards its coming into existence and maintaining itself within existence, on an affirmation being extended to it by an other (that other, in order to be able to extend such an affirmation, must of course also constitute itself as a Thou entity). For in all likelihood this assertion would strike many as being very problematic, inasmuch as they would argue that the ascription of dependency to the divine entity must, of necessity, undermine its status of divinity. This is so because a good case can be made that the very status of divinity is defined by the notion of ultimacy (an entity is divine by virtue of being the ultimate expression of the dimension in which it is placed); and this being the case, ascribing dependency to an entity should indeed deprive it of the status of divinity, seeing that dependency of necessity implicates limitation and that limitation, in turn, of necessity undermines ultimacy.

But is this argument really valid? Clearly, for the argument to be valid, all three claims that it puts forth, namely, that the status of divinity is defined by the notion ultimacy, that dependency of necessity implicates limitation and that limitation of necessity undermines ultimacy, must be valid and this, we would submit, is, in the last analysis, not really the case. For while the first and third claim, namely, the claim that the status of divinity is defined by the notion of ultimacy and the claim that limitation of necessity undermines ultimacy, are indeed valid (thus as regards the first claim, not only is it valid because it impinges upon the formulating of a definition and as such, in principle, it should be valid irrespective of what particular formulation it puts forth but because a good case can be made that the particular formulation it puts forth, i.e., the formulation whereby the status of divinity is to be defined in terms of the notion of ultimacy, is, in the light of the phenomenology of religion, a very persuasive and thus valid formulation; and as regards the third claim, it should be self-evident that the very signification of the notion of limitation and that of the notion of ultimacy would bar the possibility of an entity being limited in some sense and at the same time being ultimate in the context of the same sense), the second claim, i.e., the claim that dependency of necessity (which is to say, always and everywhere) implicates limitation, is, in our judgment, manifestly not valid. True, the claim is valid and does apply in the context of the It-dimension, i.e., in the context of a dimension that constitutes itself in terms of power, seeing that power by its very essence lends itself to being quantified (it is always and everywhere a question of the degree of power, always and everywhere a question of more or less power) and in such a context dependency does indeed implicate a diminution, a limitation, in the level of power which, in turn, necessarily undermines the status of ultimacy inasmuch as the status of ultimacy in a quantified context necessarily implicates the possession of an infinite degree, the most, of that in terms of which the dimension constitutes itself. Thus, indeed, with respect to an It-god, i.e., to the god encountered in paganism, dependency would indeed undermine its ultimacy and as such its divinity. An It-god has to be an Aristotelian god (and, by the way, it is not accidental that within the context of the dimension-of-power the tendency, in the last analysis, is inescapably toward a pantheistic and not a theistic formulation).

But the It-dimension, the dimension-of-power, is not the sole, exclusive, dimension through which reality expresses itself. Reality also expresses itself through the Thou-dimension, i.e., through a dimension that constitutes itself in terms of consciousness, and consciousness, in contra-distinction to power, is not quantified—it does not lend itself to being more or less but rather it is all or none. In such a context, ultimacy does not implicate the greatest degree, the most, of that in terms of which the dimension constitutes itself and consequently dependency (notwithstanding its implicating limitation) would not implicate here the undermining of the status of ultimacy. Rather, in the context of the dimension-of-consciousness the status of ultimacy implicates the exclusive belongingness of an entity to the dimension-of-consciousness—for ultimacy, and thus divinity, to be ascribed to an entity in the context of the dimension-of-consciousness, the entity must ontologically constitute itself exclusively in terms of consciousness to the complete exclusion of power; the ultimate, the divine in the context of the dimension-of-consciousness is the pure Thou entity, the Buberian pure Thou-god. Indeed, far from undermining divinity, dependency is a condition *sine qua non* for a divine entity to arise here inasmuch as a divine entity constitutes itself here exclusively as a Thou entity and a Thou entity can come into existence and maintain itself within existence only when a dependency is implicated, a dependency on the affirmation extended by an other. In the absence of such dependency, a Thou entity, and even more poignantly, a Thou entity that is divine, cannot come into existence or maintain itself within existence. By the way, this was intuited by the rabbis of old when they elaborated upon the verse in Deutero-Isaiah, "Thus said the Lord: This day you are my witness," and suggested that God was saying to Israel, "As long as you are witnessing to me I am God, when you cease to witness to me I am, so to speak, no longer God" (the introduction of the qualification "so to speak" is, however, the rabbis' attempt to somehow mitigate the radical conclusion that is necessarily implicated in their elaboration, namely, that God would actually cease to be god—an understandable though nonetheless unfortunate failure of nerve on their part).

27. This observation may perhaps lend additional support to the claim made above that animals (i.e., entities possessing only consciousness as such but not self-consciousness), in contra-distinction to humans, cannot be ascribed a right to life, namely, a right to request/demand that they be affirmed. For clearly, it would not seem valid to claim that animals act under the constraint of obligation. But if obligation cannot be ascribed to animals, then right too cannot be ascribed to them, which is to say here specifically that they cannot be endowed with a right to life.

28. It may be objected with respect to this claim that animals can extend affirmation to others, e.g., to humans or to other animals, even though they do not possess self-consciousness. It would seem to us, however, that we can overcome this objection by pointing out that the affirmation which animals can extend (and this would apply not only to wild but to domesticated animals who are often taken as substitutes for other humans as sources of affirmation) is an affirmation of the other not as an end-in-itself but, in the last analysis, only as a means to some further ends (thus, for example, as provider of food or shelter to domesticated animals). But the issue before us here, namely, the issue of what an entity possessing self-consciousness requires in order for it to come into existence and maintain itself within existence, is precisely the issue of affirmation as end-in-itself and not of affirmation as a means to some further means. This is so because, in the last analysis, the question before us here is the question of validation, i.e., the validation of the actuality of self-consciousness, and this can be established, we would submit, only by an affirmation that is based on a direct, unmediated intuition.

29. As such, incidentally, in contrast to the first way delineated above which may be characterized as diachronic, seeing that the right to be affirmed is established there first and only then subsequently, on the basis of fairness, the obligation to extend affirmation is established, the way here would clearly be synchronic, seeing that it claims that the right to be affirmed and the obligation to extend affirmation are placed in one and the same act.

30. This relation between the formulation given in the context of the dimension-of-power, a formulation which expresses itself primarily in terms of the entity, and the formulation given in the context of the dimension-of-consciousness, a formulation which expresses itself primarily in terms of the

relation, may reflect, perhaps, by way of analogy, the relation between the formulation given in classical physics which also seems to express itself primarily in terms of the entity (i.e., the atom) and the formulation given in quantum physics which seems to express itself in terms of the relation (i.e., the unceasing flux, the process). Indeed, if this analogy has any merit, then perhaps the duality of power and consciousness (matter and soul) may ultimately reduce itself after all to a monism in terms of power only which at different speeds of its movement may present itself as different "worlds," i.e., as reality behaving itself in terms of different rules.

31. When we say that the pole arises secondarily, we mean to say that ontologically its status is secondary to that of the relation but not that temporally it is subsequent to the relation. Clearly, temporally, the poles, being part and parcel of the relation, arise at one and the same time as the relation. The poles, and thus the entities (inasmuch as the poles constitute themselves as entities) arise simultaneously with the relation, seeing that the arising of a relation necessarily implicates its limitation on either end, which is to say, its limitation by its poles on either end, the poles constituting themselves as entities. This, by the way, would clearly also account for the claim that, ontologically speaking, the entity arises not only secondarily but inescapably in a twosome.

32. The mechanism which operates here is clearly a consequence of the refraction of the dimension-of-consciousness through the dimension-of-power, a refraction which does away with a relation of authentic simultaneity and introduces in its place a temporal sequence of before and after.

33. Of course, as we have seen above, in the traditional formulations of the biblical religions (i.e., in Judaism, Christianity and Islam), power is also ascribed to the biblical God, thus constituting it as an It/Thou entity, i.e., as man writ large, and with respect to such an entity the capacity and option to act/relate in more than one way is reinstated, thus fully qualifying this biblical God to be encompassed within the ethical enterprise on all levels. But now, within this context, the ethical integrity of the biblical God can be safeguarded only by adopting axiomatically the assumption that although having the option and capacity to act/relate in ways that would be ethically evaluated/judged as wrong, the biblical God in fact always acts/relates in ways that would be ethically evaluated/judged as right. Namely, the biblical God would differentiate itself from the human in that while the human can and does misuse the option and capacity it has to act in different ways, the biblical God can but never does misuse the option and capacity it has. Specifically, with respect to what is of concern to us here, that is to say that the adopted assumption is that with regard to humans, the biblical God would always act/relate towards them in ways that are just, which is to say that, in exercising its infinite power, the biblical God would always allot to them what they deserve.

But it should be underlined again that this assertion that the biblical God constituting itself as an It/Thou god would always act/relate towards humans in ways that are just is established only as an axiomatic assumption. It is not and indeed cannot be established on rational grounds. What can be established on rational grounds is that the ascribing of power to the Thou-god thus transforming it to an It/Thou-god precipitates the problematic of theodicy, seeing that the problematic of theodicy cannot arise with respect to a god which is either exclusively an It-god or exclusively a Thou-god but only with respect to a god that is an It/Thou-god. This is so inasmuch as neither the purely It-god nor the purely Thou-god has an option or a capacity to act in different ways (and, indeed, with respect to the purely It-god, even more fundamentally, the very notion, and thus the issue, of justice cannot arise to begin with; for, in order for the issue of justice to arise, two conditions must be satisfied: 1) The Thou-dimension must be present and 2) the option and capacity to act/relate in different ways must be available, and these two conditions can be satisfied only when power is ascribed to a Thou-god thus transforming it to an It/Thou-god). So, one can establish on grounds of rationality that the constituting of the biblical God as an It/Thou-god would allow the problematic of theodicy to be precipitated. We should note, however, that this is not to say that rationality can also provide us with a way of solving the problematic of theodicy. Indeed, we would want to argue that it cannot; though to be more precise, we should elaborate and say that it cannot not because it has no way to offer within its parameters by which the problematic of theodicy could be overcome but rather because the only way that suggests itself within its parameters is really not acceptable. For, the only way within the parameters of rationality by which the problematic of theodicy can be overcome is to maintain that whenever the human is the recipient of suffering, the suffering is to be seen as punishment meted to the human for his/her misdeeds. This is so because if God, so to speak, runs the show and He is just, then if suffering is inflicted on someone, it is that someone who must be held responsible for the suffering inflicted upon it—the suffering has to be seen as a punishment commensurate with the sins it must have committed. But all too often such a claim flies in the face of our experience, making the assumption/charge that the someone upon whom suffering is inflicted must have sinned and, indeed, sinned commensurately with the degree of suffering inflicted upon it, not only preposterous but downright obscene.

III
Some Issues Implicating the Ethical Right to Life

Having delineated in the preceding two chapters what in our view constitutes the proper nature and parameters of ethical enterprise and having established which entities can possess an right to life (or, to put the matter somewhat differently, by virtue of what ontological aspect can an entity be endowed with an ethical right to life), we can now proceed to apply the conclusions arrived there to some of the specific issues that implicate the question of an ethical right to life, i.e., such issues as that of abortion, of suicide and assisted suicide, of euthanasia and of capital punishment.[1] Now, in light of our considerations above, it should be evident that of all the various expressions belonging to the religious dimension it is the expression of Prophetic Judaism, which would best lend itself to an interesting and instructive comparison with the ethical formulation.

Now, on a certain level, applying the conclusions established in the preceding two chapters to the issues enumerated here should be a fairly simple and straightforward undertaking. For on the basis of these conclusions we can clearly claim that the criterion by which one can establish whether or not an entity possesses an ethical right to life is whether or not the entity is endowed with self-consciousness. Namely, an entity that is endowed with self-consciousness will possess an ethical right to life while an entity that is not endowed with self-consciousness will not possess an ethical right to life. And to determine whether or not an entity is endowed with self-consciousness should be a fairly straightforward and uncomplicated task. Thus, we would submit that a fetus and a full-fledged human who has lost his/her consciousness and medical prognosis is quite certain that the loss is irreversible are clearly entities that are not endowed with self-consciousness (in the former it is not yet and in the latter it is no longer, but in either case it is not a present reality) and consequently, according to our formulation, neither would seem to possess an ethical right to life thus seeming to imply that neither abortion nor euthanasia, in the specific delineation given to it by us here, should be condemned from the vantage point of ethics as delineated in our formulation. As against this, the entities implicated in suicide and capital punishment are clearly entities that retain their self-consciousness and therefore it would appear that they would hold on to their ethical right to life which, in turn, would suggest that suicide and capital punishment should be condemned from the ethical vantage point as it is delineated in our formulation.

But evidently we are not stating our conclusions here with finality but rather with a marked degree of hesitation. The reason for this lies in the fact that the issues here may implicate additional aspects which as such would complicate the picture and preclude an immediate conclusion that bases itself exclusively on the consideration which we introduced here as our criterion by which to assess the implication of these issues with respect to the question of an ethical right to life, to wit, whether or not the entity in question here is endowed with self-consciousness. Clearly, before being able to present our conclusions regarding these issues with greater finality, we have to address these additional aspects and weigh to what extent and in what manner they may impinge upon the conclusions based exclusively on our criterion of whether or not the entity in question is endowed with self-consciousness. So, let us proceed to this task and let us begin with the issue of abortion, seeing that it is by far the most widely and heatedly discussed issue in our society today which implicates the question of an ethical right to life.

Abortion

Clearly, in view of our analysis above, the crucial and decisive question before us here is not whether or not the fetus is alive in the biological sense but rather whether or not the fetus is a person, i.e., an entity that carries consciousness in its fullest expression, which is to say an entity which is self-conscious. And the answer to this question is equally clear and unambiguous. Namely, while it is quite true that the fetus is alive in the biological sense from the very early stages of pregnancy if not, indeed, from the very moment of conception,[2] it is equally clear and certain that the fetus is at no time during pregnancy a person.[3] In view of this, it would seem that the issue of abortion should indeed present a simple, open and shut case. It would seem that the logic and facts of the situation should force us to take a pro-abortion position all the way, namely, allowing abortion at any point during pregnancy, for the fetus at no time during pregnancy has a rightful claim not to have its existence terminated.[4]

Now, in view of the above, it would appear that one could clearly argue that the case can be closed at this point and if so, it would certainly go against the position of the anti-abortion proponents. For if we have successfully established that the only legitimate criterion for providing the justification for prohibiting the termination of an entity's existence is the personhood of the entity in question, then since the fetus is clearly not a person it can at no time and under no circumstances place a rightful claim not to have its existence terminated. This would seem to be a valid argument and, as such, it would certainly seem to bring the case to a close.

And yet one may well argue that far from bringing the case to a close, this argument, being fully valid, really succeeds in merely clearing the ground so that the problematics that this issue presents can really come to the fore. For one could now argue that the justification for the fetus having a rightful claim not to have its existence terminated ought to be based, in the last analysis, not on its being a person but rather on its being a *potential* person. Namely, the argument would now maintain that not only an entity that is actually a person but also an entity that is merely a *potential* person has a rightful claim not to have its existence terminated. And if this is so, then we are clearly back into the fray. For if the fetus is clearly not an *actual* person, it is equally clear and indubitable that it is a *potential* person.[5] So by the mere shift from actual to potential as regards the status of the personhood of the fetus, namely, by merely shifting our position from claiming that the fetus is actually a person (an actual "baby") to claiming that it is only potentially a person (only a potential "baby"), the issue of abortion must be reopened.

Now, in this context in which the issue is reopened, the first and, indeed, the crucial and decisive question is the question whether an entity that is only *potentially* a person has any claim at all or, if it does, has the same rightful claim not to have its existence terminated as an entity that possesses *actual* personhood. In our judgment the answer is clearly no. Indeed, not only does it not have a rightful claim of the same strength as an entity that is an actual person, it cannot have any rightful *claim* at all. Namely, it is not that it does have a rightful claim but of a weaker strength; it cannot have any rightful claim to begin with. For to have a rightful claim at all, an entity *qua* person must be actually present so as to be able to give an affirmation to another entity *qua* person and claim in return an affirmation of its own being from that other. This situation, which alone constitutes the possibility of there being such, a claim for affirmation (and therefore for not having its existence terminated) does not obtain with respect to an entity that is only *potentially* a person. Thus, the fetus as merely a potential person cannot have a rightful claim not to have its existence terminated.

Indeed, the very notion of potentiality can apply, i.e., make sense, here only when the fetus is viewed as a biological entity, as an It entity, but not when it is viewed as a personal entity, as a Thou entity. This is so, seeing that a continuum and thus the possibility of gradation and therefore also the possibility of meaningfully speaking of potentiality in contra-distinction to actualized realization is available only with respect to an It entity, i.e., only with respect to the fetus as a biological entity. Indeed, a biological entity can go through different stages of development remaining in essence the same entity thus allowing us to speak of the entity in its earlier stages as being potentially the entity of the later stages, being in the earlier stages merely the potential of itself as it constitutes itself in the later stages. A personal entity, a Thou entity, on the other hand, does not lend itself to gradation, i.e., to maintaining its identity as one and the same entity while going through different manifestations of itself. A personal entity, i.e., an entity that defines itself in terms of self-consciousness, as the bearer of self-consciousness, either exists fully actualized or it does not exist at all; it does not lend itself to being more or less—it can only be all or none.

Now, fully actualized humans are entities that are both biological, i.e., It entities, and personal, i.e., Thou entities. However, as argued here, it is only with regard to their being biological entities that they can be taken as potential, i.e., as not as yet fully realized, humans. With regard to their being personal entities, they are either fully present as persons or they are not; no gradation and thus no potentiality is available. Thus, referring to the fetus as a potential human can be meaningful only when the fetus is taken as a biological entity but not as a personal entity. But the ethical right not to have one's existence terminated can be arrogated only to an entity that is a personal, but not a biological, entity. Thus, strictly speaking, seeing that the fetus can be taken as a potential human only in terms of its being a biological, but not a personal, entity, it cannot be arrogated the right not to have its existence terminated. Still, inasmuch as in the human entity the personal dimension is inextricably linked to the biological dimension in the sense that the personal dimension, i.e., the Thou-dimension, in the human can express itself, come into existence, only in conjunction with the biological dimension, i.e., with the It-dimension, the fetus can be taken in a way as a potential human not only *qua* its being a biological entity but also *qua* its being a personal entity and thus being endowed in some measure with a right not to have its existence terminated.

But this right that could be arrogated to the fetus by virtue of its being a potential person is not ethical in the sense of our delineation above of the ethical enterprise, to wit, a right that is grounded in the ontological constitution of its claimer. Rather, it is ethical in the sense of the delineation of the ethical enterprise in terms of ethos or mores, to wit, a right that is grounded in the dictates of one's society reflecting the kind of conduct that this society deems proper and laudable. Thus, for example, the ethos of most societies would dictate that the conduct accorded to our dead fellow humans prior to their burial, even though they are now inanimate entities and no longer personal entities, be the conduct we accord personal entities, e.g., live fellow human beings, and not the conduct we accord inanimate entities, e.g., putrefied vegetables. Now, in the same way, *mutatis mutandis*, the ethos of a society may dictate that the fetus, even though in its present state it is not a personal entity, should be accorded, by virtue of the fact that at a certain point in the future it may become a personal entity, the right not to have its existence terminated if there are no other overriding considerations to the contrary. Namely, the ethos of a society may dictate that the fetus, by virtue of its being potentially a personal entity, should be granted in advance the right not to have its existence terminated if there are no other overriding considerations to the contrary. Thus, the task to which we have to turn now is to examine the various possible scenarios to see if we can indeed identify overriding considerations that would cancel the fetus's right not to have its existence terminated.

Before proceeding to such an examination, however, a few general observations that are pertinent to our concern here may be in order. First, we should be clear that while the fetus *qua* merely a potential person, a potential human being, has standing within the ethical domain, it does not likewise have a standing within the legal domain. For in being merely a potential, and not a fully actualized, human being it is not a *bona fide* entity for the concern of the law. True, in the last analysis, the parameters of the law are a matter of convention and as such, they can be extended or constricted at will. But in actuality, thus far the law has been perceived, by and large, as an instrument that regulates the relations and transactions between actual human beings; the law is perceived as the instrument by which to protect the rights of actual human beings. Namely, the law applies only to the domain of humankind and does not extend beyond that to other domains; furthermore, in the domain of humankind it applies only to actual and not hypothetical entities (and a potential entity is, in the last analysis, a hypothetical entity). Thus, any discourse regarding the way fetuses are to be treated should not really pertain to the concern of the law but rather to ethical or religious concerns.[6] Thus, since society undertakes to protect the claims, interests and rights only of its actual present members (and not if its deceased members or if its possible future members), doing this through the instrument of the law, the problematics of abortion should not concern the law but only morality. So, even if society strongly disapproves of abortion, it should express this disapproval in education, preaching or even social ostracism but not in legislation. The fetus has no standing in the context of the law and its claim cannot have the support of the law. If a case is to be made for the fetus and its claims then we must move from the context of the law to that of morality.

Secondly, although it is true that the fetus by virtue of its being a potential person has been granted a presumption not to have its existence terminated, it is important to underline that this presumption is greatly weakened by the qualification added to it, i.e., the qualification that "there being no other consideration to the contrary." For with regard to the fetus the possibility of there being a consideration to the contrary must always be present (and, indeed, all too often present not merely as a potentiality but as an actuality). This is so because the fetus cannot exist by its own power; it is a dependent entity—an entity that, for its very existence, is dependent on the mother. And the mother can clearly be the source for "there being a consideration to the contrary." Indeed, the very problematic of abortion arises because a conflict arises between the wishes or interests of the mother and the claims of the fetus.[7] The whole problematic of abortion is constituted by the conflict between the wishes, needs and interests of the mother on the one hand and the claim of the fetus not to have its existence terminated on the other. And the only way to resolve this problematic is by weighing these conflicting claims and deciding which has the ethical priority. And this being the case, there are, quite clearly, any number of different scenarios in which a conflict between the interests of the mother and those of the fetus may arise and our ethical evaluation and judgment may well vary greatly from one instance to another. Thus, there may be instances where the mother's position, i.e., her wish to have an abortion, would clearly seem to take precedence; on the other hand, there may be instances where the mother's position would by no means seem to be persuasive and abortion would not seem to be justified (but keep in mind, in view of what we said above, that this may only lead to moral and social disapproval but not to legal sanctions). The only way to decide such instances is on an *ad hoc* basis after considering all the factors that enter the picture. And clearly, there can be many variants that may enter the picture and influence the decision. As such, it is to be expected, as indeed we shall presently see, that there will be some instances in which the decision would be very clear-cut, unambiguous and decisive, and other instances which would fall into a "gray area" where the decision could very easily go either way.

Thirdly, we need to elaborate somewhat further upon the claim made above that the fetus is inescapably, by the very nature of its being, a dependent entity, namely, that it is inescapably dependent on the support and sustenance provided to it by another specific entity, to wit, its mother. For of course, in a sense, we are all dependent entities. However, our dependency, i.e., the dependency of fully fledged human beings on one another, is essentially and in principle different from the dependency of the fetus on its mother. For the dependency of fully fledged human beings on one another is due to the complexity of the industrial/commercial world that human beings have created for themselves (and the more complex this world becomes the more interdependent we become as is clearly seen in the emerging phenomenon of the "global village"). But in principle, the fully fledged human being should be able to sustain his physical existence in isolation (thus, for example, he can fish, hunt small animals or eat fruits without the help of any others). The fetus, on the other hand, is not capable of sustaining its physical existence without the support of another human being, i.e., its mother (or in the later stages of its gestation the mother's support may be substituted by that of an incubator).[8] And this being the case, the issue that confronts us here is not just whether or not an entity has a rightful claim to demand not to have its existence terminated, but rather whether or not it has a rightful claim to demand receiving support and sustenance from another entity. The claim that the fetus is making on the mother (or, for that matter, to the extent that the incubator can be substituted for the mother, on society) is far more far-reaching. It is not merely claiming the right to be left alone, not to be interfered with, not to have things done to it; it claims for itself the right to utilize and exploit another entity—it claims the right to use the mother's womb and to be nourished and sustained by her body. But is there really a right to such a claim? Do we really want to say (can we really defend the proposition) that one entity may indeed have the right to such a claim on another entity? It seems to us that the answer to this question must be in the negative. The world, which is to say, other human beings, does not owe us a living. Strictly speaking, there is no ethical rationale that could support the proposition that we have a rightful claim on others to support us.[9] Thus, the fetus does not have an innate right to place a claim on the mother or, for that matter, on society to provide for it. The only way in which such a claim can be justified is if it can be shown that the other party, i.e., the mother or society, has incurred a commitment and/or a responsibility to this effect. Now, it is very difficult to see how society could possibly incur such a commitment and/or a responsibility and consequently no claim can be placed on it.[10] With the mother, however, it may be argued that in bringing the fetus into existence, a commitment and/or a responsibility of some sort to provide for it has been incurred. Thus, the question here is no longer whether or not the fetus has a right to claim that its existence be not terminated, but rather it becomes whether or not a commitment and/or a responsibility has been incurred by the mother towards the fetus, and if yes, how binding is such a commitment and/or responsibility when it collides with other factors and other considerations.

Fourthly and lastly, we would submit that in dealing with the fetus as being only potentially a person, a case can be made that the closer the fetus gets to abandoning its status as being merely potentially a person and becoming a fully actualized person the greater weight must be given to the claim made on its behalf not to have its existence terminated. Of course, this case cannot be made with respect to the legal domain or, for that matter, to the ethical domain as delineated by us above, to wit, the ethical domain delineated in terms of the ontological constitution of the agent, which is to say specifically with respect to the right of an entity not to have its existence terminated, that it is endowed with such a right by virtue of its being a bearer of self-consciousness. For in both of these domains gradations and thus also potency cannot arise. In the context of the legal domain there is no place for such considerations as "getting closer" or "getting farther away" from a fixed point of reference; the legal domain must establish itself on an either/or resolution. Thus, from the legal vantage point there can be no distinction between an entity that is very close and an entity that is far removed from becoming a personal entity. In the context of the legal domain, as long as an entity is not *actually* a personal entity, such an entity can have no right to claim that its existence be not terminated.

Likewise, in the ethical domain that formulates itself from the vantage point of the ontological constitution of the agent gradation and thus potentiality are not feasible inasmuch as self-consciousness, as argued above, is an all-or-none proposition. The only domain where potentiality and, indeed, gradation regarding such potentiality is operative is (as already claimed above) the domain of ethics which formulates itself from the vantage point of the ethos or the mores of the society to which the agent belongs. For from this vantage point the human agent is viewed not only as a personal entity, i.e., as an entity that bears self-consciousness, but also as a biological entity. Now, it is precisely because the human fetus is constituted (at the very least in part of its being) as a biological entity, i.e., as an It entity, that gradation and potentiality can be arrogated to it. And in such a context, the closer the fetus gets to becoming a fully actualized human entity (i.e., no longer constituted merely as a biological entity but now constituted also as a personal entity), the greater weight must be given to the demand made on its behalf not to have its existence terminated.[11] The closer one approaches the goal, the more inclined we are to arrogate to it the status associated with the goal—we are more inclined to extend the title doctor to a senior medical student than to a freshman medical student; we are more likely to grant 100% (of whatever may be the case) to one who already has 90% than to one who has only 20%. Granted, such inclination, willingness, is to a considerable extent psychologically motivated (in reality the senior medical student is no more a doctor than the freshman medical student). But in the enterprise of the ethics *qua* ethos/mores the psychological dimension does play an important and indeed a legitimate role and consequently in the context of such an enterprise, i.e., the enterprise of ethics *qua* ethos/mores (and this after all is the kind of enterprise, as we have argued above, which is applicable here), the ethical evaluation/judgment will be influenced by how far along in its gestation the fetus is—the farther along in its gestation is, the weightier will the demand made on its behalf not to have its existence terminated become.

There is yet another ramification to the point under consideration here and that is that the farther along its gestation the fetus is, the stronger becomes the presumption of the mother incurring a commitment and thus a responsibility towards her fetus. This is so because the longer the mother does not resort to abortion, the more indicative it is of her acceptance of her fetus—clearly, a stronger presumption of commitment and thus of responsibility can be arrogated to a woman who carries her fetus for eight months than to a woman who carries her fetus for only one month. Now, to the extent that we would want to argue that incurring commitment and thus responsibility towards an other (e.g., the fetus) does place a restraint on what the agent incurring the commitment and responsibility (e.g., the mother) can do to that other, establishing the presence and strength of such a commitment and responsibility would clearly have a bearing on our stance regarding the ethical permissibility of abortion in these circumstances. The presence and strength of the commitment and responsibility towards the fetus incurred by the mother would clearly impinge upon determining the advantage between the right made on behalf of the fetus not to have its existence terminated and the right of the mother to pursue her interests and inclinations. Thus, to the extent that the length of gestation implicates strength of commitment and responsibility and to the extent that the strength of commitment and responsibility has a bearing on our evaluation/judgment of whether the fetus or the mother is given the advantage in the conflict that obtains between them, the factor of the length of gestation of the fetus has a direct bearing on where we would come down regarding the claims of the fetus *qua* potential person vis-à-vis the wishes and desires of the mother. Finally, it should be pointed out that this aspect of the point under discussion here, unlike the foregoing aspect, is not grounded in psychological factors. Rather, it is grounded in factors that impinge directly on *bona fide* ethical concerns. As such, unlike the foregoing aspect which was amenable to being formulated only in the context of an ethical enterprise where the ethical constituted itself in terms of ethos/mores, the aspect here readily lends itself to being formulated in the context of the ethical enterprise as it was delineated by us above.

Now, with the foregoing four general considerations to guide our deliberations, we can turn to consider some possible scenarios of concrete situations implicating the issue of abortion to see where we would come down with regard to the ethical permissibility of abortion in these concrete situations when, for the sake of argument, we concede that the fetus in these scenarios is a potential person (or even when we concede, with regard to some scenarios, that the fetus is a fully actualized person).[12] There are four scenarios that suggest themselves to us. These scenarios fall into a descending order as regards the ethical permissibility of abortion moving from a situation where, in our judgment, abortion should be clearly ethically permissible to a situation where the ethical permissibility of abortion becomes rather questionable and dubious.[13]

Thus, let us start with the scenario in which the strongest case, i.e., the least ambiguous or uncertain case, can be made for abortion—the scenario where the fetus threatens the mother's life. It would seem to us that in this scenario there could be no circumstances that would undermine or cancel out the moral right of the mother to abort in order to save her life. For seeing that what is at stake here is the rightful claim of an *actual* person not to have his/her existence terminated, no other claims or considerations could possibly take precedence over this claim. Certainly, the fetus being only *potentially* a person, there can be no conceivable circumstances in which its needs or requirements could possibly take precedence over the right of the actual person, i.e., the mother, to preserve her life. Thus, at any time during the pregnancy when the mother finds out that going on with the pregnancy may threaten her life, she has the moral right to abort. For inasmuch as one puts the highest value on preserving the life of an entity that is *actually* a person (or, put in religious terms, inasmuch as such a life is sacred), one cannot make or expect that entity to abdicate or in any way compromise its life for any other value, certainly not for any need or requirement of an entity that is not an actual but only a potential person. Nor would the giving of a commitment, even of a clear-cut commitment, alter this conclusion in any way. Namely, even if the mother, knowing full well that pregnancy will threaten her life, decides nevertheless to go on with the pregnancy or even to intentionally and willfully conceive (i.e., even if the mother in full knowledge of the facts makes a clear commitment to the fetus), she has every right at any time, even to the very last minute, to change her mind, putting aside any commitment that may have been made and giving preference to the preservation of her life. For no commitment, no matter to whom or for what purpose, can take precedence over a person's right not to have its existence terminated by forcing it to give up its life in order to honor a commitment.[14] To give preference to the honoring of a commitment over the preservation of life is the height of rigidity and stupidity; and this is so even when the commitment is made in full knowledge and awareness and acceptance of the consequences.[15]

So, there can be no question that if the life of the mother is in any way threatened, abortion should be allowed at any time. Indeed, even if one were to grant that the fetus is a fully *actualized* person (and not merely a potential person), a strong case can be made that abortion should be allowed if the fetus threatens the life of the mother. For in these circumstances abortion should certainly be viewed as an instance of a killing in self-defense and one would certainly want to defend this principle (unless, of course, one is an absolute pacifist). Killing in self-defense is not murder and it is justified.[16]

True, the case for the right to kill in self-defense is made when the attacker is *willfully* intending to kill his/her victim and this is certainly not the case here. The fetus is certainly not a *willful* killer of its mother—it is not as if the fetus intends or wishes to kill its mother; rather, the threat to the mother's life comes about as an inescapable consequence of the mere existence of the fetus—the fetus by its mere existence threatens the life of the mother. Thus, the proper analogy here should be not to a willful intentional killer but rather to an innocent carrier of a deadly virus. The fetus is like a person who through no fault of its own contracted and is now the carrier of a deadly virus.[17] Of course, there is no question that there is a fundamental difference between the situation where the threat is brought about by an innocent carrier and that where it is brought about by a willful intentional agent. But, we would want to argue, the legitimate difference here ought to be with respect to how we morally evaluate the threatening agent and consequently how we feel about the action that has to be taken against it but not with respect to what action ought to be taken. Namely, it is quite clear that there can be no moral reprobation with respect to an innocent carrier as there clearly is with respect to a willful intentional agent and that consequently we may be considerably more bothered and upset by what has to be done when it is done to the innocent carrier rather than to the willful intentional agent. But no difference arises, it seems to us, when it comes to the issue of what can rightfully be done to the threatening agent. In either case action against the threatening agent can rightfully be taken in order to remove the threat (and in either case this applies to whatever action may be necessary in order to remove the threat). Thus, for example, there is no question that quarantining is fully justified with respect to an infectious disease no matter how innocent and blameless the carrier may be. And if we stipulate, for the sake of argument, that we are confronted with a situation in which quarantining is not effective and the *only* way to remove the threat is by killing the agent then, it would seem to us, that one would be justified in doing so no matter how innocent and blameless the agent is. Sure, it is a very difficult thing to say and it is certainly a thing that one would dread doing and if done would no doubt be done with a very aching and troubled heart; but it is nonetheless, in the last analysis, an act that can be ethically justified.[18]

Clearly, this is one more instance illustrating the fact that we do not base our consideration on any utilitarian calculation, i.e., calculating what might be the greater good to the greater number of people or the lesser evil to the fewer number of people. As such, our argument with respect to what action can be rightfully taken against the innocent blameless carrier was not formulated in terms of what threat he may carry for the society as a whole. For in this context one may easily slip into considerations that are based on utilitarian calculations as, for example, that the death of one innocent person is a much lesser evil than the death of a great many innocent people and therefore justified. We are trying to make our case on different moral grounds and therefore very intentionally want to argue that even when it is a one-on-one situation, i.e., when it is the life of the innocent carrier against the life of the innocent victim, the victim has every right to defend his/her existence at the cost of the existence of the innocent carrier.

Actually, the case for the right of the mother to abort at any time in these circumstances, i.e., in the circumstances where the fetus threatens the mother's life, is considerably stronger than we have made it thus far. For in our analysis thus far we have equated abortion with the active act of killing. But this is really not precise. More precisely, we should equate abortion with the withholding of the support for life; it is really tantamount to the removal of a life-support system. True, in both alternatives the end result is the same—the victim, i.e., the fetus in this case, will die. But the means by which it is brought about are significantly different and this difference is all-important in the ethical evaluation of the situation. Thus, telling the mother in these circumstances not to abort is by no means tantamount to taking the position, as some have maintained (e.g., the Catholic church), that we should not interfere and choose the life of one entity over the life of another. For it is not as if the threat to life is emanating here from the outside, i.e., from a third source, to which the two possible victims, i.e., the mother and the fetus, are related in equal innocence and in which case it may well be ethically right to say that it is not for us to play "God" and choose or decide who shall be saved and who shall be sacrificed.[19] Rather, the situation that confronts us here is one in which one of the two parties, i.e., the fetus, is the agent, i.e., the instrument, albeit not willfully so, through which the threat to the mother's life is mediated. Thus, mother and fetus are not situated equally with respect to the issue of the threat to life. The fetus, again albeit not willfully, participates in the setup constituting the threat to life as it pertains to the mother while the mother in no way participates in the setup constituting the threat to life as it pertains to the fetus. So, mother and fetus are not equally innocent victims of a threat to life emanating from a third party. Indeed, the case of those who would want to maintain that mother and fetus are equally innocent parties is further weakened (and, in our judgment, weakened significantly) by the fact that in the context of the situation obtained here abortion is not tantamount to an actual act of killing the fetus but rather it is tantamount to discontinuing the provision of life-support to the fetus. And this being the case, when one opposes abortion in these circumstances one is, in effect, saying to the prospective victim of a killing that, from the ethical vantage point, not only can it not kill its prospective killer in self-defense but that indeed it is under obligation to continue providing life-support to it. We are saying to the mother that, ethically speaking, not only can she not kill its fetus in self-defense but that she is under obligation to extend to it its hospitality and its sustenance.[20] One last point. We have not as yet presented our position regarding the evaluation of the act of suicide from the ethical vantage point. Still, irrespective of what our position may turn out to be, i.e., whether or not it finds the act of suicide ethically reprehensible, there can be no question that here when it is not a question of the person him/herself committing suicide but rather a question of a prescription being imposed from the outside upon the person to commit suicide, such an imposition is ethically reprehensible. It is one thing for one to opt to terminate one's life, it is altogether a different matter, as far as its ethical evaluation is concerned, for one to prescribe to an other to terminate his/her life. Of course with regard to religious traditions, as for example Judaism, which equate suicide with murder, the very possibility of a difference in ethical evaluation between one opting to commit suicide and the prescription of suicide to an other cannot arise—both acts are equally acts implicating murder and are consequently equal in their ethical reprobation. Indeed, with regard to religious traditions, again for example Judaism, in whose view the life of the person does not belong to its human bearer to begin with but rather belongs to God (the human being merely entrusted with it), a case can be made that in the situation confronting us here, where the fetus is threatening the life of the mother, abortion is not only ethically allowed but ethically required and is to be carried out even if it goes against the wishes of the mother. We must admit that such a stance strikes us as sheer madness. If society were to adopt this stance, namely, not allowing the mother to have an abortion in these circumstances, it would perpetrate not only an immoral act but a heinous crime—it would be plain legalized murder. And if we now resort to our original position (a position we believe to have established) that the fetus is not an actual person but, at most, only a potential person, then it is not only a murder, it is an act of senseless murder, it is madness.

The next scenario where, it would seem to us, a justification for abortion is clearly indicated (though perhaps not as pressing as in the previous scenario where the life of the mother is threatened, but then nothing can compare with a threat to life) is where the pregnancy is brought about as a result of rape. For if the fetus is to be viewed as an entity that is biologically alive but only as a potentially, but not fully, actualized person (the only view, as we have argued, that is, in a certain sense, legitimate and corresponds to reality), then the claim made on its behalf not to have its existence terminated cannot possibly take precedence and priority over the wish of the mother to abort. This is so because the state of pregnancy is brought about here through a criminal act, i.e., an act that is morally most reprehensible, an act that resorts to force against the wishes of the mother. There are two considerations that, in our judgment, are most telling in supporting our claim that the mother's wish to abort must prevail in these circumstances.

The first consideration is that it is clear that in the case of rape there is no commitment whatsoever extended by the mother to the fetus. Clearly, there is no possible way to argue that the mother could possibly be presumed to have incurred in any shape or manner any responsibility for bringing the fetus into existence and thus assuming some degree of moral commitment towards sustaining this existence. But clearly, the only way in which a claim not to have one's existence terminated can be placed on behalf of an entity that is not actually but only potentially a person is if the entity towards which the claim is directed has in some way incurred a responsibility towards bringing it into existence in the first place. For in such circumstances a case can be made that the entity here towards which the claim is directed has incurred some ongoing moral commitment towards the entity which it brought into existence (and which is only potentially a person) not to terminate its existence. In the case of rape this clearly does not apply and so there is no ground whatsoever on which to make any moral claim on the mother to sustain the existence of the fetus. The second consideration is that in the case of rape the fetus, as noted, is brought into existence through an act that is ethically most reprehensible, to wit, it is forced upon the mother against her will in an act that violates her freedom and thus personhood. Now, we would submit that since the entity, i.e., the fetus, and the set of circumstances precipitating the dilemma before us has originated in an act that was evil and morally unjustified, it, in turn, can have no moral force to support any of its interests. In more general terms, our argument here is that one cannot disregard or close an eye to the genesis, the origin, of the set of circumstances or of the entity that precipitates the problem before us. One cannot close an eye to this and say, now that it has been brought into existence and is before us we will forget and disregard its past and will deal with it exclusively in its own terms, as it is before us. A morally reprehensible act, an illegitimate act, can have no right to claim that its consequences and fruit be considered as if it were legitimate and morally acceptable. It is morally offensive to suggest that evil should be able to expect that its propagation would receive the support and protection as if it were not evil at all. Even more so, it would clearly be morally offensive to suggest that we, i.e., society, may have the moral right to expect a woman who was raped (or, indeed, coerce her against her will) to go on sustaining the fruit of the rape and so, for all intents and purposes, assist in bringing the consequences of the rape to fruition.

Of course, we have arrived at this judgment only because we have pitted the various considerations for abortion against the claims of the fetus when the fetus is being viewed merely as a *potential* person and not as an *actual* person. The balance of judgment may well be different, however, if the fetus is viewed not just as a potential but as an actual person. For in such circumstances we may well want to argue that even though the fetus is brought into existence through an evil act of injustice that in no way can be condoned, being however already in existence as an actual person means that it is already in an existence that places a rightful claim on one and all not to have its existence terminated and this means that it precludes any moral sanctioning of killing it. If what is involved here is the killing of an actual person, then no consideration can justify it except one consideration and that is that this other actual person is about to kill me. Only the threat to life but nothing else can justify the killing of an actual person. Rape, however, horrible as it is, is not a threat to life.[21] Of course, the presumption in the argument here is that abortion is to be viewed as an act of direct killing and, as we have tried to argue above, such a view is questionable. Indeed, we have suggested that the more valid view of abortion is to view it not in terms of doing or inflicting something on an other (i.e., killing the other) but rather in terms of withholding, of not extending or giving something to an other (this something is not being itself life, albeit its withholding may well result in bringing about the cessation of life). The apt, valid analogy for abortion is the refusal to provide a "home" or sustenance to an other. Indeed, the best analogy for the act of abortion is the act of eviction where the evicted party in all probability would be unable to sustain itself in life. And in this context it is not at all clear that abortion is to be viewed as morally reprehensible in the case of rape even though one views the fetus as an actual person.

Perhaps, the best analogy to the situation confronting us here (in the sense of bringing out more clearly the moral dimension involved) is the hypothetical case where a person, indeed an innocent and helpless person, is thrust by a third party through violence and against my will into my house and that if it were to be evicted it would in all probability not be able to survive in the outside environment and consequently die, so that eviction means here, for all intents and purposes, certain death. Now, in these circumstances, is it morally incumbent upon me to keep this person in my house and, indeed, not only keep but also feed and provide for that person? There is no question that it would be a very decent thing for me to do so, seeing what the consequences of conviction would be. But am I morally obliged to do it, i.e., to keep and provide for that person, so that if I do not, I would be doing something that is morally reprehensible? Admittedly, this is not an easy shot to call. For, on the one hand, one would certainly want to argue that the entity by virtue of being a person has a morally rightful claim on me (and for that matter, on any other person) not to terminate its existence, and this regardless of any other considerations that may enter the picture. So, regardless of the circumstances, we would most probably want to say that morally (and certainly legally) it would be reprehensible of me to pick up a gun and shoot the person. But, on the other hand, as we have already argued above, what is involved here is not a direct killing of the other party but rather the withholding of support and sustenance which in all probability would result in its death. The question is not whether it is morally reprehensible to shoot the other person but whether it is morally reprehensible to evict him/her. Granted, that I do not have the moral right, regardless of the circumstances, to kill the other person, does it follow from this that I also have the moral obligation to provide for that person? Namely, granted that the person has a morally rightful claim on me, regardless of the circumstances, not to terminate his/her existence, does he/she also have a morally rightful claim on me to provide him/her with shelter and sustenance? We don't think so. As said, it would certainly be nice and decent to do so, but there is no moral obligation to do so. A person has a morally rightful claim on his fellow humans not to kill him/her but he/she does not have a morally rightful claim on them to sustain him/her in life. And it is certainly morally questionable to claim that a third party, i.e., society, has the right to make one, a totally innocent and, indeed, an aggrieved an injured party in the situation, foot the bill, so to speak, for the crime committed against it. So it would seem to us that although the decision in the case of rape, when one views the fetus as a fully fledged actual person, is very difficult and therefore, in a sense, to a degree uncertain (certainly, much more difficult and uncertain than in the case in which the fetus is threatening the life of the mother), nonetheless the morally right decision must be, in the last analysis, to allow the mother the right to abort. The balance of the various considerations involved in this case, though admittedly close, is nevertheless in favor of this position. And needless to say that if we come down here in the case of rape on the side of accepting abortion as ethically permissible when the fetus is taken as being a fully fledged actualized person, the case would be much stronger for our coming down on the side of accepting abortion as ethically permissible when the fetus is taken as being only potentially a person.[22]

Thus, in the two scenarios that we have thus far examined, i.e., the scenario based on threat to the life of the mother and the scenario based on rape, we could state our position in a fairly clear-cut and assured manner—we come down on the side of the mother's right to abort. In contra-distinction to this, in the remaining two scenarios, i.e., the scenario where the pregnancy (i.e., the existence of the fetus) is brought about inadvertently and the scenario where the pregnancy, which initially is brought about intentionally, is to be aborted because of the mother subsequently changing her mind, we can state our position in a somewhat less assured and more circumspect manner. This, perhaps, can be accounted for by the fact that, unlike in the preceding scenarios, in the two remaining scenarios we are not faced either by the consideration that the mother's life is being threatened by the presence of the fetus or by the consideration that the existence of the fetus was forced upon the mother against her will, both being considerations which clearly would significantly tilt our assessment of the conflict between the wishes of the mother and the rights of the fetus (when taken either as a fully actualized person or merely as a potential person) in favor of the mother and against the fetus. Also, it can perhaps be accounted for by the further fact that a number of additional considerations which can favor the cause of the fetus or, indeed, mitigate such favoring and which did not play any part in the preceding two scenarios come to the fore to play a significant role in the remaining two scenarios. And, clearly, in such a situation where opposing considerations may vie with each other, different people may arrogate different strength to these opposing considerations and consequently arrive at different assessments as to whether the mother or the fetus (again, the fetus when taken either as a fully actualized person or merely as a potential person) has the advantage. And, given this situation, it is to be expected that many people (as, indeed, is the case with us) would end up holding their assessments somewhat more tentatively and less assuredly.

Now, there are in particular three such considerations that may impinge significantly upon our assessment in the remaining two scenarios. First, we have the consideration of whether the mother incurs any commitment and/or responsibility towards the fetus, seeing that she brings the fetus into existence. Secondly, we have the consideration of whether there are circumstances that would mitigate any incurred commitment and/or responsibility. Thirdly, we have the consideration of how persuasive and/or compelling is the reason on the part of the mother for wanting to abort.[23] It is in the light of these considerations and the relative weights we arrogate to them that we propose to assess the following two scenarios (But, as said, other people may, of course, arrogate different weights to these considerations and therefore arrive at different assessments).

So, let us turn to the first of the remaining two scenarios (i.e., the third scenario in the total count). In this scenario the crucial aspect is that the fetus is brought into existence, i.e., that pregnancy is brought about, inadvertently, to wit, it is brought about by accident or because of ignorance or negligence. Clearly, the common denominator in these three possible ways by which the fetus is brought into existence (and, indeed, as such constituting the factor with respect to which our assessment will be decided) is that in all of them there is no intention on the part of the woman to bring the fetus into existence. And, this being the case, there is clearly no commitment towards the fetus incurred by the woman.[24] In the absence of intention no commitment can be arrogated.

But this is not to say that no responsibility towards the fetus is incurred by the woman. True, if the pregnancy is brought about by pure accident, i.e., by something that normally could not have been foreseen or known, no responsibility can be arrogated to the woman. But if the pregnancy is brought about because of ignorance and, even more so, because of negligence, a case can be made, it would seem to us, that responsibility for the fetus can be arrogated to the mother. For one may well argue that there is no excuse, particularly in our time, for a woman to be ignorant or negligent about these matters and, therefore, there is ethical justification to hold the woman responsible and consequently to see an abortion in these circumstances as being, from an ethical perspective, unacceptable. Still, granting that the woman has or has not done things she should not have or should have done, is it ethically justified to have her pay such a high price for her failing, to wit, to saddle her with such an onerous burden as to carry and provide for an unwanted fetus (and consequently for an unwanted child) because she was ignorant or negligent when she should not have been? Even more, should not her failing, particularly in the case of negligence, be mitigated by the consideration of how strong the sexual drive is in the human and how weak and fragile is the human's capacity to resist temptation? Is it ethically right to have a woman pay such a high price of having to care for an unwanted fetus/child because in a moment of passion she did not have the strength of character or the state of mind to resist or postpone temptation and consequently finds herself guilty of negligence?

There is yet another consideration that should enter our deliberations here, indeed a consideration that arises not only when pregnancy is brought about because of ignorance or negligence but also when it is brought about by accident. Namely, irrespective of how pregnancy is brought about, whether it be because of ignorance or because of negligence or by accident, a case can be made that if the woman, upon learning that she is pregnant, allows her pregnancy to proceed and does not abort, one would be justified in presuming that the woman acquiesces in her pregnancy and this, in turn, would clearly implicate that the woman incurs a commitment towards the fetus so that if later the woman wishes to abort this would have to be assessed in a context where a commitment towards the fetus has been incurred by the woman. On the other hand, however, one can persuasively argue that the woman's failure to immediately decide to abort cannot be taken as implicating her acquiescing in her pregnancy and thus incurring a commitment towards the fetus, that it would not be justified to presume that the delay in moving to counteract the pregnancy signifies its acceptance by the woman. For after all, we must realize that a decision to abort must be emotionally a very difficult decision for the woman—it is one thing not to want to become pregnant, it is quite a different thing to abort. One cannot expect the decision here to be immediate. A certain period of time may well be required here before one can presume that the woman accepted her pregnancy. Thus, the issue here is reduced to the question of how much time would qualify as the sufficient time for one to accept the presumption that the woman accepted her pregnancy and consequently incurred a commitment towards the fetus.

Clearly, neither the question of how much time should qualify as the sufficient time for one to accept the presumption that the woman accepts her pregnancy nor the question of what relative strength is to be assigned respectively to the commitment towards the fetus incurred by the woman and to such mitigating considerations as the human's sexual drive and the human frailty in resisting it are questions in which we have objective ways by which to assess them. Their assessment inescapably implicates subjective evaluations/judgments and consequently different people may arrive at different conclusions or even, indeed, one and the same individual may at different times arrive at different conclusions. And this being the case, all we can do here is give our assessment in the context of how we evaluate/judge the various considerations in the present time. So, let us proceed to briefly state our assessment regarding the three possibilities by which pregnancy can be brought about in the context of the scenario that is before us here.[25]

Thus, beginning with the situation where, for the purpose of covering all conceivable situations, we grant that the fetus is a fully fledged actualized person, it would seem to us that when the pregnancy is brought about by accident, a case can be made that abortion can be ethically sanctioned even though the fetus is taken to be a fully fledged actualized person. The justification for this lies in the consideration that the woman does not incur here any responsibility (and certainly no commitment) to the fetus for its coming into existence and in the further consideration that, strictly speaking, abortion is to be seen as being essentially an act of eviction and not an act of direct actual killing. True, the eviction here would in all probability result in the death of the fetus which is tantamount to saying here that it would result in the death of a fully fledged actualized person, an entity that is endowed with the ethical right not to have its existence terminated. As such, there is no denying that we find ourselves here in a somewhat "gray area." Still, in the last analysis, what the woman is doing, strictly speaking, when she decides to abort is to evict the entity that is a fully fledged actualized person and not to terminate its existence. It would certainly be laudable if, in these circumstances, the woman decides not to abort but such a decision would be grounded in compassion but not in ethical obligation. In terms of the analogy used before, the owner of the house, this being the woman, has no ethical obligation to provide shelter and sustenance to an intruding guest, this being the fetus, if she in no way incurred any responsibility for bringing the intruding guest into her house. As said, it would be very laudable and humane for the owner of the house (i.e., the woman) not to evict the guest (i.e., the fetus), seeing that eviction in all probability would result in the death of the guest (i.e., the fetus). But there is no ethical obligation placed on the owner of the house (i.e., the woman) to refrain from evicting the guest (i.e., the fetus).[26]

There is, however, one consideration that could change this conclusion, namely, that would place an ethical obligation on the owner of the house (i.e., the woman) not to evict the intruding guest (i.e., the fetus)—or, in other words, that would deny ethical sanctioning to the act of eviction, i.e., to the act of abortion—and that is when the owner of the house (i.e., the woman) fails to evict (i.e., abort) the intruding guest within a reasonable period of time. For, in such a case one would be justified in surmising that the owner of the house (i.e., the woman) has acquiesced in the presence of the intruding guest (i.e., the fetus) within her house, such acquiescence, in turn, being tantamount to the owner of the house (i.e., the woman) incurring a commitment/responsibility towards the intruding guest (i.e., the fetus) and inasmuch as the intruding guest (i.e., the fetus) is taken here as a fully fledged actualized person, such a commitment/responsibility would in all probability outweigh any other consideration to the contrary.

Now, this last consideration clearly presages what our position would be regarding the two remaining possible sets of circumstances connected with the bringing on of the pregnancy that are encompassed within this scenario, namely, the sets of circumstances whereby the pregnancy is brought about either because of ignorance or because of negligence on the part of the woman. For, as argued above, while in these two sets of circumstances no commitment towards the fetus can be arrogated to the woman, a responsibility for the fetus is nonetheless incurred by the woman, and this incurred responsibility outweighs, in our judgment, such mitigating considerations as the sexual drive in the human and the frailty of its willpower, particularly in view of the fact that the fetus here is taken to be a fully actualized person and as such an entity that is endowed with an ethical right not to have its existence terminated. The considerations of the sexual drive and of the frailty of the human will are not strong enough to cancel an ethical right to life. So, we must conclude that in the case where the woman incurs a responsibility for bringing the fetus into existence and the fetus is taken to be a fully actualized person, it would be problematic to ethically sanction the abortion of the fetus.

However, quite understandably, our assessment would tilt towards the sanctioning of abortion, i.e., towards favoring the wishes of the woman over the claims of the fetus, if the fetus is taken to be not a fully actualized person but only a potential person. For certainly, in the case where the pregnancy was brought about by accident the woman cannot be placed under an ethical obligation to keep and sustain the fetus—if, as we concluded above, the woman is not placed under an ethical obligation to keep and sustain the fetus when the fetus is taken to be a fully actualized person, how much more so is it the case when the fetus is taken to be only a potential person. But even in the case where the pregnancy is brought about because of ignorance or of negligence on the part of the woman, it is now, when the fetus is taken to be not a fully actualized but only a potential person, not all that clear that the woman is to be placed under an ethical obligation to keep and sustain the fetus. Here it may well seem that the mitigating considerations of the sex drive in the human and the frailty of its willpower would prevail over the consideration of the ethical right of the fetus not to have its existence terminated, seeing that the fetus here is taken to be only a potential but not a fully actualized person. Clearly, we are here in a gray area where the assessment would ultimately depend on whether or not one would want to maintain that an entity which is only a potential but not a fully actualized person possesses an ethical right not to have its existence terminated and if it does, whether or not its claim is strong enough to prevail over other considerations that oppose its claim. Different people may well come down on different sides of this question.

Lastly, our fourth scenario is the scenario where the pregnancy is initially intended by the woman but where the woman later changes her mind and wishes to abort. Clearly, this is the scenario where the case for ethically sanctioning abortion is the weakest. For in this context, the claims of the fetus would by far outweigh the wishes of the mother than in any of the other contexts that we have examined, seeing that here the woman incurs not only a responsibility but also a clear commitment towards the fetus. As such, a case can be made here that abortion would be ethically unacceptable not only when the fetus is taken to be a fully actualized person but also when it is taken to be merely a potential person. Indeed, when the fetus is taken to be a fully actualized person, the only situation where abortion could be ethically acceptable is when the fetus directly threatens the life of its mother. And even when the fetus is taken to be only a potential person, the ethical acceptability of abortion, while in principle it is available here, its applicability is clearly limited—it is limited to there being a persuasive reason for the woman to have changed her mind and wishing the fetus to be aborted. The acceptability of abortion here is contingent on whether or not the reason for aborting is deemed valid by us, namely, on whether or not we deem the reason for aborting good enough to justify the abortion. Thus, for example, the threatening of the mother's life by the pregnancy would constitute, in our judgment, a valid and persuasive reason/justification for aborting—the threat to the mother's life overrides any commitment she may have undertaken towards the fetus.[27] On the other hand, the desire of the woman to go skiing or scuba-diving (i.e., activities that would be precluded by her pregnancy) would not constitute, in our judgment, a valid and persuasive reason/justification for aborting—the gratification (or even more to the point here, the immediate satisfaction of the gratification) of the woman's desire to go skiing or scuba-diving does not override the commitment towards the fetus that she had incurred. In both of the foregoing instances the validation (in the first instance) or the lack of validation (in the second instance) of the reasoning for abortion is, in our judgment, clear-cut and unwavering in its persuasiveness.

But clearly, there may be instances where the validation or the lack of validation of the reasoning for abortion is by no means all that clear-cut and unwavering in its persuasiveness. Thus, what about the instance where the reasoning for aborting is that after becoming pregnant the finances of the family collapse and the addition of another child to the family would greatly strain the ability of the parents to provide for the children they already have? Or what about the instance where the reasoning for aborting is that after becoming pregnant the woman realizes that her marriage (or, alternatively, that her relationship with her lover) has disintegrated beyond repair and that in these circumstances having the child would place a serious psychological strain upon her? Finally, what about the instance where the reasoning for aborting is that after becoming pregnant the woman finds out that continuing the pregnancy, while not being fatal, would impair her health for the rest of her life? Now, in all these instances, different people can no doubt arrive at opposite conclusions, some validating while others disvalidating the reasoning. It would seem to us, however, that whether one validates or disvalidates these reasoning would, in no small measure, depend on whether one takes the notion of "potential person" as it is applied in the situation here (i.e., as it is applied with reference to the fetus' ethical right not to have its existence terminated) in a maximalist or minimalist sense. If it is taken in a minimalist sense, then in all likelihood the reasoning here would be validated while if it is taken in a maximalist sense, then in all likelihood the reasoning here would be disvalidated. Since we take the notion of "potential person" as it is applied to the fetus in its minimalist sense (as will be recalled we made the case that the notion of potentiality can apply to the fetus only when it is taken as a biological entity but not when it is taken as a personal entity, and that if this be the case, then an ethical right not to have one's existence terminated cannot pertain to the fetus when it is taken as a potential person because the establishment of such an ethical right is feasible only with respect to an entity that is constituted as a personal entity and not with respect to an entity that is constituted as a biological entity), we indeed find the reasoning for aborting in these instances to be valid and persuasive.

In summing up, we may note that when we grant that the fetus is to be taken as a fully actualized person or even when it is to be taken merely as a potential person, our assessment, as we proceeded through these scenarios in the order presented here, tilted in favor of the fetus' claim not to have its existence terminated and against the woman's wishes to abort (though, of course, needless to say, the progressive tilt in each scenario towards the fetus' claim over the woman's wishes is much more pronounced when the fetus is taken to be a fully actualized person rather than merely as a potential person). What is, however, even more significant for us here to note is that even when the fetus is taken to be merely a potential person or even when it is taken to be a fully actualized person, there are situations in these scenarios (in all four of them when it is taken to be merely a potential person and in the first three but not in the fourth when it is taken to be a fully actualized person) where the woman's wishes to abort outweigh the fetus' claim not to have its existence terminated. For after all, the whole point of the exercise here where we granted that the fetus be taken as a merely potential person or as a fully actualized person was precisely to see whether in these circumstances such situations could arise where the woman's wishes to abort would prevail over the fetus' claim not to have its existence terminated. Still, as was already stated above any number of times, this is in no way to be taken as intimating that we can accept either of these two alternatives as authentic representations of the ontological status of the fetus. Given our delineation of the notion of personhood in terms of self-consciousness, i.e., a person is an entity that possesses self-consciousness, and our claim that such a notion does not lend itself to gradation, i.e., it either manifests itself fully or not at all, the possibility of the fetus being a fully actualized person must be clearly excluded and the status of potentiality can be attributed to it only in a minimalist but not in a maximalist sense, i.e., only in terms of its being a biological but not in terms of its being a personal entity. And this being the case, our position must be that, in the last analysis, abortion is ethically acceptable in all conceivable situations.[28]

Infanticide

Given our claim above (i.e., in chapter 2) that it is solely by virtue of possessing an ontological constitution that implicates self-consciousness that an entity is endowed with an ethical right not to have its existence terminated, we must conclude, if we are to be consistent, that newly born infants in the first few months of their life are not endowed with an ethical right not to have their existence terminated. This is so inasmuch as a newly born infant, till about its seventh or eighth month, does not seem to possess self-consciousness even in its most minimalist manifestation, i.e., when it manifests itself merely in the capacity to acknowledge and extend affirmation.[29] Thus, there is a short period after birth where consistency requires us to concede that a validation of the feasibility of infanticide is possible.

It must be emphasized, however, that this feasibility of infanticide with respect to the newly born infant during the first few months of its life is, and indeed can be, validated here only because it is viewed and assessed from the vantage point of the ethical perspective (ethical, needless to say, as delineated by us here). It is not, and indeed cannot be, validated when it is viewed and assessed from the vantage point of the perspective of the law. For while in the context of the ethical perspective the criterion for the assessment, i.e., the point where the capability to acknowledge and to extend affirmation first arises, may vary from one infant to another (for example, arising in the sixth month of life in one infant and in the eighth month of life in another) and, indeed, where the ascertainment of the criterion does not have to be objectively delineated and universally acceptable (namely, ascertaining the occurrence of the acknowledgment and extension of affirmation is per force subjective to a degree and may well vary from one observer to another), in the context of the perspective of the law the criterion must be fixed at the same point for all infants and must lend itself to being ascertained objectively and accepted universally. In other words, while in the context of the ethical perspective the criterion for the assessment can be established conditionally (namely, if this and this be the case then the ethical evaluation would be thus and so, to wit, whenever the capability to acknowledge and to extend affirmation manifests itself in an infant, terminating its existence would be evaluated negatively as murder) and its ascertainment can be subjective (namely, one can ethically evaluate terminating the existence of an infant as murder because in his/her judgment the capability to acknowledge and extend affirmation did manifest itself in the infant while another can ethically evaluate the same termination of existence as not being murder because in his/her judgment the capability to acknowledge and extend affirmation did not manifest itself in the infant), in the context of the perspective of the law the criterion for assessment must be established factually and as such unconditionally and it must be ascertained objectively and be applicable in the same way universally (we cannot have a situation where one can claim the presence of the criterion while another can deny it and where there is no way of resolving the contradiction; nor can we have a situation where it is possible for one to claim that the termination of the existence of a certain infant in its sixth month of life is to be viewed as murder while the termination of another infant's existence at precisely the same time of its life, i.e., in the sixth month of its life, is not to be viewed as murder). This is so because in the perspective of law the assessment necessarily implicates practical application while in the ethical perspective the evaluation is theoretical and need not have practical application, and practical application, unlike theoretical pronouncement, requires a criterion that is definitive and universal in its applicability. Unfortunately, as seen, the original manifestation of the capability to acknowledge and extend affirmation in the newly born infant does not provide the perspective of the law with a criterion that is definitive, objective and universal. The perspective of the law, therefore, must seek an occurrence that is temporally closest to the occurrence where the capability to acknowledge and affirm first manifest themselves but which, in contradistinction to it, can provide the perspective of the law with a criterion that is definitive, objective and universal. Such an occurrence is evidently the birth of the infant and, indeed, within the perspective of the law it is taken as the occurrence from which point the infant is taken to be a person, thus clearly foreclosing the option of infanticide.

And while, by and large, we would want the law to adapt itself to the ethics, namely, we would want the prescriptions of the law to reflect and concur with the evaluations of the ethics thus, in other words, have the perspective of the law defer to the ethical perspective, with regard to the situation confronting us here a good case can be made that the ethical perspective should defer to the perspective of the law, which is to say that the infant should be viewed as a personal entity from the very moment of its birth. There are, in the main, two reasons for taking this position. First, although we have maintained that with respect to this issue the notion of potentiality can really apply to the entity in question only with regard to its biological dimension and not with regard to its dimension of personhood and that therefore the infant prior to its manifesting self-consciousness is, strictly speaking, not really a potential person, the appearance of self-consciousness in the infant is so close at hand and so certain to appear that even though the infant cannot claim not to have its existence terminated on the grounds that it is a potential person, its existence should not be terminated. Secondly, and perhaps even more persuasively, it is, by and large, difficult to think of a situation that would implicate the possibility of having to terminate the existence of the newly born infant. For in contra-distinction to the previous issue considered here, i.e., the issue of abortion, the issue of infanticide (as indeed the other issues involving the termination of existence which will be considered below) does not present us with a situation in which we are confronted with a conflict between the interests/wishes of two personal entities. There is no other personal entity here (e.g., the mother) whose interests/wishes clash with those of the newly born infant. True, the newly born infant needs to be fed and sheltered. But these needs impose a burden on the parents or on society that in today's world (certainly in the Western world) can be easily afforded and would, by no stretch of the imagination, implicate the need to terminate the existence of the newly born infant. So, why terminate the existence of the newly born infant? What consideration would be sufficiently persuasive to lead us to do such a thing? Indeed, the question of terminating the existence of the newly born infant (as indeed of any other personal entity, as we shall see in the issues discussed below) can arise only if the interests/wishes of the personal entity in question (i.e., the entity with respect to which the question of the termination of existence is raised) can establish that terminating its existence would be better for it than its continuing in existence. Such a situation may indeed arise with respect to the newly born infant, namely, a situation where its interests (one cannot really speak here of its wishes) would clearly weigh in in favor of terminating its existence. We shall consider such a possible situation in conjunction with the next issue to which we now turn, to wit, the issue of euthanasia.

Euthanasia

To begin with, we must clarify our position with respect to some issues that arise in conjunction with the phenomenon of euthanasia. Thus, first we must clarify what we take the term euthanasia to signify. Now, the word euthanasia literally means a good death (i.e., a death which, given the circumstances, is an act of kindness) or, in common usage, a mercy killing. As such, it should not be surprising that many people use the term to signify a killing when the killing is to be taken as an act of mercy. Namely, they delineate the phenomenon of euthanasia solely in terms of mercy killing, which is to say that they define the phenomenon in terms of the kind of death it implicates, to wit, a good in contra-distinction to a bad kind of death. Now, there is no denying that the factor of mercy killing is included in the signification of the term and that, indeed, it is an essential ingredient in the phenomenon. The question, however, is whether it alone suffices to adequately define the phenomenon. It is here that we must differ from those who delineate the phenomenon of euthanasia exclusively in terms of mercy killing. For us the delineation of the phenomenon must in addition also signify that the decision to bring about death is not made by the prospective object of the decision, namely, by the party to which the decision is directed, but by an outside party as, for example, by a physician or by a next of kin. Thus, for us a satisfactory definition of the term must include in its signification both stipulations, i.e., the stipulation that the implicated act of killing be an act of mercy killing and the stipulation that the agent making the decision to bring about death be not the prospective victim of the decision but a third party. Indeed, we would submit that only be delineating the phenomenon of euthanasia in this way, i.e., by making the delineation contingent on these two stipulations being satisfied, can it be clearly distinguished from all alternative phenomena implicating the bringing about of death, more specifically, given our immediate concerns here, from the phenomena of suicide, assisted suicide and capital punishment. For, if the delineation of the phenomenon of euthanasia is to be solely in terms whereby the decision to terminate one's existence is arrogated to an outside party, then, although suicide and assisted suicide could indeed be distinguished from euthanasia by virtue of the fact that the decision to bring about death is not made here by an outside party but by the party that is the object of the decision, capital punishment could not be distinguished from euthanasia because here too the decision to terminate one's existence is arrogated to an outside party. On the other hand, if the delineation of the phenomenon of euthanasia is to be solely in terms of mercy killing, then, although as such it could be distinguished from capital punishment (seeing that capital punishment does not implicate mercy killing), it could not, however, be distinguished either from suicide or from assisted suicide inasmuch as these two phenomena may very well (albeit not necessarily) implicate mercy killing.[30]

Secondly, we have to clarify our position with regard to the distinction that can be made with respect to the phenomenon of euthanasia whereby death can be brought about either by an act of killing the party designated for euthanasia or, alternatively, by not undertaking acts that could save such a party from death, namely, with regard to the distinction that can be introduced into the phenomenon of euthanasia between active and passive euthanasia. Now, there can be no question that such a distinction can be validly introduced with respect to the phenomenon of euthanasia itself—clearly, the party can receive its mercy killing, its good death, either by being actively killed or by passively being allowed to die by not providing it with the required sustenance or medication. The question, however, which remains (and it is after all this question which is of central concern to us here) is whether a distinction can also be validly introduced with respect to how these two modes of bringing about euthanasia are to be ethically evaluated. And here, we would submit, the answer would depend on how one chooses to view the ethical enterprise. Thus, for example, if one chooses to view it from the utilitarian vantage point where the ethical evaluation is to be determined by the consequences that would ensue from the act that is to be ethically evaluated, then clearly a distinction cannot be validly introduced. For clearly the consequences in both modes of bringing about death are the same—the bottom line in both modes is that death is brought about and the aspect of how it is brought about is inconsequential.[31] By the way, the introduction of the further distinction between the obligation to apply ordinary measures and the obligation to apply extraordinary measures to sustain the patient in life, whereby the former is expected but not the latter, is also beside the point as far as our position here is concerned. And this is so not only because, as pointed out above, the obligation of the physician to sustain the patient in life bases itself on professional and not on ethical grounds. For even if it did base itself on ethical grounds, it would not be applicable here, seeing that for us the ethical obligation to sustain a person in life, like the ethical obligation not to terminate a person's life, is to be established in terms of rights derived from the ontological constitution of the entity in question and this being the case, it cannot be said that the entity in question comes to possess an ethical right to be sustained in life only when ordinary measures but not when extraordinary measures are to be used—if an ethical right to be sustained in life is established, then whatever the measures required to effect such sustenance are, they must be provided. On the other hand, however, if one chooses to view the ethical enterprise from the vantage point of the rights and obligations inherent in the very ontological constitution of the parties involved where the ethical evaluation is to be determined by whether or not the act respects, i.e., does not violate, the rights possessed by its object (the view embraced by us), then there would be a telling distinction in the ethical evaluation that would ensue depending on which mode of bringing about death was implicated. For while we have established (at least to our own satisfaction) that any entity that is ontologically constituted as a person (i.e., per our definition above a person is an entity that possesses self-consciousness) possesses an ethical right not to have its existence terminated (and correspondingly it possesses an ethical obligation not to terminate the existence of any other entity that is ontologically constituted as a person), this in no way implicates that an entity that is ontologically constituted as a person possesses also an ethical right to be sustained in life (or, correspondingly, an ethical obligation to sustain in life any entity that is ontologically constituted as a person) and the prospects of independently establishing such a right do not seem to us to be promising.[32]

Indeed, similar skepticism as to the validity of equating the ethical evaluation of the active act of killing another person with that of the passive act of not saving such a person may well underlie the offering of an alternative formulation by which the relation between these two ethical evaluations is to be established. According to this formulation the ethical evaluation here is not to be established on the basis of what kind of act is involved, namely, whether it is an active act or a passive act is to have no bearing on determining the ethical evaluation of these acts. Rather, the ethical evaluation is to be determined here exclusively on the basis of what kind of intention is involved, namely, is the intention to have the other person dead or not? If it be the former, then the ethical evaluation would be negative, while if it be the latter, then the ethical evaluation would not be negative, and this is irrespective of whether the death of the other person is effected through an active act of killing or through a passive act of not saving. As such, we can have a case of killing another person where the ethical evaluation would not be negative inasmuch as there was no intention to have the other person dead (the killing being, for example, accidental), and we can have a case of not saving another person where the ethical evaluation would be negative inasmuch as there was an intention to have the other person dead (as, for example, seeing the other person drowning and my not saving him/her, even though it involved no risk to myself, because I wished to have that other person dead).

Now, we must concede that this alternative formulation has considerable merit on its side. For it cannot be denied that ethical evaluation necessarily and inescapably implicates intentions, that it is carried out in terms of intentions. The question arises, however, whether the evaluation can be carried out in terms of the intentions taken in themselves (so that the mere internal possession of an intention would suffice for the ethical evaluation to be applicable) or whether it can be carried out only with respect to intentions that express themselves in concrete acts. Namely, should we maintain that ethics really evaluates concrete acts/relations but that it evaluates them exclusively in terms of the intentions that they implicate or that it evaluates intentions taken in themselves irrespective of whether or not they are implicated in any concrete act/relation?[33] Given the way we formulated the ethical enterprise above, we must opt for the former delineation whereby ethics evaluates acts/relations and not intentions as such, and this being the case, we cannot accept the alternative formulation proposed here, seeing that the evaluation in this formulation is not directed towards acts/relations. We should note, however, that the claim for equivalence in the ethical evaluation of actively killing another person and passively not saving such a person can be rejected not only in terms of the latter delineation (i.e., the delineation whereby ethical evaluation is directed to intentions as such and not to concrete acts/relations) adopted by the alternative formulation presented here but equally so in terms of the former delineation (i.e., the delineation whereby ethical evaluation is directed to concrete acts/relations and not to intentions as such) adopted in our formulation of the ethical enterprise. This is so because passively not saving another person does not constitute a concrete act and therefore it cannot be ethically evaluated, which is to say that it is neutral as regards ethical evaluation.[34] Thus, in both formulations, namely, in the formulation in which ethical evaluation is directed towards concrete acts and in the formulation in which it is directed towards intentions as such, the difference as regards ethical evaluation between killing and not saving another person is retained, though the rationale for retaining this difference, which operates in these two formulations, is different (in the latter formulation it operates by removing ethical evaluation from being directed towards concrete acts while in the former evaluation it operates by excluding not saving another person from being a concrete act). As such, even though we cannot accept as valid the alternative formulation presented here which directs ethical evaluation exclusively to the intentions as such, this does not affect our ability to maintain a distinction between killing and not saving, i.e., between what has been referred to respectively as active and passive acts, as regards their ethical evaluation.[35]

Having tried to make our position clear with respect to some questions that impinge upon the issue of euthanasia, we can now proceed to state how the act of euthanasia will acquit itself when evaluated from an ethical perspective. This can be done fairly briefly, seeing that the criteria by which the ethical evaluation is established have been clearly set and the act of euthanasia has been clearly delineated. The only thing that needs still to be introduced into the picture before the ethical evaluation can be validly established is the relevant set of circumstances, the relevant situation, in which the act of euthanasia takes place. Once this is done, the ethical evaluation can be clearly established.

Now, there are, we would submit, three distinct situations in which an act of euthanasia may be resorted to and the ethical evaluation of the act may well differ, depending on the situation in which the act is resorted to. Thus, we can have a situation where the resort to euthanasia is motivated by the fact that a fully fledged personal entity, e.g., an adult human, due to severe brain damage, loses completely its consciousness and it is quite clear that there can be no expectation that it could ever regain its consciousness.[36] We can also have a situation where the resort to euthanasia is taken as the means by which to eliminate humans who are deemed not to measure up to the standards taken as the ideal, desired standards by which the human species is to characterize itself—in short, a situation in which euthanasia is resorted to in order to effect eugenics. Lastly, we can have a situation where the resort to euthanasia is in response to learning upon the birth of a child that it is afflicted with an incurable disease (which may or may not result in eventual death) that inflicts intolerable continuous suffering (e.g., cystic fibrosis) or that dramatically diminishes the quality of life (e.g., Down's syndrome) or that without involving unusual physical suffering leads inescapably to a relatively early death (e.g., Tay-Sachs disease). And, as already noted, the resort to euthanasia in these three situations may well elicit different ethical evaluations.

Thus, resorting to euthanasia in the context of the first situation cited here would be, in our judgment, ethically justified. For after all, the victim of the act is no longer and will never again be an entity that possesses consciousness, leave alone self-consciousness, in other words, a person and as such it can neither extend affirmation nor possess an ethical right to request/demand that it be affirmed. It is, for all intents and purposes, like a dead corpse, nothing else but a collection of molecules, except that here with respect to this collection of molecules the physical process of putrefaction has not set in. As against this, resorting to euthanasia in the context of the second situation cited here would be, in our judgment, ethically unjustified, indeed, ethically reprehensible. For the ethical right possessed by an entity not to have its existence terminated is contingent on one and only one consideration, namely, that the entity should possess self-consciousness, in other words, that it be a person. No other consideration, be it whether or not the entity possesses certain physical, mental or character attributes (as, for example, possessing blonde hair or blue eyes, an unusual talent for mathematics or music, courage or honesty), can have any bearing on whether or not the entity possesses an ethical right not to have its existence terminated. A dim-wit just as much as a genius, a six-footer just as much as a midget, a tone-deaf person just as much as a Mozart, has an ethical right not to have its existence terminated. As long as an entity is a person, i.e., is endowed with self-consciousness, it possesses an ethical right not to have its existence terminated. Thus, inasmuch as the prospective victim of the act of euthanasia is a person, an act of terminating its existence is but an act of murder, an act that, in no uncertain terms, is ethically reprehensible.[37]

Now, the foregoing two situations, not withstanding that the ethical evaluation of the act of euthanasia in them comes down at opposite poles (i.e., as ethically acceptable in the first situation and ethically unacceptable in the second situation), do share in common the fact that in both the ethical evaluation of the act of euthanasia can be determined in a clear-cut and decisive manner. We have no ambivalence or nagging doubts in having determined the act positively in the first situation and negatively in the second situation. When we turn, however, to the third situation, the determination of the ethical evaluation of the act of euthanasia becomes more problematic and uncertain for us (and indeed we must concede that different people may very well arrive, in the last analysis, at different evaluations).[38] The determination, therefore, of the ethical evaluation of the act of euthanasia that arises in the context of the third situation delineated here is offered by us with less certainty and more circumspection.

Actually, there are three determinations to be made, seeing that there were three sets of circumstances that we identified within the third situation. Thus, with regard to the first set of circumstances exemplified by the prognosis of cystic fibrosis, we are inclined to think that a resort to an act of euthanasia would be ethically acceptable. For, would it not be an act of mercy to spare the baby intolerable pain in the future by killing it now when it is not capable of knowing or understanding what death signifies?[39] As against this, with regard to the second set of circumstances exemplified by the prognosis of Down's syndrome, a resort to an act of euthanasia would not be, in our judgment, ethically acceptable. For in this case there is no suffering involved as far as the victim of the syndrome is concerned. On the contrary, the victims are, by and large, happy and content. True, there is a marked deficit as far as the quality of life is concerned inasmuch as the intellectual capabilities of the victim are greatly reduced. But this should not have any bearing on whether or not the victim possesses an ethical right not to have its existence terminated (see our discussion with regard to the second situation cited here, i.e., the situation where euthanasia is to be carried out for the sake of eugenics). The only consideration that has a bearing on this question is whether or not the victim possesses self-consciousness, and this the victim here clearly possesses (as is manifested in its capacity to extend affirmation and in return request/demand to be affirmed). So, even though there may be considerable suffering and hardship inflicted on the parents of the victim (and possibly considerable cost to society), this cannot override the ethical right possessed by the victim not to have its existence terminated.

Lastly, with regard to the third set of circumstances exemplified by the Tay-Sachs disease, we are inclined to hold that resorting to an act of euthanasia, if so chosen by the parents of the victim, would be ethically acceptable. At first sight, this may seem strange, seeing that this set of circumstances is similar to the second set of circumstances with respect to many of the factors that may count in determining our stance (in particular we have the similarity that in both suffering may devolve on the parents but not on the victim). Indeed, if anything, the set of circumstances here should lend itself even more to finding the resort to an act of euthanasia ethically unacceptable inasmuch as here we do not even have a deficit in the quality of life to contend with (if anything, the baby here is more developed and agile than run-of-the-mill babies). However, a moment's reflection would show that there is also a difference between this set of circumstances and the previous one, and it is this difference that accounts for the change in our stance. The difference is that, in contra-distinction to the previous set of circumstances where the person with the Down's syndrome attains adulthood and has a full span of life, albeit shorter than that of unafflicted persons, the baby here is doomed to die in a matter of a few years. Thus, we have here a situation where the parents have to live for a number of years with the knowledge that their baby, who is bright, active, and quite likely beautiful (what baby is not?), carries a death sentence. This is something parents having a child with Down's syndrome do not have inflicted upon them. And for some parents of children having Tay-Sachs disease, the suffering may be too great to take. With respect to such instances a case can be made that the suffering of the parents may override the ethical right of the baby not to have its existence terminated. For after all, one can argue, the baby is doomed to die (and in a span of time that, relatively speaking, is not too protracted, though for suffering parents it may well seem like eternity), so that resorting to the act of euthanasia merely means advancing the clock. Also, although we generally treat here the newly born baby as a person (for the reasons given above), strictly speaking the newly born baby, by the time a diagnosis of the disease can be made, is not yet a person. In other contexts we opted to close an eye to this fact. But in the context here, when we are dealing with the kind of suffering the parents will, in all probability, have to undergo day in and day out, closing an eye to this fact may not be justified.

True, there is also the possibility that some parents may opt against resorting to an act of euthanasia, preferring to keep and care for the child notwithstanding the suffering that they know lies in store for them; and coupled with this there is, no doubt, also the hope in many parents that a cure will be found in the interim so that their suffering would have justification after all. Now clearly, this stance, in contrast to the foregoing stance, avoids a clash with the ethical right of the child not to have its existence terminated. But, just as clearly, it does not overcome the suffering of the parents, a suffering that must come about when one lives with one's child who is doomed to die. Thus, in the foregoing course of action, where one resorts to the act of euthanasia, the suffering emanating from living with one's child who is doomed to die is indeed eliminated, but the clash with the ethical right of the child not to have its existence terminated is not. On the other hand, in the course of action presented here, where one does not resort to the act of euthanasia, a clash with the ethical right of the child not to have its existence terminated is avoided, but the suffering emanating from living with one's child, who is doomed to die, is not overcome. Ideally, of course, one would want to have a course of action that would satisfy both requirements, i.e., avoid a clash with the ethical right of the child not to have its existence terminated and overcome (or, more accurately, mitigate) that suffering of the parents that is brought about by their having to live day in and day out with their child who is doomed to die.

Now, it would seem that such a course of action may indeed be provided by a stance that would hold that the ethically acceptable thing to do for parents who cannot accept the prospect of the suffering resulting from their having to be in continuous contact with their doomed child would be not to resort to an act of euthanasia but rather to give the child to an outside party as, for example, a communal or a private institution (or even, perhaps, another family) to be looked after (and, needless to say, that if in the interim a cure becomes available, our dilemma here would be resolved and the child, of course, is to be returned to its parents). For such a course of action certainly avoids a clash with the ethical right of the child not to have its existence terminated, and it does abrogate the continuous, day in and day out contact between parents and child. But can the giving away of the child to an outside party mitigate the suffering of the parents to the same extent as resorting to an act of euthanasia would do? (It is important to keep in mind that we are not talking here about the suffering brought about by the tragedy of having a child afflicted with this fatal disease—this suffering can be assuaged, if at all, only by time—but about the suffering that is brought about by being in continuous, close contact with one's child who is doomed to die.) It would not seem so. For while giving away the child would clearly reduce the contact, it does not stop it completely as resorting to an act of euthanasia would do. Presumably, it would be very difficult for parents not to come periodically to visit the child, and even if they were to be prevented from visitation, nothing could stop them from thinking and wondering how their child was doing, something that would not apply if there was a resort to an act of euthanasia. Giving away the child certainly reduces the suffering in comparison to keeping and caring for it at home, but it does not reduce it to the same extent as resorting to an act of euthanasia would.

Moreover, there is a further consideration here that is of considerable significance and should not be overlooked in estimating the advantages and drawbacks of the various options. Namely, when the child's death is effected by resorting to an act of euthanasia, the child would in all probability be only a few days (or, at most, a few weeks) old and consequently would not have as yet developed a distinctive personality that, in tern, would limit, in all probability, the strength of the parents' bonding to it. In contrast, if the child's death is effected by the disease running its course, the child at death would, in all probability, be already a few years old and thus possessing a distinctive personality that, in turn, would per force greatly strengthen the parents' bonding to it. There is bound to be a difference as regards the parents' suffering between losing a child that is only a few days or a few weeks old and losing a child that is a few years old. There is a more effective closure for the parents by turning to an act of euthanasia than by giving the child away and having it die a few years later. As far as the parents' suffering is concerned, the least suffering is incurred, in the long run, by turning to an act of euthanasia, then by giving the child away to an outside party, and only then by keeping and caring for the child at home. But, of course, in opting to keep and care for the child at home and also in opting to give the child away to an outside party, but not in opting to resort to an act of euthanasia, we avoid a clash with the ethical right of the child not to have its existence terminated. Thus, if the evaluation of the options is to encompass as criteria not only the parents' suffering but also the ethical right of the child not to have its existence terminated, then we may well have to conclude that the option of giving the child away to an outside party would be the least bad course of action in a situation that is admittedly a bad situation. On the other hand, however, seeing how excruciating the suffering of the parents must be in this situation, should we not suspend in this instance our concession that infants should be taken as being persons from the very moment of their birth and resort to the original and indeed, pedantically speaking, more valid claim that infants in the first few months (certainly, in the first few days) of life cannot be taken as persons and consequently as entities possessing an ethical right not to have their existence terminated; and this being the case, committing an act of euthanasia with respect to such infants would not precipitate a clash with the ethical right of an entity that is ontologically constituted as a person not to have its existence terminated. And yet, should we really retract our concession that infants are to be taken as persons from the very moment of their birth, seeing what seriously disturbing implications may ensue from such a retraction? Should we not after all be better off, in the last analysis, to revert to our original position, which acknowledged both the infant's ethical right not to have its existence terminated and the suffering of the parents, and which in this context could validly maintain that the least evil solution available to us is to give the child to an outside party?

Clearly, in the scenario presented here, we, for one, cannot come up with a clear-cut, decisive prescription as to which course of action is to be followed. We are like the proverbial sick person who cannot be comfortable in whatever posture he turns to. Obviously, the stance one would adopt here towards the act of euthanasia would depend on the relative weight one would place on the two considerations that we have acknowledged as factors playing a legitimate role in determining one's stance towards the act of euthanasia, i.e., the consideration of the ethical right possessed by the infant not to have its existence terminate and the consideration of the parents' suffering. And this being the case, one has to concede that different people or the same person at different times may place different weights on these two considerations and consequently arrive at different stances as regards the application of the act of euthanasia here. In this relativistic context there are only two claims that we can maintain in a clear-cut and decisive manner, namely, first, the claim that in this situation the decision of which course of action is to be pursued must be left exclusively in the discretion of the parents, and secondly, the claim that a decision by the parents to resort to an act of euthanasia would not be ethically unacceptable.

One last brief observation impinging on the issue of euthanasia may be in order here. Namely, our position argued above, in contrast to many utilitarian ethicists, that there is a significant difference as regards ethical evaluation between terminating one's existence in an active act and allowing one's existence to terminate by passively not doing anything to save it, is particularly applicable in ethically evaluating the act of euthanasia. For in all likelihood the preponderant instances involving the act of euthanasia would implicate a passive rather than an active act whereby the person's existence is terminated.

We say this because it seems to us that observation would substantiate the claim that the preponderance of instances where an act of euthanasia is likely to be applied are instances in which the person has totally lost consciousness and there is no prospect of him/her ever regaining it, or instances in which a newly born infant is so deformed physiologically that it can survive in existence only when placed on life support, and in both kinds of instances existence would be terminated not by an active act of killing but rather by a passive act of not providing life support. The other instances where an act of euthanasia may be applied and where indeed the act, in all likelihood, would have to be carried out in an active act of killing are instances of eugenics or of infants born fully normal but who are doomed to die in the span of a few years, e.g., infants afflicted with Tay-Sachs disease. But these instances, fortunately enough, are not very common, and anyway as regards instances of eugenics, our stance has clearly rejected their ethical validity and, therefore, they cannot be counted among instances in which a legitimate act of euthanasia has been applied (they are instances where acts of murder rather than of euthanasia are being applied) and as regards instances of Tay-Sachs disease, we have been of a divided mind and very uncertain in our position and they are really very few, exclusively confined to a certain segment of the Jewish population.

True, in most of the instances here, not providing life support would in all likelihood consist not of withholding life support, i.e., of not providing life support to begin with, but rather in withdrawing life support, i.e., discontinuing life support that is already being given, and this in a way does implicate an active rather than a passive act which as such may lead one to believe that it would clash with a person's ethical right not to have its existence terminated. But closer examination would show that this is not really the case. For although withdrawing life support is indeed an active act, it is an active act with respect to sustaining a person in existence but not with respect to terminating its existence (the termination of existence here as, indeed, in the case of passively withholding life support, although it implicates a termination of existence as an ensuing consequence, it does not implicate it as a direct one-to-one consequence—the termination of existence is due to another factor that albeit is not blocked by the active act of withdrawing or by the passive act of withholding life support). As such, an act of withdrawing life support, just like an act of withholding it, does not really clash, in the last analysis, with a person's ethical right not to have its existence terminated. For the ethical right, as delineated by us here, does not require of us to maintain the other, if it be a person, in existence but only not to actively terminate its existence. And if this be the case, then the act of euthanasia would indeed not be, in the last analysis, ethically unacceptable.

Capital Punishment

The first thing to note with respect to the issue of capital punishment is that here, in contra-distinction to the issues of abortion, euthanasia and even infanticide, we must clearly concede that the entity whose existence is to be terminated, i.e., the object of the prospective act of killing, is a fully fledged actualized person, i.e., an entity that fully bears self-consciousness, that clearly participates in the Thou-dimension. And the second thing to note, again in contra-distinction to the issues of abortion, euthanasia, infanticide, and also the issue we will consider next, i.e., the issue of suicide, is that the act of killing is carried out here as a punishment, namely, for the sake of putatively satisfying the requirements of justice rather than satisfying the interests or the wishes of the object of the act or of an outside party.[40]

Now, with regard to the first observation, it would seem that inasmuch as the murderer is a fully fledged person executing him/her would be ethically unacceptable. Just because the murderer committed an act that is ethically unacceptable does not mean that society can likewise commit an act that is ethically unacceptable. As against this, however, one can argue (as, indeed, we have argued above) that by virtue of committing the act of murder the murderer negates and thus loses his/her personhood and consequently his/her execution by society is not an act that is ethically unacceptable—killing an entity that is not a person is not ethically unacceptable.

But is the application here of this counter-argument really valid? True, what this counter-argument can validly maintain (as, indeed, was made clear above) is that in the specific act of murdering the murderer abdicates his/her personhood—in murdering another person, seeing that this is an unmitigated, all-embracing act of utilization, the murderer acts exclusively as an It entity, an entity devoid of personhood. But what is being claimed here is that the very ontological constitution of the murderer is changed in consequence of committing the act of murder to cancel out his/her personhood permanently (for only by assuming such a change in the very ontological constitution of the murderer can we claim that the murderer at a different point in time and space and in a different context that he/she was when committing the act of murder is nonetheless an entity that is devoid of personhood). This is quite a different claim and we have no substantiation for this transformation in an entity from canceling out its personhood in a particular act to undergoing a change in its ontological constitution in which personhood is canceled out on a permanent basis. Indeed, it is quite clear that the murderer after committing his/her murder has not lost, as far as his/her ontological constitution is concerned, his/her personhood—he/she still requires and is capable of extending affirmation to other persons.[41]

But if a persuasive case for capital punishment cannot be made from the vantage point of the ontological perspective, it can be made, we would submit, from the vantage point of the ethical perspective, a perspective as validly applicable to the issue of capital punishment (if indeed not more so) as is the ontological perspective. For as we have seen, in the context of the ethical perspective right and obligation go hand in hand—they are inextricably linked together. An entity cannot be endowed with an ethical right to something without at the same time being saddled with an ethical obligation towards that same something and, vice versa, an entity cannot be saddled with an ethical obligation towards something without at the same time being endowed with an ethical right to that same something. In the case before us here this means that an entity that is a person cannot be endowed with an ethical right not to have its existence terminated without at the same time being saddled with an ethical obligation not to terminate the existence of any other entity that is a person. The abrogation of the one necessarily implicates the abrogation of the other. And this being the case, a murderer, inasmuch as he/she clearly abrogates in the act of murder his/her ethical obligation not to terminate the existence of another person, cannot claim an ethical right not to have his/her existence terminated, which is to say that capital punishment would be ethically acceptable.[42] Now, the significant thing to note here is that this claim is not affected by the above consideration that the murderer may continue to be ontologically constituted as a person (irrespective of the fact that in the act of the murder itself he/she abrogates his/her personhood) and consequently continues to possess an ethical right not to have his/her existence terminated. The validity of this claim rests not on whether or not there is a transformation in the ontological constitution of the murderer but rather on the universalizability of the claim that without an ethical obligation not to terminate the existence of other persons there cannot be an ethical right not to have one's own existence terminated, so that abrogation of the ethical obligation in the act of murder necessarily implicates the abrogation of the ethical right not only with respect to the act of murder itself but beyond it for the duration, thus making the execution of a murderer ethically acceptable.

Lastly, one further consideration should be addressed here, and that is that the act of killing implicated in capital punishment is to be evaluated not for its own sake, i.e., as the final object of the evaluation, but rather as the means through which punishment is carried out. Thus, what is ultimately to be evaluated here is not the act as such, i.e., the act in its own terms, but rather the punishment that effects itself through the act. Now, in the context of the ethical enterprise (as it was delineated by us above) the evaluation of the punishment has to be grounded in and thus reflect the basic, defining criterion of the enterprise, namely, the criterion of justice which dictates that for the punishment to be ethically acceptable it must be commensurate with the crime—the punishment must fit the crime.[43] And in such a context a good case can be made that for the crime of a premeditated murder of an innocent person, where no extenuating circumstances enter the picture, the commensurate punishment and thus the punishment that would be ethically acceptable is indeed capital punishment. It should be noted, however, that the rationale underlying our position applied capital punishment to all cases of premeditated murder where no extenuating circumstances enter the picture and did not limit its application to cases of exceptionally heinous murder, thus implying that capital punishment is the most severe punishment at our disposal. Indeed, a persuasive case can be made that capital punishment is not necessarily the most severe punishment at our disposal, but rather that life imprisonment in solitary confinement with no possibility of parole may well be a more severe punishment than capital punishment (and as such implying that, if anything, the punishment for the cases of exceptionally heinous murder should be life imprisonment in solitary confinement with no parole rather than capital punishment).

This consideration, by the way, may suggest perhaps a way by which the contradiction between the demand of justice that a premeditated murder of an innocent person where no extenuating circumstances are present should be punished by capital punishment and the demand of ontology that an entity possessing self-consciousness, i.e., an entity ontologically constituted as a person, has an ethical right not to have its existence terminated can be overcome. Namely, the conflict could perhaps be overcome by, on the one hand, excluding the resort to capital punishment and instead imposing life imprisonment in solitary confinement without the possibility of parole (namely, resorting to what, in our view, is the more severe punishment) but, on the other hand, introducing the provision that at any time that the murderer decides that he/she prefers death to this kind of imprisonment (proper precautions being, of course, taken that such a decision is not but a passing whim but an unshakable, deeply entrenched conclusion), his/her wish will not be blocked by society. In this way society does not violate the ethical right of an entity that is a person not to have its existence terminated while at the same time the demand of justice to have the punishment be commensurate with the crime is being satisfied. True, the punishment is imposed here not by an outside party, i.e., society, but by the recipient of the punishment, i.e., the murderer, and as such it is, in a way, a self-imposed punishment that may not be, strictly speaking, a fully *bona fide* punishment. Indeed, what we really end up with here is an act of suicide committed by the murderer with society being placed in the role of assisting the suicide. And, of course, the question here is now whether this kind of state of affairs which the proposed solution to the problematic encountered in conjunction with the issue of capital punishment can satisfy the basic requirement underlying our handling of all the other issues here, namely, the requirement of being ethically acceptable. This is indeed the next and last undertaking to which we must now turn.[44]

Suicide and Assisted Suicide

Let us first address the issue of suicide. Suicide is to be delineated as an act undertaken by an entity that possesses self-consciousness (thus an entity that is a fully fledged actualized person) with the clear intention (thus not by accident or by mistake) to terminate its own existence. And this, in turn, means of course that the entity here whose existence is to be terminated is an entity that is endowed with personhood. As such, the case of suicide is similar to the case of capital punishment (and like the case of capital punishment it stands in clear contrast to the cases of abortion, euthanasia and infanticide), seeing that like in the case of capital punishment here too, in the case of suicide, the entity whose existence is to be terminated is an entity endowed with personhood. At the same time, however, there is also an important difference between the case of suicide and that of capital punishment. The difference lies in the fact that, unlike the case of capital punishment, in the case of suicide the entity that is the subject of the act, the acting agent who is to terminate the existence of the entity that is the recipient, the victim of the act, is not an outside, third party but the very same entity whose existence is to be terminated. Unlike the case of capital punishment, where the entity whose existence is to be terminated and the entity which is to terminate this existence are two different entities (and in this respect, by the way, the situation here in the case of capital punishment is the same as the situation that obtains in the cases of abortion, euthanasia and infanticide), in the case of suicide they are one and the same entity. This is an important point that has, as we shall see presently, a significant bearing on the ethical evaluation of the act of suicide.

Now, there are many people who view suicide as nothing else but an act of murder pure and simple and as such, of course, as an act that is ethically reprehensible. Those, however, who maintain this view whereby suicide is taken to be tantamount to an act of murder can evidently do so only if they focus exclusively on that aspect of the phenomenon whereby the entity whose existence here is to be terminated is an entity that is a fully fledged actualized person and completely ignore the other aspect of the phenomenon whereby the entity that is the perpetrator of the act is one and the same entity that is the victim of the act, that we have in the act of suicide not an act of killing an other but an act of self-killing. For clearly, it cannot be denied that if the entity whose existence is being terminated is a fully fledged actualized person, it is an entity that is endowed with an ethical right not to have its existence terminated and therefore terminating its existence, when it is innocent of any wrong doing, is indeed an act of murder, an act that is ethically reprehensible.

But the other aspect of the phenomenon whereby the perpetrator and the victim in the act of suicide are one and the same entity must surely throw into serious question the conclusion that the act of suicide is an act of murder pure and simple. For, firstly, we would surely want to maintain that for an act of killing (i.e., an act of terminating one's existence) to be categorized as an act of murder, an essential and inescapable condition must be that the act serve the interests (i.e., the intentions, the wishes, the advantages) of the perpetrator and not of the victim, the interests of the perpetrator being different from the interests of the victim (indeed, if the act is to serve the interests of the victim and not those of the perpetrator, we would have an act of euthanasia and not of murder) and such a condition, stipulation, must clearly presuppose the presence of two entities, i.e., that of the perpetrator and that of the victim, and not of one entity as is the case in the act of suicide. Consequently, the act of suicide, while clearly implicating an act of killing, the killing implicated is not murder and therefore, whatever its ethical evaluation may turn out to be, it cannot be evaluated on the basis that it is an act of murder, which, of course, as such would yield a negative evaluation, i.e., an evaluation whereby the act is to be taken as ethically reprehensible.[45] Secondly, and on a more fundamental level, one can validly argue that the act of suicide is not a legitimate object for ethical (and, for that matter, legal) evaluation/judgment. For a good case can be made that the evaluation/judgment implicated in the ethical enterprise (and, for that matter, in the legal enterprise) impinges upon acts/relations that take place between individuals and not upon acts/relations that take place within the confines of a single individual. The ethical (and the legal) enterprise requires that at least two individual persons be implicated and as such this would exclude the act of suicide, seeing that this act takes place within the confines of a single individual, between the individual and itself. Lastly, and perhaps on the most fundamental level, a case can be made that the act of suicide in taking place within the confines of a single individual cancels out the very criterion in which an evaluation that is to be ethical must ground itself. For the ethical enterprise would evaluate acts/relations here on the basis of whether or not they convey affirmation, seeing that an entity's ethical right not to have its existence terminated is based on its ethical right to claim that it be affirmed. And this being the case, all acts/relations directed towards an entity, if they are to be ethically evaluated, would be evaluated on the basis of whether or not they convey affirmation (acts/relations conveying affirmation would be evaluated positively while acts/relations denying affirmation would be evaluated negatively). But for an affirmation to be an effective, *bona fide* affirmation, it must be conveyed from the outside, i.e., from an other (an affirmation given to an entity by itself is a sham). Thus, for a *bona fide* affirmation to become available and thus allow for an ethical evaluation to take place, at least two individuals are required and therefore an act of suicide inasmuch as it implicates only a single individual must exclude itself from being ethically evaluated.

This problematic arising from the fact that the act of suicide, when taken in isolation in its own terms, implicates a single, one and the same, entity for both the perpetrator and the recipient of the act is overcome in an alternative formulation that also rejects the act of suicide as ethically unacceptable but that does that by introducing God into the picture, thus introducing an other, alterity, into the evaluation of the act of suicide and as such rendering the act available to the ethical evaluation—the evaluation is redirected from impinging upon a single individual, i.e., the human entity that is both perpetrator and recipient of the act, to impinging upon the interaction between two individuals, i.e., the relation that subsists between the human entity committing the act and the divine entity. Thus, according to this formulation the act of suicide is rejected because it is a taking away of something, i.e., life, that belongs not to the taker, i.e., the human committing the act, but to someone else, i.e., to God. Namely, the life that the human entity possesses is given to the human as a gift (according to one version) or in trust (according to an alternative version) by God and, therefore, its annihilation by the receiver, i.e., the human, is an offense against the giver, i.e., God, inasmuch as the receiver annihilates something that does not belong to him/her but to the giver. Essentially, so would the argument here run, the situation in this case is really the same as that encountered in the case of murder pure and simple—in both cases it is the annihilation of something, i.e., life, that belongs to someone else, except that in the case of murder that someone else is another human entity while in the case here that someone else is the divine entity (both entities, however, are endowed with personhood and consequently any acting/relating towards them would be validly subject to evaluation that is ethical evaluation). And this being the case, an act of suicide must be ethically evaluated in the same way that an act of murder, pure and simple, would be, which is to say that it must be ethically evaluated as reprehensible and unacceptable.[46]

But this formulation presents us with difficulties of its own. Thus, first, we have the difficulty that inasmuch as the human individual who is the recipient of the life extended to him/her as a gift or in trust has not been consulted as to whether or not he/she wished to receive it (and thus did not give his/her consent), it would be offensive to our sense of fairness and justice to castigate his/her rejection of the gift or the trust as ethically reprehensible and unacceptable. And indeed, even if the human individual did consent to receive the gift or the trust, he/she should surely have the option to change his/her mind and return the gift or the trust without this act being evaluated/judged as ethically reprehensible. Secondly, and more seriously, we have the difficulty that this formulation, when carried out consistently to its logical conclusion, deprives the human individual of all its freedom. For inasmuch as the human's life does not belong to the human but to God, the human should not be able to do anything with his/her life (and not only terminating that life) that would be ethically approvable if it were not sanctioned or dictated, in the first place, by God. But as such the human becomes a marionette and this, in turn, undermines any possibility of the human being endowed with personhood, seeing that the possession of freedom to decide and consequently to assume responsibility for one's actions is essential for an entity that is to be endowed with personhood. And, of course, if the human is not endowed with personhood, then the whole undertaking here of submitting all acts/relations to and from him/her to ethical evaluation is not applicable (and more specifically to our concern here, if the individual committing the act of suicide is not a person, then the act of killing implicated in the act of suicide is not an act of murder and therefore should not be evaluated as ethically reprehensible). Lastly, and just as seriously, we have the difficulty that, as pointed out above, any formulation that grounds itself in the religious dimension as such (and not only in a particular religious tradition), namely, that introduces an entity that transcends the world of our sense experience (to wit, that introduces the God of biblical religion), is necessarily limited in the range of its acceptability, seeing that there are quite a few people for whom such an entity does not exist. And of course, this, in turn, means that the ethical evaluation implicated in such a formulation is not embraced universally; neither can we have any ground for expecting to ultimately persuade the totality of humankind to adopt such a formulation, seeing that with respect to a formulation that grounds itself in the religious dimension we, in principle, lack a common denominator that runs through the totality of humankind. Clearly, the presence of such a limitation is a serious weakness for the formulation grounding itself in the religious dimension and places in a marked disadvantage to alternative formulations that do possess valid prospects of ultimately being universally adopted.

Thus, the formulation that grounds itself in the religious dimension is, in the last analysis, also, like the formulation that preceded it, not a viable formulation that can provide us with a valid justification for evaluating the act of suicide as ethically reprehensible. True, this formulation, unlike the formulation that preceded it, does provide us with an other that, as we have seen, is necessary in order to make feasible that an evaluation of the act of suicide would be an evaluation that is incontrovertibly an ethical evaluation. But, as we have also seen, because that other, which this formulation provides, is an entity that transcends the world of our sense perception, this precipitates a number of difficulties that, in our judgment, invalidates, in the last analysis, this formulation. But this, in turn, means that we do not have a formulation that can provide us the necessary other that is needed for us to be able to have a *bona fide* ethical evaluation of the act of suicide, and this means, of course, that the possibility of rejecting the act of suicide as ethically reprehensible would not be, in the last analysis, available to us.

Before accepting this conclusion as final, however, there is one more formulation that we must examine, seeing that if this formulation proves to be valid it may give us the possibility of evaluating the act of suicide as ethically reprehensible after all. Indeed, this formulation has the distinct advantage for us that while it too, like the foregoing formulation, provides us with an other that is introduced into the process of evaluating the act of suicide (thus making it feasible for the evaluation to be an ethical evaluation), that other which it provides is, unlike the other provided by the foregoing formulation (an other that was an entity that transcended this world), a this-worldly entity, an entity that is totally available to our sense-perception and which as such allows this formulation to escape the difficulties encountered in the foregoing formulation.[47]

The formulation to which we are referring here is the formulation that was first promulgated by Aristotle but adopted by many others over the centuries. Now, this formulation puts forth as the other, in terms of which the act of suicide is to be ethically evaluated, the society to which the individual belongs rather than the divine entity. Basically, it maintains that the individual owes his/her society a debt for the various benefits he/she has derived from the society. In committing an act of suicide, however, the individual, instead of benefiting his/her society in return (as the ethical dimension, as it expresses itself in the sense of fairness, would require), inflicts upon his/her society injury in that (as Aquinas put it) he/she deprives it of one of its members. And this being the case, it must call forth an ethical evaluation of the act of suicide that is negative.

What is one to say regarding this formulation? To begin with, if the benefits that the individual is supposed to be receiving from society are to be material benefits, then while one would indeed have to concede that society extends such benefits to the individual and that the individual, therefore, is in debt to society for them, a good case can nevertheless be made that the extent to which these material benefits are extended is, in the last analysis, quite minimal and that the average, run-of-the-mill member of society would have in all probability repaid them in full, if not indeed in excess of what he/she owed. Also, it is not at all clear that the individual in committing suicide can inflict harm upon his/her society. The harm spelled out above, to wit, that by committing suicide one is opting out of one's society, thus reducing its membership, and this is tantamount to inflicting harm upon one's society, is at best a claim whose validity is contingent on place and time. Namely, it may indeed be the case that in olden times the strength of a society was dependent on the size of its membership and that, by and large, membership was low, but this is certainly not the case today. Today, the dependence of the strength of a society upon the size of its membership is minimal, if at all, and our problem is not being underpopulated but, just the opposite, overpopulated. In the context of modernity, therefore, one may well argue that committing a suicide may not be seen as inflicting a harm upon society (indeed, if anything, it may well be seen as being a helpful, beneficial act towards society).

But even with respect to olden times, the claim is not all that persuasive, seeing that the act of suicide merely advances the time of exiting from life and thus diminishing the membership of society. It is not as if without committing the act of suicide there would have been no exiting from life and the individual would not have had to deprive society of one of its members. Exiting life and thus diminishing the membership of society through natural death is inescapable. Committing suicide merely hastens the occurrence of death, which would have taken place sooner or later regardless.

But aside from these difficulties, a much more serious difficulty arises in connection with this formulation, so much so that even if these or any other difficulties did not exist, this formulation would still be incapable of providing us with a valid justification for rejecting the act of suicide as being ethically reprehensible. For in deriving its rejection from a linkage between the individual and his/her society, which is based on an exchange of goods, this formulation implicates the individual and the other members constituting his/her society as entities that are ontologically constituted in terms of the dimension-of-power, which is to say, they are ontologically constituted as It entities. But as such, an ethical evaluation of the act of suicide on the basis of a linkage between the individual and his/her society in terms of the exchange of goods is not really feasible. This is so, because, as we have seen, an ethical right not to have one's existence terminated, on the basis of which the ethical evaluation of the act of suicide is made possible, can be established only with respect to entities, in our case here specifically human entities, that ontologically constitute themselves in terms of the dimension-of-consciousness, i.e., as Thou entities (and if the ontological constitution in terms of the dimension-of-consciousness does not comprise the totality but only a part of the entity's ontological structure, as indeed is the case with the human entity, then the ethical right not to have one's existence terminated can be established only with respect to this aspect of the ontological structure of the concerned entity). The linkage between the individual and his/her society can be used as the basis for the ethical evaluation of the act of suicide only if the individual and the others constituting his/her society are entities which ontologically constitute themselves, at least in part, in terms of the dimension-of-consciousness, i.e., as Thou entities, and when, therefore, the linkage is in terms of an exchange of affirmations rather than of material goods.[48] Now this is in stark contrast to the situation that obtains when the individual human constitutes itself ontologically in terms of the dimension-of-power, i.e., as an It entity. True, here too there is a dependence of the individual human on a collectivity of other humans constituting his/her society, but the dependence here, while it contributes (and, indeed, contributes significantly) to facilitating the material hardships of existence and helps in advancing its technological and material progress, does not impinge upon the entity's coming into existence nor upon its ability to sustain itself within it. An individual human that ontologically constitutes itself as an It entity can, in principle, exist in isolation from his/her society—a Robinson Crusoe, if stranded long enough on the island, may well lose his personhood but not his physical existence. And this being the case, the linkage of an individual human to his/her society/community when he/she ontologically constitutes him/herself as an It entity is on a secondary, less fundamental level of significance than when he/she ontologically constitutes him/herself as a Thou entity. A linkage that is in terms of an exchange of material goods cannot provide us with a valid ground on which to ethically evaluate the act of suicide. To have a valid ground on which to ethically evaluate the act of suicide we must turn to the linkage that is in terms of an exchange of affirmations, i.e., to the linkage between the individual human when he/she constitutes him/herself as a Thou entity and his/her community, i.e., the collectivity of other human individuals as they constitute themselves as Thou entities. So, it is to the examination of the ground for ethically evaluating the act of suicide, which the linkage in terms of the exchange of affirmations between the individual human and his/her community provides, that we must now turn.

Now, as we have just seen (in note 48), there can be no denying that the individual human as he/she constitutes him/herself in terms of his/her Thou-dimension is very much in debt to his/her community. For after all, it is from his/her community that he/she receives the required affirmation that would bring him/her into existence and sustain him/her within it. One cannot think of any set of circumstances that would exact a greater debt, the repayment of which, it is reasonable to surmise, would require no less than the extension of affirmation in return to the givers of the original affirmation, i.e., to the members of the community to which the receiver of the original affirmation belongs. In such a context, the act of suicide may, indeed, be seen as an act which allows the receiver of the original affirmation to escape having to pay back his/her debt by removing him/her from the scene so that he/she cannot extend in return his/her affirmation to the members of his/her community and, as such, the act of suicide would indeed have to be viewed as ethically reprehensible.

But this conclusion is, in our judgment, flawed in that the view of the process of the receiving and the giving of affirmation that underlies it assumes that the receiving and the giving of affirmation take place consecutively in time so that one can receive affirmation at point A in time, incurring a debt for it that would be expected to be paid back at point B in time. For, as will be recalled, in our analysis above of the mechanism by which affirmation is exchanged between two entities we have argued that the receiving and the extending of affirmation take place simultaneously, that when viewed from the vantage point of the relation of affirmation itself, i.e., when viewed from within the relation itself, the receiving and extending of affirmation take place at one and the same time—it is one and the same act outside the flux of temporality. Thus, there is never a situation when affirmation has been received but not extended. Indeed, even when we enter temporality by shifting the vantage point, from which the process is to be viewed, from the "in-between," i.e., from within the relation itself, to one of its poles, thus "refracting" the one and the same act encompassing both the receiving and the extending of affirmation into two consecutive acts, the two acts, i.e., the act of receiving and that of extending affirmation, are inextricably linked together. Indeed, as we have tried to show above, the mechanism by which an act of affirmation is received is for the potential receiver to extend an affirmation to an other, its acceptance, i.e., acknowledgment, by that other constituting itself as an act of extending affirmation, in return, by that other to the potential receiver. In other words, if we view the process as it manifests itself in the flux of temporality, i.e., if we take the acts as occurring consecutively, the act of extending affirmation precedes the act of receiving it. Thus, not only is there always an act of extending affirmation coupled with the act of receiving it (i.e., the bill being, so to speak, paid upon receiving the merchandise), but the act of extending affirmation precedes the act of receiving it (i.e., the bill being, so to speak, prepaid in advance of receiving the merchandise). The all-important bottom line of all this is, however, that there is never a situation here where a debt is left, so to speak, unpaid. The balance is always zero—there is no credit nor is there any debit left in the account. Thus, when an individual human decides to take leave of the "game" through an act of suicide (or, for that matter, when he succumbs to natural death), he/she leaves the "arena" without leaving behind any unpaid debts. His/her exiting is, therefore, in no way harmful to his/her community. True, he/she would no longer contribute his/her affirmation to the others constituting his/her community, but, by the same token, he/she would not be receiving any affirmation from them either. There is a closing of the account but with the books balanced and the slate clean and, therefore, the closing of the accounts, i.e., the act of committing suicide, should not carry any ethical evaluation that is negative. Thus, this formulation, when it implicates the linkage between the individual human and his/her community in terms of an exchange of affirmations rather than in terms of the exchange of material goods, also fails, in our judgment, to establish a negative ethical evaluation for the act of suicide.

We must conclude, therefore, that the arguments which attempt to establish that the act of suicide is ethically reprehensible are not really persuasive or, for that matter, valid. We may well think, as indeed we do, that the act of suicide is an ill-advised act on the part of the person committing it, for no matter how disillusioned and unhappy with life the person may be, there is no hurry to leave it—the end will come soon enough by itself. The one set of circumstances where resorting to an act of suicide may make sense and may be exonerated is when the person is continuously suffering horrific pains that cannot be sufficiently mitigated by medication and death is inevitable and imminent. In all other circumstances, our disillusionment and unhappiness could be greatly minimized, if not indeed completely obliterated, if we could but bring to the fore in our consciousness the realization that soon enough it would all disappear without us having to hasten the end. But all these considerations clearly have no bearing on the ethical evaluation of the act of suicide. With respect to no set of circumstances can we condemn the act of suicide as ethically reprehensible. The act is between the person and him/herself and, no matter how ill advised it may be, ethical evaluation of the act is not legitimate.

Finally, in turning to the related issue of assisted suicide, the first thing to note is that while this issue shares in common with the issue of suicide as such (but in contra-distinction with the issues of euthanasia and capital punishment) that the *decision* to terminate one's existence is placed with the entity that is to be the victim, the recipient, of the decision, i.e., the entity whose existence is to be terminated (and because of this it is indeed very proper to link it with the issue of suicide as such), it differs with the issue of suicide as such (but now being in agreement with the issues of euthanasia and capital punishment) in placing the *perpetration*, the carrying out, of the act not with the entity that is to be the victim, the recipient, of the act but with an entity that is an other, an outside agent.

Now, this state of affairs, i.e., placing the perpetration of the act of terminating one's existence not with the entity that is to be the victim of the act but with an outside agent, means that the issue of assisted suicide, unlike the issue of suicide as such, is a legitimate object for ethical evaluation. For now the act to be ethically evaluated is no longer an act that takes place between an entity and itself (an act that, as we have seen above, does not lend itself to a legitimate ethical evaluation) but it is an act that takes place between two discrete entities and as such it is an act that is a fully legitimate object for ethical evaluation. Still, one may object that while the case of assisted suicide may well be a legitimate object for ethical evaluation, the ethical evaluation here will per force have to remain vacuous. For after all, the ethical evaluation in the case of assisted suicide is directed towards the agent that perpetrates the act of terminating one's existence (it is the perpetrator of the act that is, so to speak, in the dock) but what, in the last analysis, it is supposed to evaluate with respect to the agent is the decision to terminate one's existence. In the case of assisted suicide, however, this decision is not in the hands of the agent—it is relegated to the victim of the act and not to its perpetrator. Thus, inasmuch as the evaluation here is to be with respect to the decision to terminate one's existence and at the same time is to be directed to the agent who perpetrates the act, the evaluation must remain vacuous, seeing that the decision to terminate one's existence in no way implicates the agent who perpetrates the act—it implicates the victim of the act. The agent perpetrating the act is but the means, the tool, by which a decision made by someone else, to wit, the prospective victim of the act, is effected.

This objection, however, may lose its persuasiveness when it is considered more carefully. For while it is true that the agent here cannot be ethically evaluated with respect to the decision to terminate one's existence, it can be ethically evaluated with respect its decision to provide itself as the means, the tool, by which the decision to terminate one's existence can be effected. Indeed, the concern with the decision of a person whether or not to help another person effect his/her decision to commit suicide is the only legitimate concern, and indeed the only concern that can be, strictly speaking, ethically evaluated within the context of the case of assisted suicide (if the ethical evaluation is directed to the decision as such to commit suicide, then we are back in the context of the case of suicide as such).

So, how are we going to evaluate the decision of a person with respect to whether or not to assist another person in his/her resolve to commit suicide?[49] Shall we say that since the person extending the assistance is not the person to have made the decision, his/her complying with the request from the person who is to be the victim of the act should not be ethically condemned? After all, we do not ethically condemn the person who makes the decision and is to be the victim of the act so why should we ethically condemn the person who abides by a request from the concerned party to be of assistance in carrying out the decision? But it would seem to us that although this argument may seem at first sight reasonable, in the last analysis it is not really persuasive. For while we cannot ethically condemn the person who commits suicide because it is an act between him/her and him/herself and such acts are not subject to ethical evaluation, here, in the case of a person who assists in an act of suicide, we can ethically condemn the act (and, in turn, the agent who perpetrates the act) because it is an act from one person to another and such an act is subject to ethical evaluation. Thus, a person who extends assistance towards effecting a suicide act is (and this, in contra-distinction to the prospective victim of the suicide act when it is he/she, i.e., the prospective victim, who effects the suicide act) open to ethical evaluation for the assistance he/she extends, even though he/she extends the assistance at the bidding of the prospective victim so that the original decision to effect the act is made by the prospective victim and not by the outside person who extends the assistance. This is so because the outside person who is to extend the assistance retains the decision of whether or not to abide by the prospective victim's request (he/she always has the option not to abide by the victim's request—just because one is asked to do something does not mean that he/she has to do it) and this being the case, he/she remains accountable for the acts contained in the assistance extended by him/her to the prospective victim and therefore any ethical evaluation of these acts would devolve on the person extending the assistance.

Now, the acts that would be contained in any assistance that is extended would clearly be acts that implicate the killing (though, strictly speaking, not the murdering) of another person, which, in the absence of any mitigating circumstances, would clearly have to be ethically evaluated as reprehensible.[50] And, of course, the more proactive the person extending the assistance is and the more directly does his/her assistance impinge on the prospective victim of the suicide act, the more ethically reprehensible they will be.

Now, there are, in the main, three levels of proactivity by which assistance can be extended that suggest themselves to us. The lowest level (a level that actually shifts from activity to passivity) is when the assistance to the act of suicide expresses itself in having the person extending the assistance refraining from stopping the prospective victim from carrying out the act of suicide. Its assistance to the act of suicide consists in refraining from stopping an act that would have stopped the act of suicide (a minus plus a minus gives a plus). And with respect to this level one could argue that such a refrain from acting, such a non-act, should escape altogether being ethically condemned. For after all, the person extending assistance is merely refraining from imposing his/her views and judgment on those of the prospective victim—after all, it is the prospective victim's life and the prospective victim should be allowed to do with it as he/she pleases (this argument being similar to the one used above in rejecting ethical condemnation of the act of suicide as such). Who are we, i.e., any one of us who is not the prospective victim, to decide regarding another person's life? The only consideration that would undermine this position and would ethically sanction intervention by an outside party is when it is abundantly clear that the prospective victim is not of sound mind or is acting impulsively on the spur of the moment without considering carefully enough all the implications of his/her intended action. Excluding, however, this consideration, the stance of not intervening would be ethically exonerated. But even more fundamentally, as we have seen above, the ethical enterprise (granted, as we have delineated it above) confines ethical evaluation to acts that have actually been carried out. If no act that has actually been carried out is available, ethical evaluation has nothing to evaluate and, as such, a negative ethical evaluation is clearly not feasible. Thus, with respect to this level we have to conclude that no negative ethical evaluation is applicable.

The remaining two levels, however, do implicate acts that are actually carried out and are, therefore, subject to ethical evaluation, which, in turn, means that an ethical evaluation that is negative is feasible with respect to these two levels. Thus, in the first of these two levels (i.e., in the second of the three levels mentioned above, the middle level of proactivity), the person's assistance extends only to providing the means by which the act of suicide can be carried out, but the actual carrying out of the act is left in the hands of the prospective victim (for example, a doctor knowingly prescribing a pharmaceutical product or a person providing a loaded gun so that the prospective victim can terminate his/her life by using it). In the second of these two levels (i.e., in the third of the three levels mentioned above, the highest level of proactivity), the person's assistance extends much further in that it is that person who, albeit at the bidding of the prospective victim, actually terminates the prospective victim's life (and not merely provides the means by which he/she can carry out such a termination). While in the preceding case the person extending assistance is but an accessory to the killing, in the case here he/she is the direct agent carrying out the killing. Now clearly, as we have just observed, in both cases ethical evaluation is possible (seeing that in both cases there is an act that was actually carried out), and furthermore, since in both cases an innocent person's existence is terminated (the fact that the existence is terminated at the behest of the prospective victim does not exonerate the person who extends assistance to the act of suicide, seeing that, as we have argued above, he/she certainly has the option to reject such a behest and, therefore, in accepting it he/she must assume responsibility for his/her action), the ethical evaluation would have to be, at least *prima fascia*, negative (although, since we hold that there is a valid distinction between being an accessory to a killing and being the one who actually carries out the killing, the latter being more culpable than the former, the ethical condemnation of the person extending assistance to an act of suicide should be more severe in the last, i.e., in the third, case than in the case preceding it, i.e., in the second case). But, of course, this conclusion will have to be mitigated or indeed canceled out if there were to be any mitigating circumstances.

So, are there any mitigating circumstances that could counteract and cancel the negative ethical evaluation in these two cases? It would seem to us that there is one situation that offers such mitigating circumstances that would justify the claim that, in these two cases, extending assistance to an act of suicide should not be evaluated as ethically reprehensible and this is when the killing implicated in extending assistance to an act of suicide is a "mercy killing," namely, a killing where the prospective victim is doomed to an imminent and inescapable death and where in the meanwhile he/she is subjected to insufferable pain that cannot be sufficiently mitigated.[51] In this situation only extending assistance to an act of suicide is, in our judgment, not to be evaluated as ethically reprehensible. In all other situations, extending assistance would, in all probability, have to be evaluated as ethically unacceptable.

A Concluding Remark

We have now covered, we believe, all the main cases in which terminating the existence of another person is implicated and have made a case, hopefully in a persuasive manner, for the kind of ethical evaluation that can be justified in each one of them. The on omission that is bound to be noticed is the case of war. Our justification for not including it is that in the case of war the decisions and acts that are implicated are decisions and acts that are made by collectivities of human persons, i.e., by nations, and not by individual human persons and, as such, it is really a case that belongs in the domain of political philosophy rather than in the domain of ethics.

Notes

1. Of course, these issues implicate not only the ethical dimension but also the social/political dimension (a dimension that expresses itself most authoritatively in the legal domain) and the religious dimension. As such, the assessment of these issues in these two dimensions would readily lend itself to being compared with their assessment in the ethical dimension. However, such a comparison would be particularly instructive and interesting only with respect to the religious dimension and not so much with respect to the social/political dimension. For a good case can be made that the social/political dimension as it expresses itself in the legal domain should ultimately ground itself in the ethical dimension, i.e., express the assessment posited in the ethical dimension (or, at least, not contradict it), and this being the case there is, in the last analysis, not much point in comparing the assessment in the two dimensions. As against this, the religious dimension does not ground itself in the ethical dimension; it has its own independent grounding, to wit, a grounding in divine revelation, in commandments emanating from God. And as such, a comparison with the ethical dimension can be interesting and instructive.

But even so, this does not mean that comparison with all the particular concrete historical expressions within the religious dimension would prove to be interesting and instructive. For in order for a comparison with a particular expression to be interesting and instructive, that particular expression has to be an expression that formulates itself in terms of the ethical dimension as, for example, an expression that takes the failure by humanity to establish itself as a righteous community as the fundamental predicament and consequently sees the striving towards the establishment of a righteous community as its main undertaking and its attainment as the act of redemption (in other words, an expression for which the relations and interactions between human and fellow human constitute the focus of its concern). But most concrete historical expressions within the religious dimension do not actually formulate themselves in terms of the ethical dimension. Rather, the preponderant majority of the concrete historical expressions formulate themselves in terms of the ontological dimension, which is to say that they are expressions for which the fundamental predicament lies in the finitude of the human and commensurate to this salvation would consist in the ontological transformation of the human to a "new being," to a human who would transcend its finitude (or, short of this, would diminish its finitude).

Indeed, only the expressions commonly referred to as biblical faiths, i.e., Judaism, Christianity, and Islam, encompass within their formulation the ethical dimension. (By the way, the expressions formulating themselves in terms of ontology may be referred to as non-biblical or as pagan. Also it is worth noting that this bifurcation between biblical and pagan expressions on the basis of whether the expression formulates itself in terms of the ethical dimension or in terms of the ontological dimension follows directly from the fundamental alternative which accounts for this basic bifurcation in the typology of religion, to wit, from the alternative of whether the ultimate, i.e., the divine entity, is seen/encountered as blind power, an It entity, as is the case in the expressions of paganism, or whether it is encountered/seen as a person, an entity possessing self-consciousness, a Thou entity, as is the case in the expressions of biblical faith.) But even these concrete historical expressions of biblical faith do not formulate themselves exclusively in terms of the ethical dimension. True, they all do contain a strand that formulates itself in terms of the ethical dimension and, indeed, it is by virtue of this strand that they come to possess their distinctiveness. But at the same time, these expressions, without exception, also contain a strand that formulates itself in terms of the ontological dimension (i.e., taking the ontological finitude of the human as a fundamental predicament).

As such, one can, indeed, differentiate these expressions with respect to the relative predominance of the two dimensions. Thus, for example, a case can be made that in Christianity (more specifically, Pauline Christianity) we encounter an expression of biblical faith in which the ontological dimension plays, relative to the role it plays in the other expressions of biblical faith, the most pronounced role. Still, even so, Christianity remains an expression of biblical faith. This is so inasmuch as although its main concern is with the ontological finitude of the human as manifested, par excellence, by its focusing on the human's constitution as flesh and on the event of its inevitable death (thus clearly reflecting its linkage with the ontological dimension), it expresses its concern with the ontological finitude of the human in terms of the acting/relating which characterizes human conduct (thus, clearly retaining its linkage with the ethical dimension). Namely, Christianity encounters the ontological finitude of the human in the human's predicament of original sin—the inevitability of and the inescapability from sin. And this, in turn, is so inasmuch as sin is grasped as a falling short of perfection and finitude does indeed signify lack of perfection. To the extent, therefore, that the human is finite in his ontological constitution, all his acts are finite too and thus imperfect, which is to say, sinful. Thus, while, in the last analysis, it is the ontological finitude of the human that constitutes the fundamental predicament for Christianity (hence its linkage to the ontological dimension), Christianity confronts and addresses it in terms of the human's sinfulness (hence its linkage to the ethical dimension). And as such, Christianity can indeed be seen as the great attempt at synthesizing biblical faith with paganism, Jerusalem with Athens.

At the same time, an equally persuasive case can be made at the other extreme that in Judaism (more specifically in Prophetic Judaism) we encounter an expression of biblical faith in which the ontological dimension plays no role.

Indeed, the finitude inherent in the ontological constitution of the human is not perceived here as a predicament; on the contrary, it is fully accepted as a given which, if anything, is valued positively inasmuch as it is established in the divine act of creation. The fundamental predicament is located here in the flaunting of injustice by humans in their acts/relations among themselves and commensurate to this the redemptive task is seen to lie in the striving towards the establishment of a righteous society. Clearly, in the expression of biblical faith that is Prophetic Judaism we have an expression where there is a sole and exclusive linkage to the ethical dimension (indeed, it may not be all that far fetched, perhaps, to suggest that we have here an expression that really belongs to the ethical dimension but articulates itself in terms of the religious dimension).

2. Certainly if biological life is determined by the presence of DNA the fetus is alive from the very moment of conception. But if biological life is to be determined not by the presence of DNA but rather by physical movement or by metabolic processes, then the fetus cannot be taken as alive from the moment of conception though it can still be taken as alive from a fairly early moment in pregnancy.

3. Indeed, a good case can be made that even at birth personhood is not yet attained. It is not until well into the first year of life that the human baby becomes a person—it is not until the sixth or seventh month that the human baby becomes conscious of an other and not until much later that it becomes self-conscious. This observation clearly carries unsettling implications as regards the issue of infanticide. But as we shall try to show below our position by no means grants carte blanche permission for infanticide. On the contrary, we will try to show how our position would strongly prohibit infanticide, except that the rationale and justification for this strenuous prohibition must be somewhat different from that which underlies the prohibition of terminating the existence of an adult human person.

4. Thus the anti-abortion proponents are quite disingenuous when they shift back and forth between talking about the fetus as being alive and referring to it as a "baby." It is a clear case of their eating the cake and wanting to have it too. For on the one hand they can certainly make the case that from the very early states of its gestation the fetus possesses life in the biological sense (if we define biological life in terms of the presence of DNA then life is present from the very moment of conception, if not indeed before that, and if we define biological life in terms of physical movement or certain chemical, metabolic processes then it is present at fairly early stages of gestation), while, on the other hand, by referring to the fetus as a "baby" they clearly insinuate that by terminating its existence we are terminating not only the existence of an entity possessing biological life but rather an entity that is a person, i.e., self-conscious, and consequently perpetrating an act that is most reprehensible. Namely, the proof is made with respect to biological life (which is feasible) but the accusation is made with respect to personhood (which again, in its turn, is quite valid). In this way they pretend to base their accusation on the demonstrated facts. But this is disingenuous because they have never

established that the fetus is a person, i.e., "a baby"; they have only established that the fetus possesses biological life and this is something quite different from possessing personhood. Indeed, the fetus quite clearly does not possess personhood. So what the anti-abortionists rightfully claim to have demonstrated as scientific fact has nothing to do with their further claim that abortion is tantamount to an act of murder. This slight of hand in the argument of the anti-abortionists is, however, much more a manifestation of disingenuousness than of dishonesty for in all probability, this shift in ground is not perpetrated consciously or intentionally but rather unconsciously. But precisely as such, this shift perpetrated unconsciously by the anti-abortion opponents provides a most telling support to our contention that the crucial consideration in lending justification to the prohibition of terminating an entity's existence is whether or not the entity in question is a person. Indeed, this indicates that it should be possible to have the pro- and anti-abortionists agree on the criterion by which the conflict between them can be resolved, this criterion being the one we have suggested above, namely, whether or not the entity in question is a person, i.e., self-conscious. But if this be the case, then the anti-abortion position becomes untenable for clearly the fetus is not a person, not a "baby." Indeed, because this is so that the talk of the anti-abortion proponents of killing so many millions of "babies" every year, comparing this to the slaughter of six million Jews in the Second World War, becomes offensive demagoguery.

5. We say it is clear and indubitable because when left to itself the fetus would in the course of time become a person. But by saying "when left to itself" we don't mean to imply that its becoming a person does not depend on other factors (as, for example, being placed in a living womb or in an incubator or being properly nourished and protected). For obviously this is not the case. What we mean to state is that the fetus does not require that it join or combine with other entities before it can be actualized as a person. As such, it is potentially a person in a different sense than the male's semen or the female's unfertilized ovum may be considered as a potential person.

6. And the distinction between law, on the one hand, and ethics and religion on the other, should not be fudged. In the former, force and punishment are implicated while in the latter, only persuasion and disapproval can be implicated. Now, there are many actions that we may want to persuade our fellow humans to pursue but would strongly object to forcing them to do so; and conversely, there are many actions of which we would greatly disapprove and yet would strongly feel that they entail no punishment. And what we are arguing here is that any action with respect to the fetus fall in the former and not in the latter category, namely, that it implicates only persuasion and approval or disapproval and not forcing and punishment.

7. The only other possible sources that can provide "considerations to the contrary" as regards the fetus's claim are the father of the fetus and society. With respect to the father, it is very far-fetched. But if a woman impregnates herself without the consent of the father (and this conceivably is possible if, like Lott, the father is not fully conscious when duped into copulation or, now that sperm banks are available, that his sperm is taken without his consent by

the wrong party), a case can be made that the prospective father should have the right to demand abortion. For although he does not carry any responsibility for the fetus nor does he do anything for it, he may nonetheless claim that he does not wish his genes to be joined with those of that particular woman. And as to the case where society has the right to demand abortion, the scenario is much more likely and indeed is practiced by some societies already. For if we accept that society has the obligation to provide a certain standard of livelihood for all its members, then a case can be made that society has a right, when threatened to be deluged by a large number of people who cannot care for themselves, to control the birthrate of such people not only by means of birth control but also by means of abortion. Many may object to this claim and in a way such objection would be quite understandable. For the urge to procreate and, commensurate to this, the right to do so, is very fundamental, and consequently any interference with it from an external source is very likely to repulse us. But one is not talking here of a person's right to have a *reasonable* number of offspring but rather an unreasonable number. And here the question arises whether a person has a right to expect other people to work towards the sustenance of its offspring. Of course, the case for the right of society to require abortion collapses if we remove the demand that society has an obligation to provide a certain minimal standard of living for all its members. But do we really want to remove this demand? Thus, both the prospective father and society may come into conflict with the claim of the fetus not to have its existence terminated. Still, it is only too clear that the main and by far the overwhelming source of conflict with the fetus's claim not to have its existence terminated comes from the mother who is the entity that, by the very nature of the biological scheme of things, is most intimately connected with the fate of the fetus.

8. True, there is yet another sense in which fully fledged human beings are also inescapably dependent upon one another. Namely, as a conscious entity, as a person, a Thou, the fully fledged human being is inescapably dependent on his fellow humans, his fellow Thous. The human as a person, as a Thou, cannot arise in isolation; as such, the human can arise only from within a community, a collectivity of other human beings that are already constituted as persons, as Thous. But this dimension, the dimension of the Thou, does not apply as yet to the fetus and thus our distinction between the fetus and the fully fledged human being could not possibly be with respect to this dimension. In actuality, the fetus exists only in terms of its biological life, thus only with reference to the dimension-of-power, to its being an It. And indeed, it is precisely because of this consideration that the distinction we are trying to establish here is specifically with respect to the dimension of the It. Namely, we would want to argue that the fully fledged human being precisely *qua* It is in principle an independent entity (though practically, given the artificial complexity of the world we have constituted for ourselves, this may not be the case), while the fetus *qua* It (it cannot be anything else) is not.

9. One can argue that the world owes us a living only when our living is pursued no longer in the context of nature but in the context of an artificial

world created by humankind. It is only because humankind has placed itself in an artificial bubble created by its spectacular advances in technology and in which its members are made to be inextricably dependent on one another for their living, that there is a rationale for the claim that the world, i.e., humankind, owes a living to each one of its members. It is in this context only that there is an ethical justification for the claim of a "safety net." In the context of nature there could be no such justification. One might appeal here to compassion and empathy but not to ethical rationale.

10. Any commitment and/or responsibility that society may undertake towards the fetus in this context, will have to be established not on any innate rights of the fetus but rather on the interests of society, as, for example, its interest to increase its numbers.

11. By the way, it would seem that this consideration affects not only our evaluation/judgment regarding the fetus but also our evaluation/judgment regarding animals, namely, it affects our evaluation/judgment with respect to which animals may be killed and/or eaten. The more an animal interacts with us (in the sense that our being receives affirmation from it) and thus the closer the animal is to becoming a personal entity, the more troubled and uncomfortable we become about killing or eating it. Thus, for example, it certainly is more problematic for us to kill a monkey or a dog than to kill a chicken or a cow or to kill a dolphin than to kill a salmon. And this, by the way, shows with respect to our argument above that our position regarding the killing of animals is determined, in the last analysis, not by the criterion of biological life but rather by the criterion of personhood.

12. It is important to reiterate and emphasize that conceding that the fetus is a potential person and, even more so, that it is a fully actualized person is purely hypothetical and academic to see how far we can go towards taking the fetus as a fully actualized person and still find abortion ethically permissible. In reality, of course, our clear position is that the fetus (and, strictly speaking, even the born baby for the first six to eight months of its life) is not a fully actualized person and not even a potential person in a sense that would have a bearing on the ethical domain, more specifically, on the issue of whether the fetus has an ethical right not to have its existence terminated. It should be clear that our position is that in the context of the ethical enterprise as delineated by us above, abortion is in all conceivable scenarios ethically permissible.

13. But let us keep in mind that these degrees in certainty, ambivalence or ambiguity are not with respect to what the law should be in these instances but rather what our moral assessment should be. For as we have argued above, as far as the law is concerned the conclusion is quite clear with respect to all possible scenarios and that is that in none of them does society have the right to intervene and dictate in terms of the law to the mother what she should or should not do. The law is simply not applicable here in any of the instances (not even in those where we would be most disapproving), seeing that the fetus is not a person and consequently has no standing in the eyes of the law. The degrees in ambivalence and clarity is only with respect to our moral/social assessment of what would be the right action to pursue in the circumstances.

The question before us is not whether or not society has the right to impose its judgment on the mother by force of law (because society does not have such a right in any of these instances). Rather, the question before us is what are the morally defensible judgments that one can make in these instances.

14. We should note that throughout the discussion here and below on abortion we accept that incurring a commitment to a fetus is feasible. Now, ethically such acceptance may indeed be valid, seeing that in an ethical context we are evaluating/judging the acts of the agent irrespective of the status of their recipient and the agent here, i.e., the mother, is a fully actualized person. However, it would seem to us that legally such an acceptance may not be valid. For in the legal context the evaluation/judgment of the act must take into account not only the status of the agent of the act but also the status of the recipient of the act. Now, since the recipient of the act here (i.e., of the commitment) is the fetus and seeing that the fetus is not a fully actualized person, incurring a commitment towards it cannot be valid in a legal context. So, while in an ethical context incurring a commitment towards the fetus may well have a bearing on our evaluation/judgment, in a legal context the whole undertaking is beside the point. Since our deliberations here, however, are, as said, in the ethical and not in the legal context, considering the incurring of a commitment towards a fetus remains a valid undertaking for us.

15. One may well be justified in condemning the making of a commitment in such circumstances but certainly not in insisting that it be carried out. This is so even if there is absolutely no mitigating consideration to account for the original making of the commitment. In the case before us here, however, there is a very important mitigating consideration and that is the very strong maternal instinct to have children and protect them to the very point of sacrificing one's own life for that purpose. As such, a woman may well decide at one moment to risk her life or indeed sacrifice her life for the sake of her progeny only to change her mind at another moment. We have here the conflict of two elemental and all-powerful forces, that of giving life and that of preserving one's own life. Thus, while it is quite understandable that some people at certain times may come down in favor of the first alternative, the ethical preference, in the last analysis, should be always given to the latter alternative.

16. Indeed, most of us would generally want to say that even if I am not the threatened party but only a third party witnessing a murder that is about to be committed, I would be justified (indeed, mandated?) in killing the attacker in order to save the life of the attacked person. And on the analogy of this case, one could argue that not only does the mother have the right to abort but also a physician as a third party on his/her judgment (and not at the request of the mother) would have the right to abort. The physician is like the third party who may kill the attacker in order to save the life of the attacked. Nor is this scenario purely hypothetical; it may well arise in actual life when at the moment when the decision is made the mother is incapable of communicating her wishes or, for that matter, really know what her wishes are.

17. To push the example to its most radical parameters, let us assume that the virus is deadly to everyone else except the carrier. In the analogous case

with respect to the fetus, therefore, we are facing the situation where the fetus threatens the life of the mother but not its own. Thus, one can take as an example the instance where the fetus is sufficiently advanced in its gestation so that it can survive the death of the mother that it brings about. The reason for this stipulation whereby the carrier or the fetus are to be unaffected by the threat they pose, is to exclude the argument that since the carrier or attacker would itself sooner or later die, one may be justified in killing it first before it does additional harm. In other words, the point here is to exclude the possibility of arguing that it is not really an act of killing that we commit but merely an act of advancing the date of a death that is otherwise anyway inevitable and that given the consequences which would inevitably follow if the date were not advanced such advancement may be justified (but if it were a *bona fide* killing in the sense that the carrier would otherwise not die such a killing would not be justified). We want to consider the case in its most difficult terms and that is whether the life of the carrier is to be forfeited in order to protect the life of another person.

18. Concretely speaking, it is very difficult to imagine a situation where terminating the existence of the agent is the only way to remove the threat. In all probability such a situation does not exist. But nonetheless, it is important to raise this far-fetched (indeed, impossible) hypothetical situation in order to bring into the sharpest focus the considerations that are involved here and to face them head on. And in this context our position is that although there is clearly a difference between the different things that one can do in self-defense to an other (thus, for example, there is a difference between taking away his/her freedom, i.e., quarantining, and terminating his/her existence, i.e., killing), still if action towards an other is allowed in principle then it is only a question of degree (and as such, merely a secondary question) at which point to stop. Obviously, one would not be justified in the action taken against an other in going beyond the minimal point that is required in order to be effective. But if in order to be effective one must go all the way, i.e., one must terminate the existence of the other, we fail to see what moral reasoning could stop one from doing that. Our point is that one has the moral right to take any action that is necessary towards an other (but not more than necessary) in order to prevent the termination of his/her own existence that would result from the threat posed by that other.

19. The people who take this position, e.g., the Catholic church, would in all likelihood want to argue that since the potential killer here, i.e., the fetus, is "an innocent killer," namely, an agent who kills not intentionally or willfully but merely by its mere existence, the threat to life here is really emanating from a third outside party and consequently the case here is really equivalent to the preceding case where one may argue with much greater plausibility that we should not play "God" and decide who shall be saved and who shall be sacrificed (though some, e.g., the utilitarians, would not agree to this even in these circumstances). This may well be persuasive to some. But as we have tried to argue above, the fact that the potential killer is innocent should certainly affect our moral judgment of it and our feeling towards it but it should

not affect what the potential victim should or should not do to save itself. An innocent killer is a killer nonetheless and the potential victim has every right to relate to it not in terms of its being innocent but rather in terms of its being a potential killer.

20. In view of the above more precise description of the situation that confronts us here, it would seem that a more appropriate analogy for the case before us, i.e., the case where the fetus threatens the life of the mother, is not the rather straightforward situation of the killing of a prospective killer in self-defense but the more complex situation whereby an other to whom one extended the hospitality of one's home becomes by its mere existence and through no fault of its own (thus clearly, not willfully or intentionally) a threat to the very life of the host, a threat that can be removed only by the retraction of the extended hospitality, i.e., by the eviction of the other, an eviction that admittedly would inescapably implicate the death of that other. Now, in such a context it may well be saintly on the part of the host not to evict the other and let nature or providence take its course. But from an ethical vantage point there can be no justification for prescribing such a conduct to the host (and, of course there can be no ethical justification for prescribing to or, indeed, expecting of an other to act in a saintly way—saintly acts are acts that one can only demand of oneself but not of an other). From an ethical perspective, if a guest who finds him/herself in my house (and it is immaterial how he/she comes to find him/herself in my house, whether it came about by accident or by my invitation or, indeed, if I knew or did not know of this condition at the time of the invitation—these alternatives do indeed affect the degree of commitment that I may incur but since no degree of commitment can outweigh the consideration that my life is threatened by its existence, the variation in degree of commitment has no practical impact) and he/she by his/her mere existence threatens my life, I have every right to evict him/her regardless of the consequences that may ensue for him/her.

Indeed, prescribing to the host not to evict is tantamount to prescribing that it commit suicide. True, the prescription here does not require the host to actually take in an active way its life. Rather, it requires the host not to take the only defensive act available to it to prevent the loss of its life. But since the difference here between active and passive action is not with respect to action directed towards an other but rather with respect to action directed towards oneself, the difference here should have no effect on the ethical evaluation of the two acts—both acts are acts of committing suicide. Namely, our position, as made clear above, that from the ethical vantage point there is a valid difference between actively killing an other and passively not saving an other applies only to one's conduct with respect to an other but not to conduct with respect to oneself. With respect to conduct directed towards oneself the difference between active and passive action dissolves itself as far as their ethical evaluation is concerned—ethically speaking, it is irrelevant how an entity brings about the termination of its own life.

21. Of course, needless to say that even in terms of this position, if the fetus which is brought into existence through an act of rape presents a threat to

the mother's life, abortion should be allowed. The abortion, however, is allowed here not because of the rape but because of the threat to the mother's life. Namely, it is allowed not in terms of the case before us here but rather in terms of the case that we have considered previously.

22. We should, however, reiterate and emphasize that our coming down on the side of accepting abortion as ethically permissible both when the fetus is taken as being only potentially a person and, even more so, when it is taken as being a fully fledged actualized person is contingent, in a very decisive sense, on our claim that the act of abortion, in its essence, is to be seen not as an act of actual killing but rather as an act of eviction (or, if it were technically feasible, of withholding sustenance) which albeit, given the state of medical technology today, would in all probability result in the death of the fetus. If, however, it were to be seen as an act of active killing, a case could, most probably, be made for coming down on the side of rejecting abortion as ethically permissible. For horrible as rape is, we cannot actively kill an entity (e.g., the fetus) that is a fully fledged actualized person and is a completely innocent party as regards the act of rape (the fetus is a consequence of the act of rape but in no way a participant in carrying out the act). The act of rape, horrible as it is, cannot override the ethical prohibition against actively terminating the existence of an entity that is a fully fledged actualized person and that is an innocent party. We must accept this consequence of the horrible act as a *fait accomplis* about which, difficult as it is to come to terms with, we cannot do anything. What we can do is impose the most severe penalty on the rapist, a penalty much more severe than the one imposed on a rapist whose act did not result in impregnating the woman.

23. By the way, it is because of this third consideration that the other two considerations (i.e., the consideration regarding whether or not the mother incurs any commitment and/or responsibility and the consideration regarding whether or not there are circumstances that would mitigate any such incurred commitment and/or responsibility) were precluded from our deliberations in the preceding two scenarios. Namely, the reason on the part of the mother for wanting to abort in these two scenarios was, in our judgment, so compelling that it countermanded the other two considerations.

24. And since there is no ethical consideration (ethical as delineated by us here) that would require us to view the act of copulation as an act undertaken exclusively for the purpose of procreation, we cannot assume that any act of copulation necessarily implicates an intention to procreate and, therefore, a commitment towards the fetus on the part of the parties to the act, specifically, for our purposes here, on the part of the woman. Engaging in the act of copulation as an expression of the love existing between two persons or even for the sake of mere sensual gratification (and these motivations for engaging in the act of copulation rather than the motivation for procreation are by far the more prevalent motivations) are alternative rationales that are equally acceptable from the ethical perspective and these rationales in no way implicate the incurring of a commitment towards the fetus. Indeed, while some religious traditions would accept only procreation as a legitimate motivation for

engaging in the act of copulation, for our civilization in modern times (and, for that matter, for many other civilizations in present and past times) the other motivations are fully acceptable and thus they are acceptable not only by the ethical enterprise as delineated by us but also by the ethical enterprise as delineated in terms of ethos/mores.

25. At the risk of being very repetitious, we must emphasize here again that the act of abortion which is implicated in our assessment here is to be taken on the analogy of an act of eviction, albeit an eviction that in all probability would result in death, and not on the analogy of an actual direct act of killing. For it is only on the basis of taking the act of abortion on the analogy of an act of eviction that we can provide in some of the situations a rationale for abortion that is persuasive to us. On the basis of taking the act of abortion on the analogy of an actual direct act of killing, the only situation where, in our judgment, an acceptable rationale for abortion can be provided, when the fetus is taken as a fully fledged actualized person, is when the fetus threatens the life of its mother. And even here it may be questionable, seeing that the fetus is an innocent participant in the threat posed to the mother's life—merely a passive, non-contributing medium through which the threat is presented, it itself being devoid of all intention thus also, specifically, of the intention to kill its mother. (By the way, maintaining this position would seem, however, to be inconsistent with maintaining that the fetus is to be taken as a fully fledged actualized person—it seems inconsistent to hold that an entity is, at one and the same time, both a fully fledged actualized person and devoid of intention; likewise, but in a reverse way, a similar inconsistency would seem to arise in connection with the attribution, in Jewish law, of the status of *rodef*, i.e., of a pursuer, to the fetus when its presence threatens its mother's life—it seems inconsistent to attribute intention, which is what the status of pursuer would seem to necessarily implicate, to an entity that is not taken as a fully fledged actualized person.)

26. While this is the conclusion to which cold logic leads us, we cannot help feeling uncomfortable about it. Granted that the act implicated here is in essence an act of eviction and not an act of direct actual killing; still, the probability that this act of eviction would result in the death of the evicted entity is so great (indeed, bordering on certainty) that we may be perhaps justified in seeing the act of eviction here coalescing with the act of direct actual killing. And now clearly, when the prospective victim of this act is an entity that we take to be a fully fledged actualized person, i.e., an entity that is endowed with the ethical right to request/demand that its existence not be terminated, it is quite understandable that we should feel uneasy and uncomfortable with the conclusion to which cold logic led us. We should perhaps concede that we have here a case where the rabbinic maxim of *lifnim m'shurat ha-din* may apply, i.e., a case where blindfolded justice is bent by a more lenient, flexible approach.

27. Of course, the situation that would most clearly support this conclusion is when the threat to the mother's life becomes known after the commitment towards the fetus has been undertaken. But even if the threat to the

mother's life is known before the commitment towards the fetus is undertaken, when the fetus is taken to be an entity that is merely potentially a person, the threat to the mother's life overrides, in our judgment, the commitment towards the fetus. It may be a grayer area if the fetus is taken to be an entity that is a fully actualized person. Here it is possible that one might want to argue that the commitment should override the threat. But if the fetus is taken to be an entity that is merely potentially and not actually a person, the case for the threat overriding the commitment is, in our judgment, completely persuasive.

28. Before bringing this section to a close, one further last observation may be in order. Namely, with the advances made in medical science and technology it is by no means farfetched any more to expect that in the not too distant future it would be possible to remove the fetus from its mother's womb at any time during its gestation and bring it to term in an incubator or in a surrogate mother's womb (for our purposes here, it may be advisable to focus on the possibility of bringing the fetus to term in an incubator rather than in the womb of a surrogate mother inasmuch as there would seem to be some indication that the makeup of the fetus when it is brought to term and becomes a child is determined not only by the genes received from its biological mother but also, to some extent, by the "womb environment" (e.g., the presence of hormones and other chemicals in the womb) provided by the surrogate mother and if this be valid, then clearly the surrogate mother becomes, to some extent, a co-parent with the biological mother thus greatly complicating the picture from both the ethical and the legal perspectives, a complication that is avoided when the fetus is brought to term in an incubator). Now, having the availability of an incubator into which the fetus can be transferred at any time (no matter how early) during its gestation and brought to term can clearly impinge in a significant way upon the conflict between the woman's wish to abort and the fetus' claim not to have its existence terminated. For it clearly can resolve the conflict if the woman's wish to abort is essentially brought about because she does not want to or cannot provide shelter and sustenance to the fetus. For in such a context, having the alternative of transferring the fetus into the incubator frees the woman from this burden without at the same time having to abrogate or compromise the fetus' claim not to have its existence terminated. Thus, for example, the first scenario cited above clearly illustrates the point we are trying to make here. Indeed, having the possibility of transferring the fetus into an incubator would be a God-send here, seeing that in this context the woman wants to have the fetus come to term but her being pregnant (i.e., her providing shelter and sustenance to the fetus) poses a threat to her life or health—having the alternative of transferring the fetus to the incubator relieves the woman from her pregnancy while safeguarding her wish to have the fetus come to term. Likewise, in the first formulation presented in the fourth scenario cited above where the woman wishes to abort the fetus because the pregnancy interferes with her desire to go on holiday, the possibility of transferring the fetus to the incubator where it can be brought to term would resolve the conflict between the woman's desire and the fetus' claim—the woman now can go on her holiday while the fetus need not be aborted (though, needless to say, the

resolution of the conflict here does not elicit our sympathy and satisfaction as does the resolution of the conflict presented in the first scenario). So, if the reason for the woman's wish to abort does not lie in her not wanting to have a child but rather in some problematic that the pregnancy presents for her, having the possibility of transferring the fetus to the incubator is of great help to us.

However, if the reason for the woman's wish to abort does lie in her not wanting to have a child (for whatever the considerations may be, be they because she does not want to undertake the burden or responsibility of rearing the child or because she does not want to join her genes to the genes of that other person who would be the prospective father of the child) rather than in any problematic which her becoming pregnant may present, the possibility of transferring the fetus to the incubator and bringing it to term there is of no help to us; the availability of the incubator would not make any difference in our assessment of the situation. This can be seen with respect to the second scenario cited above, i.e., the case of rape, and with respect to the second and third formulations presented in the fourth scenario cited above, i.e., the case of the woman changing her mind regarding her having a child because of the onset of economic hardship or of psychological stress. Obviously, the possibility of transferring the fetus to the incubator and bringing it to term there would in no way alleviate the problematic that these cases present. The woman would still eventually have the child to contend with. At the very most, one could perhaps contend that a situation may arise here where having the possibility of transferring the fetus to an incubator, while not overcoming the problematic of the woman not wanting to have the fetus brought to term, may nonetheless mitigate somewhat the woman's predicament in giving her at least the alternative of freeing her from the burden of bringing the fetus to term, seeing that the incubator could now replace the woman's womb. Such a situation may, for example, be encountered in the second and third formulations of the third scenario, i.e., in the formulations where the pregnancy is brought about inadvertently due to the woman's negligence or ignorance and where we concluded that because the woman does incur here a commitment towards the fetus (and the fetus is conceded to be a personal entity) the fetus must be brought to term even though the woman does not want to have a child. Thus, having the possibility of transferring the fetus to an incubator and bringing it there to term, while clearly providing a panacea in some situations, does not encompass all the possible situations where a panacea to the problematic of the conflict between the woman's wish to abort and the fetus' claim not to have its existence terminated is sorely needed. At best, it is a partial panacea.

But aside from this consideration that the advantage which the possibility of transferring the fetus to an incubator may provide is spotty, i.e., not applicable in all possible situations, there are two further considerations that impinge upon this opinion that should be briefly mentioned. First, there is the consideration that bringing the fetus to term rather than aborting it may in all probability bring about much more serious psychological consequences for the woman. For in the context of the situation confronting us here where the woman does not wish to have the child we would be justified in assuming that upon coming to term the fetus now being a child would be put up for adoption and here a good case can be made that putting the child for adoption would be psychologically much harder on the woman than aborting it when it is still a fetus, seeing that an abortion may allow closure and the prospect that the passage of time would provide healing while a separation from one's child through adoption can provide neither—it must remain a festering wound. Secondly, there is the consideration of cost which, in all likelihood, would not be insignificant, seeing that bringing a fetus to term in an incubator only from its seventh or eighth month of gestation is a considerably costly proposition. Who is to carry the burden of the cost? Shall we expect the prospective mother and/or the prospective father to carry the burden? And what if he/she does not have the means? Alternatively, assuming that in the overwhelming majority of the cases here the born child would be put up for adoption, should we expect the adopting couple to carry the burden? And what if they could not afford such an additional expenditure? Lastly—and in all probability the approach most likely, realistically speaking, to be adopted—should society be expected to carry the burden of the expense? Now, of course, society can decide whatever it wants to decide. We would want to argue, however, that from the ethical perspective (ethical as delineated by us here) no such obligation can be placed upon society. You and I and all other third parties to the occurrence of the pregnancy (and these constitute society here) have no ethical obligation to carry the burden of expense for the parties that are directly responsible for bringing about the pregnancy. Clearly, the economic issue implicated here may place serious obstacles in making the option of transferring the fetus to an incubator viable.

29. The more pronounced manifestations of possessing self-consciousness such as awareness of self or awareness of being an entity that possesses self-consciousness appear even later, the former about the age of two and the latter only after attaining maturity. It should be noted, however, that in order to be able to attribute to an entity (in our case the newly born infant) an ethical right not to have its existence terminated, it is not essentially required for the entity to possess self-consciousness in its more pronounced manifestations. Possessing self-consciousness in its minimalist manifestation would suffice. Thus, the newly born infant after coming to possess self-consciousness in its minimalist expression, i.e., after its seventh or eighth month, give or take a month or two, is endowed with an ethical right not to have its existence terminated. It is only in the few months preceding its coming to possess self-consciousness in its minimalist manifestation that the newly born infant is devoid of the ethical right not to have its existence terminated and consequently compelling us to concede that in this period it is subject, from the ethical perspective, to infanticide.

30. It is interesting to note, however, that in the context of delineating the phenomenon of euthanasia solely in terms of mercy killing, it is possible to encounter a fudging of the distinction between it and the phenomenon of assisted suicide but not between it and the phenomenon of suicide as such. The

reason for this most probably lies in the fact that in the phenomenon of assisted suicide but not in the phenomenon of suicide as such the presence of an outside party is implicated after all and this, in turn, would suggest that even in a context where euthanasia is manifestly delineated solely in terms of mercy killing there lurks nonetheless a recognition, albeit unconsciously, that the presence of an outside party is also implicated in the phenomenon of euthanasia and thus allowing the fudging of the distinction between the two. But this may be a persuasive psychological justification for incorporating the phenomenon of assisted suicide within the phenomenon of euthanasia but not a logical justification. (By the way, the way by which the phenomenon of assisted suicide is incorporated into the phenomenon of euthanasia is by introducing a three-fold subdivision into the phenomenon of euthanasia, to wit, the subdivision of the phenomenon of euthanasia into voluntary, non-voluntary and involuntary euthanasia and whereby the phenomenon of assisted suicide is nothing else but that of voluntary euthanasia. Of course, given our delineation of the phenomenon of euthanasia, a voluntary euthanasia is a contradiction in terms and cannot be incorporated within the phenomenon of euthanasia. Only non-voluntary and involuntary euthanasia can be incorporated within the phenomenon of euthanasia though, of course, their incorporation in no way implies that they would also be ethically acceptable—indeed, as we shall presently see, while non-voluntary euthanasia may well be ethically acceptable, involuntary euthanasia, e.g., eugenics, would clearly not be ethically acceptable.) For clearly, while the stipulation that an outside party need be included within the delineation of the phenomenon of euthanasia is made specifically with respect to the issue of who is to make the decision that death be brought about (the stipulation being here that it is the outside party) and not with respect to the issue of who is to carry out the decision, in the delineation of the phenomenon of assisted suicide the inclusion of the outside party is clearly not with respect to the issue of who makes the decision (the decision being made here by the party that is to be the victim of the act) but rather only with respect to the issue of who is to execute the decision. And this being the case, the phenomenon of assisted suicide must be, from the vantage point of logic, linked to the phenomenon of suicide and not to the phenomenon of euthanasia.

31. Sometimes the code of conduct for physicians is cited in support of this claim, seeing that the physician is equally under obligation to sustain his/her patient in life as he/she is under obligation not to kill the patient. But this reference to the conduct expected of the physician (which, true, equates not sustaining in life with not killing the patient) does not really support the argument that there is no distinction between the ethical obligation not to kill and the ethical obligation to sustain in life. For the physician's obligation to sustain the patient in life is a professional—and in some instances may also be a legal—obligation but not an ethical obligation. The physician is obliged to keep the patient in life *qua* physician but not *qua* person.

32. Of course, one could argue that the same rationale mentioned above (to wit, the dependency of an entity ontologically constituted as a person, a

Thou, on the existence of another entity ontologically constituted as a person, a Thou, who as such can provide it with the necessary affirmation by which it can sustain its existence *qua* person) which imposes an ethical obligation on an entity constituted as a person not to terminate the existence of another entity constituted as a person also imposes an ethical obligation on such an entity to sustain in existence any other entity constituted as a person. For after all, what is required here in terms of this rationale is only that the existence of an entity ontologically constituted as a person should not be canceled out; how this is to be safeguarded, whether it be by prohibiting to terminate its existence or by requiring to sustain it in existence, is beside the point. What counts here is the bottom line and this is the same in both instances—both killing and not saving yield the same end result, i.e., canceling the existence of the other entity. But this rationale basing itself, as it does, on calculations in terms of the egotistic interests of an entity ontologically constituting itself as a person is not really persuasive, in the last analysis, either with respect to the killing of another person or with respect to not saving its life, seeing that the world is populated with a great many other entities constituting themselves as persons who would not be affected by either of the two scenarios and consequently the feasibility of the entity being the agent in these scenarios continuing to receive affirmation is in no way jeopardized. This rationale could have been persuasive if, and only if, the entity that is to be killed or that is not to be saved were the only remaining entity being constituted as a person (beside, of course, the entity that is the agent here). Only in such circumstances would the egotistic interests of the agent dictate against its killing or its not saving of the entity constituted as a person. But clearly these circumstances do not obtain in the reality of the situation here. The reality of the situation here is that the agent has a great many other persons that can extend to it affirmation thus sustaining its existence *qua* person and in such a context the cancellation of existence with respect to any single person would not affect the self-interests of the agent. And this being the case, this rationale cannot be, in the last analysis, fully persuasive.

A more persuasive rationale which was also mentioned above and which indeed is tied to the foregoing rationale, except that it formulates itself on a more fundamental level, is the rationale which goes beyond the rather self-evident calculations which base themselves on the self-centered interests of the agent to formulate itself in terms of the dictates which necessarily emanate from the very ontological constitution of the agent (being as such the ethical rights and obligations which devolve on the agent) and which, indeed, underpin the self-centered interests of the agent in terms of which the calculations in the foregoing rationale were carried out. Thus, this rationale bases itself on the fact, as argued above, that a person has, by its very ontological constitution, a right (an ethical right) to demand to be affirmed as an end in itself which, in turn, implicates on the basis of the golden rule that it also has an obligation (an ethical obligation) to extend such an affirmation to any other entity which is constituted as a person. Making such a demand to be affirmed and the implicated obligation to extend a likewise affirmation are inextricable expressions of personhood. Indeed, and most significantly for our concern here, the very making of the demand to be affirmed is, as was shown above, mediated through the agent extending its affirmation to any and every other entity where, however, only those entities which are ontologically constituted as persons have the capacity to, so to speak, pick up the extended affirmation which, in turn, is tantamount to extending a returned affirmation to the agent thus meeting its demand to be affirmed. We say that this mechanism by which the demand for affirmation is met is of great significance for our concern here because it follows from this that an entity which is ontologically constituted as a person can relate to another entity which is likewise ontologically constituted as a person only via the mode of affirmation. The ontological constitution of personhood limits the relation between its bearers to the relation of the affirmation—only the relation of affirmation is viable in such a context. Relating via the remaining alternative mode of relating, namely, via the mode of utilization, is not viable for entities that are ontologically constituted as persons. Indeed, the only alternative option to relating via the mode of affirmation that is available to an entity which is ontologically constituted as a person is to withhold its affirmation which is here tantamount to refraining from relating to the other. (True, this option may well implicate the disintegration of an entity which is ontologically constituted as a person, its committing, so to speak, suicide, seeing that an entity which is ontologically constituted as a person is by its very essence a relating entity, i.e., an entity that for its very existence must be in a relation, specifically in a relation of affirmation. Still, this alternative must be available inasmuch as it reflects in the most pronounced way the dimension of freedom, the dimension which is perhaps the most basic and essential expression which characterizes personhood.) Thus, an entity that is constituted as a person can relate to another entity either by extending or by withholding its affirmation but not by utilizing that entity. (Of course, the entity implicated here, i.e., the human entity, is not constituted exclusively as a person, as a Thou-entity, but rather as both a person and a physical entity, as an It/Thou-entity, and this clearly requires some clarification with respect to the claim made here. For as such a human entity can now relate to another entity not only via the mode of affirmation/non-affirmation but also via the mode of utilization, except that its relating via the mode of utilization would be viable only when directed to a physical entity, to an It-entity, but not when directed to a personal entity, to a Thou-entity. This means that while we cannot say—as we did with respect to an entity that was ontologically constituted exclusively in terms of personhood—that a human entity by its very ontological constitution cannot relate via the mode of utilization, we can and have to say that when it relates via the mode of utilization to an entity that is ontologically constituted as a person, a Thou-entity, the dimension of personhood, the Thou-dimension, in its ontological constitution is inevitably compromised.) And this being the case, it should be quite clear that in terms of this rationale there is a significant difference between killing and not saving another entity that is a person. For the act of killing an entity that is a person is an act of utilization par excellence (what can be a greater act of utilizing an other than taking away its existence?) and indeed as such it is an act that undermines in its agent the dimension of personhood and consequently is ethically reprehensible. As against this, the act of not saving an entity that is a person is not an act of utilization but of withholding affirmation and as such it does not undermine the dimension of personhood, the Thou-dimension, in the agent of the act and consequently, while the act may well be unkind and indeed cruel, it is not ethically reprehensible. Thus, there is no equivalence between the act of killing and the act of not saving which, had it existed, would have allowed us to transfer our ethical evaluation of the act of killing to the act of not saving.

33. By the way, a distinction between ethics and law can be maintained in terms of either the delineation of the ethical enterprise given here. Thus, in terms of the latter delineation, the distinction could be established in that ethics would evaluate/judge intentions while the law would evaluate/judge acts; and in terms of the former delineation, while both ethics and law evaluate/judge acts, the distinction could be established in that ethics would evaluate/judge the acts exclusively in terms of the intentions implicated in them while in the evaluation/judgment of the law, although intentions do also play a role, it is by no means the primary, essential, leave alone exclusive, role that it plays in the evaluation/judgment of ethics.

34. By the way, this concurs with our argument made above that passively not saving another person in contrast to actively killing such a person does not constitute an act of utilization—which in the circumstances here would implicate a negative ethical evaluation—but only a withholding of affirmation, and while such a withholding does not implicate a positive ethical evaluation, it does not implicate a negative ethical evaluation either, which is tantamount to saying that it implicates an ethical evaluation that is neutral.

35. We should note, however, that the notion of a passive act strikes us as being self-contradictory. For it would seem to us that the notion of an act necessarily signifies a "doing," i.e., the doing of something, while the notion of passivity necessarily signifies a "not doing," i.e., the absence of doing something. As such, an act can only be active and not passive. (Perhaps it is because of this that the colloquial expression for passivity is "doing nothing," implying a doing of a something, that something being a "nothing," rather than "not doing anything" does; it merely signifies a negation, i.e., a negation of any substantive entity that is being referred to. As such, "doing nothing" really signifies not doing anything.") Indeed, the alternative to the notion of an active act, which after all is what the notion of a passive act is supposed to provide, is not a notion signifying doing nothing, i.e., doing something that is called "nothing," but rather a notion signifying not doing something. For the opposite of doing something is not doing something else but rather not doing that something. These considerations, by the way, would seem to us to clearly buttress the argument put forth above in support of the claim that there is a clear distinction as regards their respective ethical evaluations between killing another (i.e., an active act) and not saving that person (i.e., a passive act). The fact, however, that these considerations are camouflaged for many people may

be due perhaps to the fact that for many people ethical evaluation is to be directed towards the behavior of a person rather than towards any individual act/relation and the notion of behavior, in contra-distinction to that of act/relation, can indeed encompass not only activity but also inactivity—behavior expresses itself not only in doing things but also in refraining from doing things. The trouble, however, with this position is that, in our judgment, the notion of behavior is too general and too flexible to be an adequate object for ethical evaluation. Indeed, a case can be made that when behavior is taken as the object for ethical evaluation, it is taken in the sense of being an accumulation of acts over time so that the ethical evaluation here is, in the last analysis, but a summation of ethical evaluations of individual acts.

36. Of course, it is true that in principle one can never foreclose the possibility of "miracles," (i.e., the unexplainable occurrences, occurrences that are beyond our grasp and in contradiction to everything we know) taking place or of medical breakthroughs that can radically change the prognosis occurring, and this being the case, the possibility of regaining consciousness can never be denied with absolute certainty. True, we can never have absolute certainty with respect to anything in our lives. Thus, if we were justified in acting only if we had absolute certainty, we could never act on anything. We must and do act on the basis of probability and not on the basis of absolute certainty, and the greater the probability the more justified we are in our acting. Now, in the situation confronting us here we are talking of a situation in which we would have a very high degree of probability.

37. By the way, aside from this fundamental consideration there is the additional consideration that eugenics is very relative. Different societies, cultures, may view different attributes as undesirable and consequently different societies, cultures, may apply the act of euthanasia to different kinds of humans. What in one society, culture, may be viewed as undesirable may be viewed in another society, culture, as quite desirable. Thus, while in one society, culture, short people may be viewed as undesirable and therefore terminating their existence would be ethically acceptable, in another society, culture, such people may be viewed as quite desirable and therefore terminating their existence would be ethically unacceptable. But given our understanding of the ethical enterprise, ethical evaluation must be universally applicable, which is to say that if the circumstances are the same, the ethical evaluation has to be the same. Euthanasia for the sake of eugenics fails this test.

38. This may perhaps be due to the fact that in those instances where the act of euthanasia is ethically approved in the context of this situation, the act clearly presents itself as an act of "mercy killing," something which was not the case when the act of euthanasia was ethically approved in the context of the first situation and ethically disapproved in the context of the second situation. For there is much more room for variations and differences when it comes to decide whether or not an act of killing qualifies as an act of "mercy killing."

39. Of course, one can argue against the ethical acceptability of resorting to an act of euthanasia here by maintaining that a decision of this magnitude, namely, a decision to terminate the existence of an entity that is a person,

should not be relegated to an outside party but must be left in the hands of the concerned person. Thus, according to this stance we should wait for the baby to attain adulthood and then let him/her make the decision. Instead of resorting to euthanasia we should countenance the option of suicide. There is no denying that this stance has merit—we certainly should be very leery of relegating the decision of terminating a person's existence to an outside party. Still, there are two weighty considerations that militate against this stance. First, in having to postpone the decision until the baby attains adulthood, it inevitably must allow a good many years of great suffering to elapse. And secondly, in arrogating the decision of whether or not to terminate its existence to the victim of the disease, it inescapably inflicts on the victim great psychological suffering. In view of these considerations the question must inevitably arise whether the victim of the disease would not have been better off to have been spared this suffering by succumbing in its early infancy to an act of euthanasia. Clearly, deciding between this consideration and that of relegating the termination of one's existence to an outside party is very difficult, and we can see how different people may come down on opposite sides of this decision. We came down on the side of euthanasia because we gave compassion the upper hand over the reluctance to arrogate a decision of this nature to an outside party.

40. Thus, in the case of abortion it is for the sake of satisfying either the interests or the wishes of mother (i.e., an outside party), and in the case of suicide it is for the sake of satisfying either the interests or the wishes of the person committing suicide (i.e., the object of the act). As against this, in the case of euthanasia and infanticide it is only interests and not wishes that are implicated in the act. But the interests implicated here can also be either for the sake of the object of the act (as in cases of euthanasia where the object of the act is irretrievably unconscious or in cases of infants with dreadfully painful diseases that are incurable or of infants with severe deformation or who are doomed to die in a matter of a few years) or for the sake of an outside party, to wit, society (as it would be in cases of euthanasia performed for the sake of eugenics or in cases of infanticide, though in this latter instance the outside party can be not only society but also the infant's parents).

41. It should be noted, however, that this argument would not apply to a killing that is in self-defense or in the defense of another innocent person, namely, to the killing of a human who is unmistakably about to kill me or another innocent human. Such a killing is not open to the same ethical evaluation as the killing implicated in the act of execution. For in the killing in self-defense or in the defense of another innocent human, the would-be murderer is already, for all intents and purposes, relating to its other in terms of murder, i.e., he/she is already acting as a non-person, as an It entity, towards the intended victim—for all intents and purposes he/she is already involved in carrying out the act of murder and is, therefore, an entity that has abrogated its dimension of personhood, its Thouness, and consequently is an entity that at that moment does not possess an ethical right not to have its existence terminated. The killing here is different, as far as ethical evaluation is concerned, from the killing implicated in the act of execution not because a

transformation in the ontological constitution of the killer does take place in this case and not in the case of an execution (no transformation in the ontological constitution of the killer takes place in either case) but because the killing in this case impinges upon an entity that is implicated in an act of killing (and is, therefore, presently abrogating its dimension of personhood) while the killing in the case of an execution impinges upon an entity that was but is not presently implicated in an act of killing (and therefore is not presently abrogating its dimension of personhood). By the way, our position clearly differs from that of a total pacifist who would not kill even in self-defense or in the defense of an innocent other person. From our perspective, such a total pacifist fails to recognize that in the act of killing the killer abrogates its dimension of personhood.

42. By the way, this consideration, which grounds itself in the linkage between ethical right and ethical obligation, is the same consideration that plays an important role, as we have seen, with regard to the issue of whether animals are endowed with an ethical right not to have their existence terminated. For, as seen, aside from the consideration of whether or not certain animals possess self-consciousness and as such are endowed with an ethical right not to have their existence terminated (a consideration that is open to different assessments and consequently must remain inconclusive), the consideration that is conclusive and that can persuasively establish that no animal is endowed with an ethical right not to have its existence terminated is the consideration that no animal can be saddled with an ethical obligation not to terminate the existence of other entities that are persons.

43. This after all is the point, as we had occasion to point out above, of the much maligned scriptural verse of "an eye for an eye and a tooth for a tooth."

44. We have not dealt above with the claim that capital punishment acts as a deterrent to would-be murderers, not only because the validity of such a claim is questionable but, more important, because the claim impacts the issue before us here only when it is considered in the context of a utilitarian calculus, and given the way the ethical enterprises has been delineated here, a utilitarian calculus is of no relevance.

45. One can perhaps neutralize this argument by the counter-argument that having both the victim and the perpetrator present in one single entity rather than in two separate entities does not necessarily exclude the possibility of the act of killing implicated in the act of suicide being an act of murder. For while it is true that because both victim and perpetrator are present in one and the same entity, they must share the same interests, the interests that arise in conjunction with the entity may reflect either the stance of the victim or the stance of the perpetrator, and if it be the latter, then the act of killing implicated in the act of suicide would be tantamount to an act of murder. Thus, theoretically it is possible to have a killing that is murder in an act of suicide. In actuality, however, it would seem that in the act of suicide it is the interests of the victim and not of the perpetrator that are being reflected. For the cause of the act of suicide, i.e., that which brings it on, is clearly the wish of the entity, i.e., the person, to die, not to go on living. The perpetrator here is merely the

agent that carries out these wishes. Thus, even in terms of this counter-argument we come up with the same bottom line, namely, that it would not be valid to take the act of suicide as an act of murder and thus evaluate it as ethically reprehensible.

46. It should be noted, however, that this formulation finds expression specifically within biblical religions, i.e., within Judaism, Christianity and Islam, and not within pagan religions (indeed, within cultures linked with pagan religion, suicide is very often evaluated positively, e.g., as the honorable thing to do in certain circumstances). This should not be surprising, seeing that only in biblical religion does the human encounter the divine entity, i.e., the ultimate entity, as a personal entity, as a Thou (this indeed is the fundamental change, the great innovation, that biblical religion introduces into the history of religion). In pagan religion the God, i.e., the ultimate entity, that the human encounters is an impersonal entity, an It, i.e., a blind power. Thus, only in biblical religion do we have two kinds of entity that are endowed with personhood, to wit, the human and the divine; in pagan religion only the human is endowed with personhood (as regard the gods of the pantheon they are, first of all, not ultimate but only penultimate entities and secondly, even so, they are not really, in the last analysis, authentic persons but rather personifications of the blind power as it manifests itself in nature). Now, this clearly has a significant bearing on whether introducing the divine entity into the picture can make any difference to the ethical evaluation of the act of suicide. For first, accountability can clearly be exacted only by a personal entity. If therefore the divine entity is not a personal entity, it cannot exact accountability. But the very function that the introduction of the divine entity into the picture is to fulfill is to provide for the perpetrator of the act of suicide a someone other than him/herself that can exact accountability for the act. And secondly, ethical evaluation, as has been argued above, can impinge only upon acts/relations that take place between personal entities, thus if the divine entity is impersonal, its introduction into the picture would still fail to provide us with an evaluation of the act of suicide that is an ethical evaluation. In the context of pagan religion, therefore, the human remains, in the last analysis, alone accountable only to him/herself (or, as we shall presently see, to other humans, i.e., to society) thus allowing the evaluation of his/her acts/relations to be only from the vantage point of his/her interests, and in such a context there could be circumstances where a positive ethical evaluation of the act of suicide would be indicated.

Indeed, there are any number of instances within pagan religion, both with regard to individuals (e.g., Seneca, Cato) and in philosophic formulation (e.g., those of the Cynics, the Stoics and the Epicureans), where the act of suicide far from being negatively evaluated is actually evaluated as a positive act. What is, however, more interesting to note is that even in the defining canons of such biblical religions as Judaism (i.e., the Hebrew bible) and Christianity (i.e., the New Testament), the act of suicide is not rejected as ethically reprehensible. The utterances and commandments attributed to God, i.e., the stuff constituting verbal revelation (revelation relayed through speech and received through the medium of hearing), do not address the issue at all and in the instances of suicide that are mentioned (six in the Hebrew bible and one in the New Testament), no negative evaluation is pronounced and, indeed, in some a positive evaluation is intimated. An explicit and incisive negative evaluation of the act of suicide is articulated in the case of Judaism only by the rabbis (even more precisely, only by post-Talmudic rabbis) and in the case of Christianity by Augustine (for whom one of the principal reasons for condemning the act of suicide grounds itself in the sixth commandment that, however, he takes as reading "Thou shall not kill" when in actuality it reads "Thou shall not murder," which says something significantly different from Thou shall not kill) and by a number of Church Councils in the sixth century C.E. But the notion of suicide as used in these religious traditions (certainly as used in Judaism) excludes acts of martyrdom and acts committed under duress or as a result of an unbalanced mind and this, in turn, means that, practically speaking, not too many acts, if indeed any, are left that would qualify as acts of suicide. Thus, while in their theoretical formulation the concrete historical religions reflecting biblical religion are very radical and unambiguous in their condemnation of the act of suicide, in their practical application their rejection is greatly restricted. Many acts that clearly appear to be acts of suicide escape condemnation by resorting to these exceptions (particularly, seeing that the exception of unbalanced mind would seem to be, in the last analysis, always available when all the other exceptions fail). Thus, not only in pagan religions but even in biblical religions the act of suicide, for all practical intents and purposes, escapes condemnation.

One last observation may be in order. As we will presently try to show above, grounding the negative evaluation of the act of suicide in the claim that the life possessed by the human does not really belong to the human but to the divine (as is held by the human merely in trust or as a gift) has implications that would conflict with a fundamental and essential requirement of biblical religion (certainly as it manifests itself in Judaism though admittedly its applicability in its manifestation in Islam and in some strains of Christianity, e.g., Calvinism, may be problematic), to wit, the requirement that the human entity be endowed to some extent with free choice, and as such a grounding in such a claim presents, to say the very least, a rather serious problem for biblical religions. Thus, although the "official" position in biblical religion is to ground the negative ethical evaluation of the act of suicide in the claim that the life which belongs to the human does not really belong to the human but to the divine, it would seem to us that a better justification for such an evaluation (i.e., better in the sense that it does not conflict with any fundamental or essential requirement of biblical religion) would be to ground it in a strong affirmation of this earthly life; the act of suicide is evaluated negatively because it clashes head on with such an affirmation—cutting life short contradicts the affirmation of life.

Now, such a strong affirmation of life can indeed be readily arrogated, for example, to Judaism and consequently it would seem to us that a persuasive case can be made that, notwithstanding the "official" justification, the justification of the negative evaluation of the act of suicide is, in the last analysis, derived in Judaism from the high priority accorded to the preservation of life (the prohibition against placing one's life in danger, i.e., the prohibition against Pikuah Nefesh, takes precedence over all other commandments with the exception of committing idolatry, adultery and murder); it is this fundamental feeling for the preciousness (in a religious context one might well say sanctity) of life, rather than the "official" justification, which, in the last analysis, provides the most basic motivation in Judaism for the rejection of the act of suicide as ethically reprehensible. After all, mainstream Judaism (more specifically, prophetic Judaism) is very much a this-worldly religion—in its context the drama of religion and the redemption it envisions are confined within the world as it is given to us in the here and now. On the other hand, however, it would seem to us that such a strong affirmation of life as we encounter in mainstream Judaism cannot be arrogated to mainstream Christianity. Christianity, it would seem, is much more pessimistic about this-worldly life and commensurately its anticipated salvation is placed in the ontological transformation of the human into a "new being." In Christianity there is an underlying motif consisting of the wish to escape this-worldly life—the drama of religion and the envisioned salvation are other-worldly. In such a context the termination of human existence in the form known to us in the here and now cannot be so readily rejected as ethically reprehensible. Indeed, it is interesting to note that when alternative justifications to the "official" justification for the negative evaluation of the act of suicide are put forward in Christianity (as is the case, for example, in Aquinas), these alternative justifications would tend to ground themselves with respect to the notion of natural law (i.e., that the act of suicide violates natural law) or with respect to the Aristotelian argument (i.e., that the act of suicide goes against the interests of society)—notions and arguments that are linked to the orientation of pagan religion and not to the orientation of biblical religion. But then, after all, Christianity is the great attempt at synthesizing biblical and pagan religion and consequently we should expect to find in it elements derived not only from biblical but also from pagan religion.

47. By the way, this being the case, this formulation can be seen as the secular version in contra-distinction to the foregoing formulation, which clearly represents the religious version of an underlying formulation whose distinctiveness lies in its providing an other that can be introduced into the process of evaluating the act of suicide, allowing it thereby to become an evaluation that is a *bona fide* ethical evaluation.

48. As such, by the way, not only is this linkage, in contrast to the linkage in terms of the exchange of material goods, a linkage that can provide a basis for the ethical evaluation of the act of suicide, but it is a linkage that binds the individual human to his/her society (or, more accurately, to his/her community, seeing that the proper appellation of an aggregate of Thou entities linked by the exchange of affirmation is community rather than society) on a much more fundamental level and provides a bonding between the individual human and his/her community that is by far stronger and, indeed, more essential. For, as we have seen, for an entity to ontologically constitute itself (at least in part) in terms of the dimension-of-consciousness, i.e., as a Thou entity, namely, for

such an entity to come into existence and preserve itself in it, being affirmed from the outside, i.e., by other entities who likewise constitute themselves (at least in part) as Thou entities (these entities constituting the community for the entity to be affirmed) is a condition *sine qua non.* Thus, a linkage to an aggregate of entities that establishes itself in terms of the exchange of affirmation, in other words, to a community, is essential to the very existence of an entity that constitutes itself (at least in part) as a Thou entity. An entity, to the extent that it constitutes itself as a Thou entity, cannot exist independently of a community of other entities constituting themselves (at least in part) as Thou entities.

49. We use the word "resolve" advisedly for, in our judgment, it goes without saying that if a person's decision to commit suicide is made impulsively or in a period of depression or when his/her mind is not quite stable, in short, whenever the decision is not carefully thought through and is held deliberately and firmly, extending assistance in effecting the decision is an act that is ethically reprehensible.

50. We say that the acts contained in any assistance that is extended would implicate a killing, but not a murdering, of another person because the acts involved here are carried out not for the sake of accruing any advantage or profit to the person extending the assistance and for an act of terminating one's existence to be an act of murder, rather than of killing, it has to be accompanied by the clear intention that it be committed for the sake of accruing some advantage or profit to the perpetrator, rather than to the victim, of the act. Of course if there is an advantage or a profit accruing to the person extending the assistance (which is certainly possible as, for example, when he/she receives payment for extending his/her assistance or when he/she stands to profit from the death of the victim), the act would become an act of murder.

51. In this respect, by the way, the justification for the act of assisted suicide coalesces itself with the justification for the act of euthanasia as it expresses itself in the third scenario delineated above. This lends itself to the confusion of the two acts and to using them interchangeably. True, in both cases the motivation is the same, namely, to relieve the prospective victim of horrific pain that has no redeeming aspect. Still, as already observed above, the two acts differ from each other in one all-important respect and that is that the decision to terminate life is made in the case of assisted suicide by the prospective victim while in the case of euthanasia it is made by an outside party.

Literature Cited

Brody, Baruch. 1978a. "The Morality of Abortion." In *Contemporary Issues in Bioethics,* edited by Tom L. Beauchamp and LeRoy Walters. Encino, Calif.: Dickenson; also in 2d edition, Belmont, Calif., Wadsworth (1982).

———. 1978b. "On the Humanity of the Foetus." In *Contemporary Issues in Bioethics,* edited by Tom L. Beauchamp and LeRoy Walters. Encino, Calif.: Dickenson; also in 2d edition, Belmont, Calif., Wadsworth (1982).

Dyson, Freeman. 1988. *Infinite in All Directions.* New York: Harper and Row.

Glover, Jonathan. 1977. *Causing Death and Saving Lives.* London: Penguin Books.

Levinas, Emmanuel. 1985. *Ethics and Infinity.* Pittsburgh: Duquesne University Press.

Noonan, John T. 1968. "Deciding Who Is Human." *Natural Law Forum* 13.

Singer, Peter. 1980. "Animals and the Value of Life. In *Matters of Life and Death,* edited by Tom Regan. Philadelphia: Temple University Press.

———., ed. 1991. *A Companion to Ethics.* Blackwell Companions to Philosophy. Oxford: Blackwell Reference.

Thomson, Judith Jarvis. 1971. "A Defense of Abortion." *Philosophy and Public Affairs* 1, no. 1: 47-66.

Tooley, Michael. 1972. "Abortion and Infanticide." *Philosophy and Public Affairs* 2, no. 1: 37-65.

Warren, Mary Anne. 1982. "On the Moral and Legal Status of Abortion." In *Contemporary Issues in Bioethics,* 2d ed., edited by Tom L. Beauchamp and LeRoy Walters. Belmont, Calif.: Wadsworth Publishing.

Wertheimer, Roger. 1971. "Understanding the Abortion Argument." *Philosophy and Public Affairs* 1, no. 1: 67-95.

About the Author

Manfred H. Vogel is professor in the Religion Department at Northwestern University where he teaches Modern Jewish Thought, Jewish Ethics, Philosophy of Religion, and Comparative Religion. He received his Ph.D. in the Philosophy Department at Columbia University in 1963. He was visiting professor at the Hebrew University in 1969-70, at Tel-Aviv University in 1974, at Stanford University in 1985-86, and at the Pontifical Gregorian University in 1999. His publications include *Feuerbach: Principles of the Philosophy of the Future,* Bobbs-Merrill Company, Inc., Indianapolis and New York, 1966; *A Quest for a Theology of Judaism,* University Press of America, 1987; and *Rosenzweig on Profane/Secular History,* Scholars Press, 1996.